The PainEdu.org Manual:
A POCKET GUIDE TO PAIN MANAGEMENT

A companion to www.PainEdu.org

Lynette Menefee Pujol, Ph.D.
Nathaniel P. Katz, M.D.
Kevin L. Zacharoff, M.D.

D1516662

Produced for Inflexxion®, Inc. by:
Lynette Menefee Pujol, Ph.D.
Nathaniel P. Katz, M.D.
Kevin L. Zacharoff, M.D.

Reviewed by:
Robert Jamison, Ph.D.
Pain Management Center
Brigham & Women's Hospital
Boston, MA

Acknowledgment
The authors would like to acknowledge with deep appreciation and gratitude, the work of Evelyn Corsini, M.S.W. This project only came to be successfully completed through Evelyn's perseverance and successful management of this project at every level. Evelyn's vision of this revised manual is apparent throughout and provided the inspiration and momentum for this project from beginning to end.

ISBN: 978-0-9740093-0-8

Supported through an educational grant from Endo Pharmaceuticals.

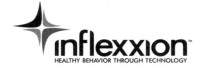

CONTENTS

Foreword

Pain management continues to become an increasingly important clinical issue and challenge for health care providers. Almost as quickly as new medications are developed, new conditions and theories about appropriate treatment are identified. The burden of unsuccessfully diagnosed and treated pain on society is tremendous, ranging from inability to perform activities of daily living, to poor emotional status and impaired relationships, to tremendous financial impact. Many health care professionals have devoted their careers specifically toward the appropriate assessment and management of pain. These health care providers often act as consultants when their area of expertise is needed.

This manual is intended to serve as a pocket reference for those physicians, health care professionals, and health care students who are not experts in the field, but who are faced with issues surrounding management of patients with pain on a daily basis. We offer this guide as a resource to physicians and health care providers who will inevitably encounter this common and difficult problem that presents in many forms. The current edition has been updated to try to keep up with modalities, approaches, and regulations as they continue to evolve. It should serve as a handy tool to quickly guide the health care provider in the right direction toward the assessment and appropriate treatment of common painful conditions.

Although it would be impossible to cover all conditions and details in a handy reference, we feel confident that this manual, in conjunction with its companion web site, http://www.PainEDU.org, will become an invaluable part of your quick-reference library for treating the common painful conditions affecting your patients' lives.

Lynette Menefee Pujol, Ph.D.
Nathaniel P. Katz, M.D.
Kevin L. Zacharoff, M.D.

I.

Basic Principles of Pain Management

BASICS OF PAIN TREATMENT

> "We must all die. But that I can save him from days of torture, that is what I feel as my great and ever new privilege. Pain is a more terrible Lord of mankind than even death itself."
>
> —Albert Schweitzer

Pain is a phenomenon that all people encounter at some point in their lives. Both a sensory and an emotional experience, *pain* is defined as being an unpleasant experience associated with actual or potential tissue damage. Pain, in both its acute and chronic manifestations, can commandeer a patient's body and mind. When improperly managed, pain can lead to decreased productivity and diminished quality of life.[1] The consequences of inadequate attention to pain reach into the professional, family, sexual, and avocational realms.

Pain is treatable, however. As the science of pain continues to unravel the mystery of its mechanisms, doctors have an increasingly large arsenal of tools to deploy against pain. There are clinically accepted methods for assessing pain in adult, pediatric, and elderly populations. Each of these measures is calibrated to elicit the most accurate self-report from a patient of a certain age group and level of cognitive ability. In addition, a review of a patient's medical history and a thorough physical and neurologic examination can be useful tools in qualifying and quantifying pain.[2]

Using these measurement tools, a health care provider is empowered to treat pain with pharmacologic, nonpharmacologic, and psychological remedies. Treatment should be tailored to the type of pain, the location of the pain, its duration, and its intensity. Other considerations include, but are not limited to, the patient's medical history and previous reactions to particular drugs. Assessment of the psychological and social consequences of pain is an important part of tailoring treatment. Multimodal treatment strategies are often necessary to achieve success. Any pain treatment needs to be fine-tuned to a patient's particular needs. There is almost invariably a trial-and-error period while the regimen is adjusted. It is also essential that the patient and his or her family understand well the limitations of pain management.

Modern society has high expectations for health care, and it is important to communicate that complete relief from pain is frequently not possible. Special considerations apply in cases of young patients, those who are cognitively impaired, those with psychiatric comorbidities, and patients at the end of life. In managing pain, the emphasis should be on effectively minimizing discomfort and maximizing function while attending to its underlying cause.

When treating pain, regardless of the modalities used, some basic "pearls" that appear in Table 1 below are worth keeping in mind.

■ Table 1.
Basics of Pain Treatment

Analgesia should be integrated into a comprehensive patient evaluation and management plan.

The emotional and cognitive aspects of pain must be recognized and treated.

There is no reliable way to objectively measure pain.

Pain is most often undertreated, not overtreated.

Pain control must be individualized.

Anticipate rather than react to pain.

Whenever possible, let the patient control his or her own pain.

(continued)

■ **Table 1.**
   Basics of Pain Treatment (Continued)

Pain control is often best achieved by rational polypharmacy.
Pain control often requires a multidisciplinary, team approach.

Adapted from Ducharme J. Acute pain and pain control: state of the art. *Ann Emerg Med* 2000;35:592–603.

BARRIERS TO THE ASSESSMENT AND MANAGEMENT OF PAIN

Despite the fact that principles and tools exist for assessment and treatment of pain today, barriers exist that may hinder successful outcomes. Improved education about appropriate assessment and treatment of pain will, it is hoped, someday conquer some of these barriers and the myths they promote.

Even though the decade beginning in 2000 was designated as the "Decade of Pain Control and Research" by the U.S. Congress, the health care system still lacks clearly articulated primary care practice standards for pain management. Other than the Joint Commission on Accreditation of Healthcare Organizations' institutional standards, there is a noticeable absence of accountability and competency for adequate assessment and management. The growth of managed care has also led to fragmentation and lack of communication among physicians, leading to less coordination of care. Obviously, financial barriers, such as lack of insurance, may lead to a lower level of care.

Clinician perception of the relative importance of pain and its management can also lead to undertreatment. Some health care professionals do not want to routinely accept the patient's self-report of his or her degree of pain as credible. Fear of regulatory scrutiny may also inhibit efforts to control pain.

The inability of the patient to report symptoms accurately, such as with cognitively impaired patients, may result in poor communication with the health care provider and a decreased likelihood of successfully understanding the patient's needs.

■ **Table 2.**
  Common Myths about Pain

Children do not feel pain to the same degree as adults.
It is not possible to adequately measure pain in cognitively impaired patients.
Physical manifestations of pain are more important than self-report measurements.
Pain does not exist in the absence of detectable tissue damage.
Pain without an obvious source is usually psychogenic.
The same stimulus produces the same degree of pain in all individuals.
Analgesic therapy should not be started until the cause of pain is established.
Noncancer pain is not as severe as cancer pain.
Knowledgeable patients have a higher incidence of drug diversion.
Use of opioids causes all patients to become addicted to them.
Aggressive pain management is synonymous with prescribing opioids.

These barriers are associated with a number of myths about pain and its treatment.

IMPORTANCE OF TIMELY REFERRAL TO A PAIN SPECIALIST

Many painful conditions may be managed adequately by the primary care clinician. However, referral to a pain specialist or a pain management team may be best for certain cases of chronic, cancer-related, or otherwise complex pain that is debilitating or refractory to treatment.[3]

Important members of the pain management team may include the following:

■ Anesthesiologists
■ Clergy

- Counselors
- Neurologists
- Nurse specialists
- Physiatrists
- Physical or occupational therapists
- Psychiatrists
- Psychologists
- Social workers

Pain clinics may bring all relevant team members "under one roof." Many pain specialists believe that referrals frequently are made past the so-called "golden hour," when their intervention may be of maximal effectiveness, especially in cases of neuropathic and cancer pain.[4] Referral to a pain specialist ideally should occur before significant disability or loss of function occurs; pain behaviors or the emergence of maladaptive coping strategies may serve as cues for referral.

REFERENCES

1. Coda BA, Bonica JJ. General considerations of acute pain. In Loeser JD, Butler SH, Chapman CR, Turk DC, eds. *Bonica's Management of Pain (3rd ed)*. Philadelphia: Lippincott, Williams & Wilkins, 2001:222–240.
2. Turk D, Melzack R. *Handbook of Pain Assessment (2nd ed)*. New York: Guilford Press, 2001.
3. Ballantyne JC. *The Massachusetts General Hospital Handbook of Pain Management (3rd ed)*. Philadelphia: Lippincott Williams & Wilkins, October 1, 2005.
4. Warfield CA, Bajwa ZH. *Principles and Practices of Pain Management (2nd ed)*. New York: McGraw-Hill Companies, Inc. 2004.

II.

The Epidemiology of Pain

DEFINITION OF PAIN

The International Association for the Study of Pain (IASP) defines pain as "an unpleasant sensory and emotional experience associated with actual or potential tissue damage."

Pain is a ubiquitous phenomenon. As clinicians know, the same set of circumstances can cause significant pain in one patient and little or none in another. The challenge, then, is not only to identify the type and source of pain a patient is experiencing, but also to assess the severity and impact that the painful condition has on the individual patient to ensure optimal treatment. Pain is somewhat of a "black box," in that only the sufferer fully understands the experience. Pain has both subjective and objective components, the proportions of which may be variable but all of which must be treated. Additionally, consideration must be given to the temporal nature of the pain, as treatment strategies for acute pain may differ dramatically from those for chronic pain.

INCIDENCE AND PREVALENCE OF PAIN

Almost everyone experiences pain at some time in his or her life. Pain is the single most common reason for patients to seek medical attention.[1] On average, 15–20% of Americans experience chronic pain each year, approximately 68 million Americans. Americans seek advice from a physician on average 3.1 times per year,[2] and the majority of these contacts are precipitated by complaints of some type of pain. In the case of back pain, one of the most prevalent forms of chronic pain, age has been found not to be a major influence on its incidence.

Surgery is the single largest cause of acute pain in the United States, with approximately 41.5 million Americans undergoing hospitalization for surgery each year.[2] The majority of patients in the United States report moderate to severe pain postsurgically, even in the face of current treatments and techniques.

As the American population continues to age, there is an increase in the burden of arthritis pain and chronic joint symptoms in people aged 65 or older.[3] In a 1999 poll, a large proportion of respondents indicated some degree of disability secondary to pain, with two out of three elderly individuals responding that pain kept them from participating in activities. Arthritis is the leading cause of disability, with approximately 39 million physician visits and 500,000 hospitalizations per year.[4] Cancer, the second leading cause of death in America,[5] is associated with chronic pain in approximately 67% of patients.[6]

BURDEN OF PAIN ON SOCIETY

Besides the physical, physiologic, and psychosocial effects of pain on individual patients, the burden placed on our society in financial terms is tremendous. In 1998, the National Institutes of Health estimated the financial burden of pain to be as much as $100 billion per year in medical expenses, lost wages, and other costs, including lost productivity. This loss of productivity is often largely invisible to employers because it includes under-performance on the job due to pain, as well as time off the job.[7]

The American Productivity Audit, a survey of 28,902 working adults, found the following in relation to pain-related work productivity[8]:

■ 52.7% of the work force surveyed reported having headache, back pain, arthritis, or other musculoskeletal pain in the prior 2 weeks.

- 12.7% of the work force lost productive time in a 2-week period due to pain.

- Headache (5.4%) was the most common pain condition prompting lost productive time, followed by back pain (3.2%), arthritis pain (2%), and other musculoskeletal pain (2%).

- Headache produced, on average, 3.5 hours of lost productive time per week.

- Overall, workers lost an average of 4.6 hours per week of productive time due to a pain condition.

- Lost productive time from common painful conditions was estimated by this study to cost $61.2 billion per year.

- 76.6% of lost productive time was explained by reduced work performance, *not absenteeism*.

PATIENT DESCRIPTIONS OF PAIN

Pain is described by patients experiencing it in words that relate to physical sensations, such as "tingling" or "aching," and in emotional words, such as "horrifying" or "terrifying." To illustrate pain, people often use vivid verbal analogies such as "I feel like someone is stabbing me repeatedly and twisting the knife," or "My head is in a vise that is being squeezed tighter and tighter." Behavioral responses, including grimacing, bracing, or rubbing the affected area, result in nonverbal communication about pain. These behaviors, and the accompanying physiologic signs and symptoms of autonomic activation (e.g., tachycardia, tachypnea), are common in acute pain but are uncommon in chronic pain, even when it is severe. Physicians and health care providers can feel challenged when called on to evaluate and treat painful sensations and the suffering they evoke.

The importance of alleviating the adverse consequences of pain and improving pain treatment globally was recognized by the World Health Organization in 1990. The United States government has officially designated 2000–2010 as the "Decade of Pain Control and

Research." Pain has now earned the official designation as the "fifth vital sign," and patients are encouraged to understand that they have the right to effective assessment and adequate treatment of pain.[9]

Much can be done to improve pain assessment and treatment, as this manual and the accompanying Web site http://www.PainEDU.org demonstrate.

REFERENCES

1. Coda BA, Bonica JJ. General considerations of acute pain. In Loeser JD, Butler SH, Chapman CR, Turk DC, eds. *Bonica's Management of Pain (3rd ed)*. Philadelphia, PA: Lippincott Williams & Wilkins. 2001:222–240.

2. National Center for Health Statistics. 1998. *Health, United States, 1998*. Hyattsville, MD: Public Health Service. 1998.

3. Centers for Disease Control and Prevention (CDC). Public health and aging: projected prevalence of self-reported arthritis or chronic joint symptoms among persons aged ≥65 years—United States, 2005–2030. *MMWR Morb Mortal Wkly Rep.* 2003;52:489–491.

4. Centers for Disease Control and Prevention (CDC). Prevalence of disabilities and associated health conditions among adults—United States, 1999. *MMWR Morb Mortal Wkly Rep*, 2001;50:120–125.

5. National Center for Health Statistics, 2000. *Health, United States, 2000*. Hyattsville, MD: Public Health Service. 2000.

6. Fitzgibbon DR. Cancer pain: management. In Loeser JD, Butler SH, Chapman CR, Turk DC, eds. *Bonica's Management of Pain (3rd ed)*. Philadelphia: Lippincot, Williams & Wilkins, 2001:659–703.

7. National Institutes of Health. *The NIH Guide: New Directions in Pain Research I.* Washington, DC: GPO, 1998.

8. Stewart WF, Ricci JA, Chee E, et al. Lost productive time and cost due to common pain conditions in the US workforce. *JAMA* 2003;190:2443–2454.

9. American Pain Foundation Pain Facts. http://www.painfoundation.org.

III.

Pathophysiology of Pain

MECHANISM OF NORMAL PAIN

In the past, it was thought that a sensory input, such as a pinprick, would cause a pain "signal" to be sent directly to the brain via a single nerve. Although not completely understood today, the science of pain reveals a much more complex process that still is continuing to evolve. New receptors, pathways, and hypotheses are being investigated every day. The following is a brief review of basic concepts important to understanding the physiology of pain. For more detailed information on this topic, as well as new developments, the reader is strongly urged to visit http://www.PainEDU.org.

THE PAIN PATHWAY

Four steps occur along the pain pathway: transduction, transmission, modulation, and perception.[1]

Transduction is the process by which afferent nerve endings participate in translating noxious stimuli (e.g., a pinprick) into nociceptive impulses. Silent nociceptors, also involved in transduction, are afferent nerves that do not respond to external stimulation unless inflammatory mediators are present. The peripheral nervous system contains primary sensory afferent neurons that have an important role in pain signaling. The axons of these afferents diverge from the cell body in the dorsal root ganglion near the spinal cord and send a short fiber centrally into the cord and a long fiber down the peripheral nerve into the tissues. Their receptors detect mechanical, thermal, proprioceptive, and chemical stimuli. There are three types of primary afferents: A beta fibers, A delta fibers, and C-fibers. A beta fibers are myelinated, large-diameter fibers that respond primarily to light touch and moving stimuli, such as vibration. A delta fibers (myelinated, small-diameter fibers) and unmyelinated C-fibers respond to noxious (potentially painful) stimuli. Fibers that respond maximally to noxious stimulation are classified as pain fibers, or *nociceptors*. These are generally A delta fibers and C-fibers. These nociceptors respond to noxious mechanical, thermal, and chemical stimuli.[2]

Noxious stimulation is first carried by the faster A delta fibers and then by the slower C-fibers. Local injury can cause nociceptors to become hypersensitive to noxious stimuli, thereby creating a condition called *sensitization* mediated by algogenic (i.e., pain-generating) substances in the periphery. A sequence of events occurs after local tissue injury, including local vasodilation, edema, and spreading vasodilation (flare), which is known as the *triple response of Lewis*. This is accompanied by *hyperalgesia* (an exaggerated response to painful stimuli) in the injured area (primary hyperalgesia) and hyperalgesia that spreads beyond the injured area (secondary hyperalgesia).[3]

Transmission is the process by which impulses are sent to the dorsal horn of the spinal cord, and then along the sensory tracts to the brain. The primary afferent neurons are active senders and receivers of chemical and electrical signals. Their axons terminate in the dorsal horn of the spinal cord, where they have connections with many spinal neurons. In turn, spinal neurons have inputs from many primary afferents. These spinal neurons project axons to the contralateral thalamus, which in turn projects to the somatosensory pathway, frontal cortex, and other areas. The somatosensory cortex is thought to be involved in the sensory aspects of pain, such as the intensity and quality of pain, whereas the frontal cortex and limbic system are thought to be involved with the emotional responses to it.

The major ascending tract is the spinothalamic tract (STT). Cell bodies of the STT are located primarily in lamina V, but also in laminae I, VII, and VIII. These neurons have axons that cross to the opposite side of the spinal cord and enter its anterolateral quadrant.

The STT divides in two different pathways as it approaches the thalamus. The neospinothalamic tract, or lateral STT, is the tract that subserves the sensory/discriminative aspects of pain perception. It synapses on the lateral thalamus and projects to the somatosensory cortex. The medial STT, or paleospinothalamic tract, synapses in the brain stem reticular formation, the medial thalamus, periaqueductal gray matter, and the hypothalamus and has subsequent projections to the cortex and limbic system. This tract subserves the affective/motivational aspects of pain perception.[3]

Modulation is the process of dampening or amplifying these pain-related neural signals. Modulation takes place primarily in the dorsal horn of the spinal cord, but also elsewhere, with input from ascending and descending pathways. Rich arrays of opioid receptors (mu, kappa, and delta) are present in the dorsal horn. In addition to an ascending tract, the nociceptive system contains descending pathways that send neurons from the frontal cortex and hypothalamus to the midbrain and medulla. These neurons inhibit nociceptive neurons and interneurons in the ascending pathway.[4] Important centers of this descending antinociceptive modulation system are the periventricular and periaqueductal gray matter, the dorsolateral pons, the nucleus raphe magnus, and the rostroventral medulla. Descending pathways project axons to laminae I, II, and V in the spinal cord. In addition to endogenous opioids, the biogenic amines (serotonin and norepinephrine) are neurotransmitters involved in this process. A variety of modalities can activate the descending antinociceptive pathways, including systemic or neuraxial injection of opioids, electric stimulation, stress, suggestion, and pain.[3]

The *gate control theory* is a popular model of pain modulation proposed by Melzack and Wall in 1965 and later revised by Melzack and Casey in 1968. These investigators proposed the existence of an endogenous ability to reduce or increase the degree of perceived pain through modulation of incoming impulses at a gate located in the dorsal horn of the spinal cord. The gate acts on signals from the ascending and descending systems and weighs all of the inputs. The integration of these inputs from sensory neurons, the segmental spinal cord level, and the brain determines whether the gate will be opened or closed, either increasing or decreasing the intensity of the ascending pain signal. The importance of psychological variables in the perception of pain, including motivation to escape pain, and the role of thoughts, emotions, and stress reactions in increasing or decreasing painful sensations is evident in the gate control theory. An example of this is when patients report more pain at night when they are isolated and less distracted from their pain than they might be during the day. The proposed gate can be opened or closed by pharmacologic manipulation, transduction, transmission and modulation, and psychological intervention.

Perception refers to the subjective experience of pain that results from the interaction of transduction, transmission, modulation, and the psychological aspects of the individual.

■ **Table 3.**
Normal Pain Pathway at a Glance

Transduction	Transmission	Modulation	Perception
The process by which afferent nerve endings participate in translating noxious stimuli (e.g., a pinprick) into nociceptive impulses	The process by which impulses are sent to the dorsal horn of the spinal cord and then along the sensory tracts to the brain	The process of dampening or amplifying pain-related neural signals, primarily in the dorsal horn of the spinal cord, but also elsewhere, with input from ascending and descending pathways	The subjective experience of feeling pain that results from the interaction of transduction, transmission, modulation, and psychological aspects of the individual

DEFINITION OF ABNORMAL PAIN

Pain associated with the functioning of the unaltered nociceptive system, such as stepping on a thumbtack or touching a hot stove, is referred to as *normal pain* or *nociceptive pain*. Pain that occurs in the context of a nociceptive system that has been altered by tissue damage or other processes may be referred to as *abnormal pain*. There are a number of different ways of classifying abnormal pain, with no universally accepted approach. Following is a classification system that appears to represent emerging consensus.

Inflammatory pain is the sensation that results from injury to a somatic tissue (e.g., skin, muscle, bone), which is invariably followed by an inflammatory reaction. For example, inflammatory pain is felt as the result of an acute injury or infection. The pain produced consequent to tissue inflammation results from a number of different processes. The release in injured tissue of so-called algogenic substances such as bradykinin and serotonin results in "sensitization" of the peripheral nociceptors, resulting in a lower threshold for firing and an increased frequency of firing compared with their resting state. Sensitization of nociceptive afferents means that these neurons now respond to non-noxious stimuli, such as a light touch or contact with clothing. So-called silent nociceptors may also be recruited; these are nociceptive nerve fibers that normally are silent, but in the setting of inflammation generate "pain" signals. After tissue healing, the pain generally resolves. However, in states of ongoing inflammation, such as rheumatoid arthritis or cancer, pain persists. In cases where inflammation may resolve but leave permanent anatomic alterations, such as the joint damage produced by osteoarthritis, chronic pain may result even though inflammation disappears or becomes inconspicuous.

What mechanisms lead inflammatory pain to become chronic or severe? One proposed mechanism is *central sensitization*, which refers to the process by which, as a consequence of excessive nociceptive nerve signals bombarding the central nervous system from the periphery, long-term changes occur in the central nervous system that result in persistent amplification of pain signals. One experimental paradigm resulting in central sensitization is known as *wind-up*; there are also other pathways to central sensitization. Central sensitization is one proposed mechanism by which in the context of inflammation or nerve injury (see below) normally innocuous stimuli produce pain, such as is seen in many cases of postherpetic neuralgia.[2] The phenomenon of normally innocuous stimuli (such as light touch) producing pain is called *allodynia*.

Central sensitization may also cause an exaggerated response to normally painful stimuli; this is called *hyperalgesia. Primary hyperalgesia* occurs at the site of injury and is characterized by a lower pain threshold, spontaneous pain, and increased sensitivity. It usually features thermal and mechanical hypersensitivity.[3] *Secondary hyperalgesia* refers to hyperalgesia occurring outside the area originally injured and is thought usually to be a consequence of central sensitization. The significance of the distinction is that to effectively treat chronic pain, hypersensitivity must be addressed during the clinical assessment of patients. Therapy that targets the mechanisms of hypersensitivity, if present, rather than mechanisms of nociception, must be used to try to alleviate symptoms.[4]

Neuropathic pain is defined as pain due to damaged or dysfunctional nerves. The pathophysiology of neuropathic pain can have both peripheral and central mechanisms. There have been multiple proposed mechanisms for both peripheral and central components to the pathophysiology of neuropathic pain; it is doubtful that a single mechanism can account for all cases. Damaged primary afferents may generate signals at ectopic or abnormal locations and their excitability increases after mechanical stimulation. In addition, nerves that are cut off from input from the periphery, as in the case of amputation, may become hyperactive. Changes in the dorsal horn after nerve injury include reorganization, modulation in sensory input, enlargement of the second-order neuron's receptive field, alteration in opioid receptivity, abnormal ingrowth of sympathetic nerve terminals, and abnormal temporal summation.[5] Thus, central nervous system changes, as well as peripheral nerve changes, may generate neuropathic pain.

Woolf and Mannion categorize peripheral neuropathic pain as either spontaneous (*stimulus-independent*) or hypersensitive (*stimulus-evoked*) because of increased sensitivity after damage to sensory neurons.[6]

Dysfunctional pain refers to a pain syndrome in which patients experience pain and abnormal sensitivity not associated with noxious stimulus, tissue damage, inflammation, or identifiable lesion to the nervous system. The conditions encompassed by dysfunctional pain may include fibromyalgia, tension-type headaches, migraines, and even irritable bowel syndrome. Individuals with these syndromes share a number of common characteristics, including hypervigilance to sensory stimuli, exaggerated experience of a diverse array of sensory stimuli (e.g., pain, but also sound, light, etc.), high prevalence of associated conditions (e.g., the high prevalence of irritable bowel syndrome in patients with fibromyalgia), and in some cases abnormal biomarkers (e.g., opioid peptides in spinal fluid).

There are many other ways of describing pain and terms that support them. An important term is *referred pain*, the perception of pain in a body part in which it did not originate (e.g., feeling pain from the diaphragm near the shoulder). The mechanism of referred pain is thought to be convergence of primary afferents from different locations (e.g., shoulder and diaphragm) onto the same spinal cord neurons. Because spinal neurons subserve both deep structures and skin, mislocation of sensations is possible. Classification of pain into different types and mechanisms is more than just academic interest. Data continue to emerge indicating that different types of pain respond to different types of treatment, so that accurate classification of the type of pain can support accurate selection of treatment options for the individual patient.

REFERENCES

1. Katz WA. *Pain Management in Rheumatologic Disorders: A Guide for Clinicians.* N.p.: Drugsmartz, 2000.

2. Fields HL, Basbaum AI. Central nervous system mechanisms of pain modulation. In Wall PD, Melzack R, eds. *Textbook of Pain*. London: Churchill, 2000:309–330.

3. Raj PP. *Pain Mechanisms. Pain Medicine: A Comprehensive Review*. St. Louis: Mosby, 1996:12–23.

4. Mannion RJ, Woolf CJ. Pain mechanisms and management: a central perspective. *Clin J Pain* 2000;16(Suppl 3):S144–S156.

5. Galer BS, Dworkin, RH. *A Clinical Guide to Neuropathic Pain*. New York: McGraw Hill Healthcare Information Programs, 2000.

6. Woolf CJ, Mannion, RJ. Neuropathic pain: etiology, symptoms, mechanisms, and management. *Lancet* 1999;353:1959–1964.

IV.

Pain Assessment

DEFINITIONS

Regardless of whether or not pain is nociceptive, neuropathic, or idiopathic, it is usually broadly categorized as either *acute* or *chronic*. Pain is also categorized based on other characteristics, such as its intensity, location, quality, and factors that alleviate it or worsen it.

Some simple distinguishing characteristics of acute and chronic pain include the following:

- Acute pain
  - Generally sudden onset, certainly recent onset
  - Obvious identifiable cause
    - Injury
    - Disease
    - Iatrogenic (e.g., surgery)
  - Short duration (less than 1 month)
  - Intensity generally variable and indicative of severity of condition
  - Characteristic behavior, such as rubbing, moaning, crying
- Chronic pain
  - Persistent (3 months duration or longer), often undetermined onset
  - Usually the result of some chronic disease or condition
  - May have no obvious cause
  - Prolonged functional impairment
    - Physical
    - Psychological

- May or may not be associated with characteristic behavior such as insomnia, anorexia, irritability, and even depression
- Often more difficult to manage than acute pain

Basic Terminology

Acute pain is pain that is the result of an injury or illness that is time-limited and of recent onset. Low back pain after an injury, acute headache, and postoperative pain are examples of acute pain. Acute pain is generally thought to have the biologic function of alerting the individual to harm and preparing for the "fight-or-flight" response to danger. Diagnosing and treating the underlying cause of pain, in addition to treating the symptomatic pain, are the critical elements of pain management. *Subacute pain* is pain that usually lasts up to 3 months.

Baseline pain is pain that is generally constant in nature and lasts at least half of the day.

Breakthrough pain is pain that increases over baseline pain to a significantly higher degree of intensity. *Incident pain* is a type of breakthrough pain that increases with activity or movement.

Chronic pain is pain that persists and does not resolve spontaneously. Chronic pain has usually been defined arbitrarily as pain that persists for 3–6 months or beyond the period of time that healing could be expected to have occurred.[1] Ongoing or progressive tissue damage may be present in some types of chronic pain, including progressive neuropathic pain and rheumatologic conditions. In other cases, chronic pain may be present when tissue damage is stable or undetectable.

Nociception is the activity in peripheral pain pathways that transmits or processes information about noxious events usually associated with tissue damage. Pain is the perception of nociception, which occurs in the brain. In some conditions, such as diabetic peripheral neuropathy, nociception due to tissue damage may occur, but the patient may not perceive, or feel, it. Conversely, the patient may perceive severe pain with no demonstrable evidence of tissue damage (e.g., trigeminal neuralgia).

Pain Categorized by Source and Related Nociceptor

Cutaneous pain is caused by injury to skin or superficial tissues. Cutaneous nociceptors terminate just below the skin and have a high concentration of nerve endings, producing well-localized pain.

Somatic pain originates from somatic nociceptors, located in structures such as ligaments, bones, blood vessels. The low concentration of nerve endings results in a dull, poorly localized pain sensation that is usually of longer duration than cutaneous pain.

Visceral pain originates from organ-level nociceptors located within the organs themselves or visceral cavities. Visceral nociceptors exist in even lower concentrations than somatic or cutaneous nociceptors, resulting in even more elusive qualities with respect to localization. The quality of visceral pain is typically more of a diffuse aching pain of longer duration.

Assessment

Careful and accurate assessment of pain is critical for successful diagnosis and treatment. Some important first steps include identifying some key points with respect to the patient's pain:

- The description of painful symptoms (e.g., burning, throbbing)
- The location of the pain
- The temporal nature of the pain
  - Acute versus chronic
  - Time of occurrence and duration
- The severity of the pain
  - Impact on activities of daily living
  - Psychological impact
  - Social impact
- Exacerbating and alleviating factors
- Steps taken before managing the pain
  - Reduction in activity
  - Medication use before visit

Pain assessment is not a one-time phenomenon. According to the Joint Commission on Accreditation of Healthcare Organizations Standards for 2001,[1] pain is now considered to be the fifth vital sign and should be assessed initially and reassessed on a scheduled and regular basis. The National Comprehensive Cancer Network guidelines of 2000 indicate that severe cancer pain should be assessed every 15 minutes for rapid titration of short-acting opioids and at least every 24 hours after administration of oral opioids. Patients can be informed of the regularity of pain assessment and informed that a score above a predetermined level will be addressed.

To begin an assessment, all patients should be asked about the presence of current pain or of pain over the past several months. Clinicians often ask, "How can I know how much pain my patient is feeling?" Unfortunately, there are no objective tests that can indicate the precise quality and intensity of pain and tease out the patient's affective and behavioral reactions to it. Because of the multiple dimensions of pain, it is considered to be a purely subjective experience. There are, however, standardized measures and clinical questions that can be used to assess pain and associated symptoms, such as sleep disturbance and functional status. These measures rely primarily on the patient's self-report, which, despite its limitations, remains the single most reliable indicator of the existence and intensity of pain. Techniques to assess pain when self-report is unavailable or unreliable are introduced in Chapter VII. In this section, several commonly used measures of pain intensity are reviewed, as are clinical interview questions that form part of the pain assessment. Important points of assessment in the physical examination and thorough diagnostic testing are also reviewed.

PATIENT HISTORY

Much of the information the clinician gleans about the patient's pain complaint is gained in a thorough history and physical examination. The following sample questions should be included as part of a thorough clinical history evaluation:

■ What is the location, quality, and frequency of pain?

In addition to pointing to the location of the pain and a verbal description, the patient can draw the location of pain on a body diagram. Primary and secondary sites should be elicited because patients often experience more than one location of pain. In addition, the patient can be asked to assign the percentages of pain in each area relative to the overall pain he or she experiences. Diagnostic information can be obtained by asking about the quality of pain. For example, neuropathic pain is often described as "tingling, burning, shooting," whereas visceral pain is often described as "dull, aching, or squeezing." The frequency of pain can be constant, intermittent, or cyclic, with exacerbations that occur over and above a consistent level of pain. The presence and timing of exacerbations may indicate the need for increased analgesic medication or nonpharmacologic interventions.

- What are the variations and patterns of pain? What factors alleviate or worsen pain?

Patterns of pain can be helpful in diagnosis and treatment. Patients with consistent patterns of morning pain can have their medication regimen adjusted to help them accomplish morning routines. The temporal pattern of pain—that is, whether it is constant or intermittent, sudden or gradual—is one of the most important elements in the medical history that leads to diagnosis. Provocative factors, such as bending forward or backward, may also be helpful in determining the differential diagnosis.

- When was the onset of pain? What is the history of pain management interventions? How did each of these interventions work?

The onset of pain, both in terms of the duration of pain and the manner in which the pain occurred (acute, accident, insidious), has implications for treatment and may hold meaning for the patient. For example, an insidious onset of pain with an unexplained etiology may have different implications in terms of seeking treatment and coping with pain. Patients should be asked about their use of pharmacologic, nonpharmacologic, and procedural interventions for pain. The patient may have used alternative or complementary medical approaches, such as the use of herbal preparations, acupuncture, or magnets. The relief experienced from each of these interventions can be measured by using a visual analogue scale (VAS) or by asking the patient to assign a percentage value of relief (e.g., 50% pain relief from the use of nonsteroidal antiinflammatory drugs) for each treatment.

- What are your physical limitations due to pain?

Patients are generally quick to describe their functional limitations due to pain. Walking, performing domestic chores, or continuing to work in their occupation may all be affected. Individuals in acute pain may be unable to turn over, cough, or breathe deeply secondary to their pain. Special attention should be paid to the ways patients compensate for their inability to perform physical tasks, such as walking. Compensation with another limb (e.g., performing all duties with one hand) can lead to overuse syndromes and/or more serious problems in previously unaffected areas.

- What are your expectations of treatment?

Patients today have high expectations for treatment. Although the probability that these expectations can be met in an acute, postoperative setting is high, the probability decreases for chronic pain conditions. The urgency of treatment and the expectations for it may be based on inaccurate assumptions or beliefs, such as that pain signifies ongoing damage or a return of a cancerous tumor. Patient education about the underlying cause of the pain and the effectiveness of medications, interventional procedures, and nonpharmacologic treatments should be explained carefully and honestly in lay language. Setting appropriate expectations of treatment can itself be of therapeutic benefit.

PHYSICAL EXAMINATION FOR PAIN

The physical examination for patients with pain should include a general physical, neurologic, musculoskeletal, and mental status of a patient and is likely to be a more complex process than that of other medical patients.[2] In addition, the examination should involve an assessment of the patient's functional abilities. A careful examination of the site of the patient's pain, including anatomic sites of commonly referred pain, should also be performed. The general appearance of the patient, including attributes of the skin, posture, and demeanor, are important aspects of the general physical examination.

Musculoskeletal Examination

The musculoskeletal examination includes an overall examination and focused palpation or manipulation at the site of pain. The examination needs to be tailored to the pain complaint. Muscle systems in the neck, upper extremities, trunk, and lower extremities, should be tested.[2] Deep or superficial muscle tenderness should be noted. The quality of the patient's response to palpation may be considered in the assessment. Vocalizations or a display of pain behavior may be part of the patient's cultural and/or ethnic background and can be of importance when a more stoic individual displays pain behavior in response to palpation.[2] Range of motion, including flexion, extension, side bending, rotating, and straight-leg raises, should be performed when relevant to ascertain whether pain is experienced on movement and to note the presence of functional restrictions. The degree to which these actions are performed and whether pain is incurred during each of these exercises should be recorded.

Neurologic Examination

A tailored neurologic examination is a key component of the physical examination for pain. The screening neurologic examination should include standard elements, with testing of the cranial nerves II–XII. Motor and sensory functioning in the limbs and an evaluation of rectal and urinary sphincter function have been recommended.[3] Sensory deficits are tested by sensitivity to light touch, pinprick, and mechanical and thermal stimuli. Light touch, pressure, or the application of hot and cold stimuli can cause *allodynia*—that is, the presence of pain from a stimulus that is not normally painful. Hyperalgesia, or extreme pain from stimuli that normally do cause pain, can be tested by single and multiple pinpricks and is evidence of pathology. A motor examination should test for motor weakness, ataxia, apraxia, and decreased endurance.[4] Reflexes should be normal and symmetric. In addition, pathologic reflexive signs, such as those of Babinski, Oppenheim, Gordon, Chaddock, Schaeferand, and Hoffman, should be tested when relevant.

DIAGNOSTIC TESTING

Diagnostic testing can be useful for some pain conditions and may not be useful in other types of pain conditions. Therefore, familiarity with general principles of diagnostic testing is important when assessing patients with pain.

Imaging Studies

Imaging studies show anatomy, not pain. Thus, there may be false-positives where "abnormalities" are revealed that are unrelated to the patient's pain or false-negatives where the anatomy is "normal" yet pain continues. Computed tomography myelogram, magnetic resonance imaging, ultrasound, and radionuclide examinations are used in patients with pain to confirm or rule out a diagnosis based on the patient's report and the physician's assessment. In the presence of certain signs and symptoms, such as an extremely severe headache or a history of malignancy, imaging can be critical to diagnosis and treatment. Imaging is appropriate for potentially serious spinal conditions, including spinal tumor, fracture, and cauda equina syndrome. Imaging studies are necessary for chronic pain conditions (e.g., unremitting cervical or back pain) for which surgery is being considered. However, imaging plays a limited role in some chronic pain conditions. Because suspected pathologic conditions, such as herniated or bulging disks and nerve root scarring, are frequently found in asymptomatic individuals, the need for imaging studies, and interpretation of results, must be carefully considered, lest they result in inappropriate interventions for irrelevant pathology or in distraction from the real cause of the pain.

Neurophysiology Studies

Electromyography and nerve conduction studies are electrodiagnostic procedures that evaluate action potentials and conduction along peripheral sensory and motor nerves. They are used to suggest the presence or absence of nerve entrapment, radiculopathy, trauma, and systemic neurologic disease.[5] These tests can provide useful information in the evaluation of the cause and extent of peripheral nervous system disease, but they are often unnecessary in the diagnosis of neuropathic pain conditions. Because they measure the functioning of large nerve fibers, they are not useful in diagnosing many neuropathic conditions that result from small-fiber damage or dysfunction.[4] Quantitative sensory testing measures the function of large and small nerve fibers in addition to pain thresholds. The technique is currently used for researching the mechanisms of neuropathic pain and is generally not needed for diagnosis and treatment. Analogous to the case of imaging, electromyography/nerve conduction studies show nerve damage, not pain; thus, electromyography/nerve conduction studies may be abnormal but unrelated to the pain, or normal in the presence of pain.

MEASURING PAIN INTENSITY

Knowledge of the patient's current pain intensity is important, as are pain intensity levels over time. Questions about pain intensity generally include a time line (week, month), a parameter (average, least, most), and a rating of pain. Asking about the least and most pain that the patient has experienced over some period of time can establish whether a range of pain exists.

Unidimensional Scales

Two common assessment instruments that can be used to measure pain intensity are the visual analogue scale and the numerical rating scale.

Visual Analogue Scale

The VAS is a 10-cm line with anchors at both ends. Common anchors are "no pain" and "worst pain." Patients are asked to draw a vertical line through the horizontal line to indicate their pain intensity. The distance from "no pain" to the point at which the patient's line intersects the horizontal line is measured in millimeters, yielding a number between 0 and 100. Research has shown the sensitivity, validity, and reliability of the VAS scale.[6] An example (not to scale) is shown below:

What is the intensity of your pain right now?

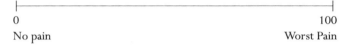

0   100
No pain   Worst Pain

Numerical Rating Scale

The numerical rating scale (NRS), sometimes referred to as a *verbal rating scale* (VRS), is an 11-point scale on which patients rate the intensity of their pain by choosing a number from 0 (no pain) to 10 (pain as bad as it could be). This rating scale is commonly used and easy to understand. The scale can be administered visually or verbally, including over the telephone, which can be useful during the dosage titration process.

What is the intensity of your pain right now?

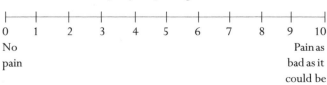

0   1   2   3   4   5   6   7   8   9   10
No   Pain as
pain   bad as it
                                                          could be

Some investigators prefer the VAS because of certain theoretical psychometric advantages. Others prefer the NRS because fewer patients fail to understand its usage, it is easier to score, and for practical purposes, the psychometric properties work well. A recent survey of 85 chronic pain patients was performed using both the VAS and verbal rating scale.[7] The results of this one survey concluded that comparatively, "the [verbal rating scale] is a simple instrument that can save time and compares favorably to the VAS." Some suggestions for increasing the ease with which patients use the numerical rating scale have been proposed[8] and are also useful in explaining the VAS. The pain scale (e.g., the NRS, VAS) should be explained each time it is administered, and patients should be taught how to use the scale. Patients can be taught that a "10" rating means the worst possible pain. This orientation can reduce the exclusive use of the higher end of the scale and increase the practical application of the measurement. Additional aids can be used to ensure that the patients with hearing or visual difficulties can use the measure with relatively little difficulty. In addition, a quiet place should be provided for the completion of this instrument, and the patient should be allowed to ask questions.[8]

Categorical Scales

Below are two examples of verbal categorical pain scales that provide a simple means for patients to rate their pain intensity using verbal or visual descriptions of their pain.

Simple Descriptive Pain Intensity Scale

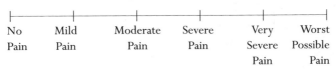

| No Pain | Mild Pain | Moderate Pain | Severe Pain | Very Severe Pain | Worst Possible Pain |

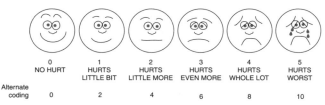

■ Figure 1.
Wong-Baker FACES Pain Rating Scale. (Adapted from Hockenberry MJ, Wilson D, Winkelstein ML. *Wong's Essentials of Pediatric Nursing [7th ed]*. St. Louis: Mosby, 2005:1259. Used with permission. Copyright, Mosby.)

These unidimensional and categorical pain rating scales remain useful screening tests that frequently should be supplemented by a more detailed assessment.

Multidimensional Tools

Multidimensional pain assessment tools provide information about the pain's characteristics and impact on daily life. The following are three examples of commonly used multidimensional tools for pain assessment in use today.

Initial Pain Assessment Tool

The Initial Pain Assessment Tool was developed for the initial patient pain evaluation. This tool includes a diagram of different body locations so that the patient can mark the areas that correspond to the location of his or her pain. In addition, the following topics are covered in the evaluation:

- Intensity of pain
- Quality of pain (in the patient's own words)
- Onset
- Duration
- Variations

- Presence of rhythmic nature
- Manner of expression of pain
- What, if anything, relieves the pain
- What causes or increases the pain
- What impact the pain has on the patient
  - Accompanying symptoms
  - Sleep
  - Appetite
  - Physical activity
  - Interpersonal relationships
  - Emotional state
  - Ability to concentrate
- Any other pertinent points
- Care plan

Brief Pain Inventory

The Brief Pain Inventory is easy to use and helps to quantify pain intensity and interference with a patient's life. Patients rate their pain severity at its worst, least, and average in the last week and at the time of assessment ("right now").

Brief pain inventory items include the following:

- A diagram of a front and back view of a human figure to identify the location of pain
- A rating of the amount of relief the patient feels that the current pain treatments (if any) provide
- A rating of the duration of the patient's pain relief after taking prescribed pain medications
- An assessment of the patient's attribution of pain to the disease, the treatment of the disease, or conditions unrelated to the disease

Patients also rate their level of pain interference in the following seven contexts from 0 ("does not interfere") to 10 ("completely interferes"):

- Work
- Activity
- Mood
- Enjoyment
- Sleep
- Walking
- Relationships

McGill Pain Questionnaire

The McGill Pain Questionnaire is one of the most extensively used pain scales. The questionnaire consists primarily of three major classes of word descriptors—sensory, affective, and evaluative—that are used by patients to specify their subjective pain experience. It also contains an intensity scale and other items to determine the properties of the pain experience.

The questionnaire was designed to provide quantitative measures of clinical pain that can be treated statistically. The three major measures are the following:

1. The pain rating index, based on two types of numerical values that can be assigned to each word descriptor

2. The number of words chosen

3. The present pain intensity based on a 1–5 intensity scale

Memorial Pain Assessment Card

The Memorial Pain Assessment Card[9] was developed as a rapid multidimensional tool in cancer patients that uses three separate VASs to assess pain, pain relief, and mood. This tool includes a set of adjectives for pain intensity as well. The major advantage of this tool is that it takes very little time to administer; the results also correlate with other, more time-consuming evaluators of pain and mood. The convenience of this card is that it can be carried easily in the clinician's pocket and conveniently presented to the patient one scale at a time.

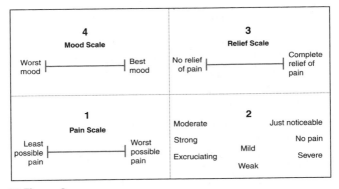

■ **Figure 2.**
Memorial pain assessment card.

PSYCHOSOCIAL EVALUATION

Pain affects the patient in many ways psychologically and socially. An overall gestalt of the most salient emotional aspects of pain can be elicited by posing a general question about the patient's well-being, such as, "How is the pain affecting your life?" or "How are you coping with your pain and its effect on your life?" Following are some of the more common areas where patients' concerns may lie.

Emotional Reactions

A variety of emotional reactions can be elicited by persistent pain. Identifying negative emotional content and assessing patients' ability to cope with these emotions are critical to improving their functioning. Asking patients, "What's your mood generally like?" may elicit some of the following:

- Anger: often expressed as frustration, irritability, disgust
- Grief: sadness, blue, loss, "I'm not me"
- Depression: anhedonia, anergia, loss of interest
- Anxiety: nervous, restless, push to be "fixed"

Patients may experience negative emotions about the following:

- Their circumstances (an injury or accident)
- Their diagnosis (cancer, chronic pain)
- An inability to perform tasks previously performed with ease
- Not being able to "handle" pain
- Treatment providers
- Insurance coverage
- The inability to return to previous job
- A terminal illness

Suicidal ideation is relatively common in patients with chronic pain conditions and should be assessed for in every patient and addressed immediately. The risk of death by suicide is estimated to be at least double for patients with chronic pain compared with controls.[10]

Warning Signs for Referral to a Psychologist, Psychiatrist, or Mental Health Professional

- Suicidal ideation with or without intent or plan
- Anergia (i.e., lack of energy)
- Persistent anhedonia (i.e., lack of pleasure)
- Loss of appetite
- Sleep disturbance
- Anxiety or panic
- Prolonged difficulty accepting the condition
- Angry outbursts toward self or others

Cognitions, Coping, and Beliefs about Pain

Cognitions, or thoughts the patient has, exert powerful effects on emotional reactions, behavioral responses, and interpretations of pain. Beliefs are a foundation for cognitions. For example, the belief that the etiology of pain can be "fixed" or "cured" affects expectations of and satisfaction with treatment. Some maladaptive beliefs and cognitions according to research include the following:

- *Catastrophizing: a cognitive and emotional process that involves magnification of pain-related stimuli, feelings of helplessness, and a negative orientation to pain and life circumstances.*[11] Examples of catastrophic statements include "I can't handle this pain," "There is nothing I can do about my pain," and "My pain is uncontrollable." The effect of catastrophizing should not be underestimated. Catastrophizing is associated with depression, decreases in physical functioning, increased pain,[12] risk of death by suicide,[10] and interpersonal distress.[13] Recent studies suggest that catastrophizing may be related to cortical responses to pain[14] and, potentially, inflammatory disease activity.[11] Catastrophizing predicts poor outcomes for patients with chronic pain and should be treated with cognitive-behavioral therapy.

- *Belief that persistent pain signals ongoing tissue damage.* This belief results in fear of movement, physical activity, and the future. Educating the patient that hurt does not equal harm and appropriate physical activity should continue may be needed.

- *Belief that if a cause of pain can be found, a treatment will fix it.* Patients are generally socialized to believe that medicine has a cure for their problems. Many believe that once a cause of the pain can be found, a treatment that results in a cure is likely (e.g., removing a problematic disk always resolves pain). For many, accepting that chronic pain can be managed but not necessarily cured is a gradual process. Encouragement to continue to be engaged in life as pain is being managed and not wait for a "cure" is often necessary.

- *Belief that pain is a signal to stop activities and movement.* Some patients believe that pain means that they should rest and be inactive. Social activities may be curtailed or stopped because they feel pain. Although patients may not be able to perform the same physical activities as before, they should be encouraged to do as much as possible because physical inactivity increases pain.[15]

Constructive coping styles, such as using coping self-statements and increasing behavioral activities, have been shown to be more effective ways to manage chronic pain[16] than passive coping strategies (e.g., resting).

The patient should be asked how he or she generally copes with pain, both cognitively (e.g., "What do you tell yourself when you are having a pain flare up?") and behaviorally (e.g., "What do you do when you are having a pain flare-up?"). Increases in drug, tobacco, and alcohol use or taking more medication than is prescribed can be other maladaptive ways of coping with pain that can lead to an exacerbation of the difficulties in the patient's life.

Behavioral Reactions

Verbal and nonverbal expressions of pain include a range of behaviors, such as the following:

- Grimacing
- Rubbing the affected body part
- Guarding or restricting movement
- Sighing
- Groaning, wailing
- Taking medications
- Resting

These behaviors are overt and are called *pain behaviors*. They can be used to do the following:

- Communicate distress
- Cope with pain
- Elicit solicitous behavior from others
- Express pain in a culturally learned or valued manner
- Express pain when verbal skills are absent or impaired

The frequency with which pain behaviors are displayed, as well as an evaluation of the environmental responses received, may be helpful in assessing whether these expressions are adaptive or maladaptive in a particular circumstance. The expression of pain behaviors may be critical when an individual is unable to express pain verbally (e.g., children, cognitively impaired individuals).

Some behaviors (e.g., resting, taking medication) are problematic when used exclusively as a pain-coping strategy. Sleep disturbance, including insomnia and middle-of-the-night awakening, initially related to painful exacerbations, can become conditioned behavioral responses over time.

Family Functioning and Responses to Pain

The family system is affected when one person becomes unable to function in the expected manner. The responses of family members have been categorized in three ways[17]:

1. Solicitous (e.g., providing assistance or special attention to the patient)
2. Punishing (e.g., becoming angry when pain is expressed)
3. Distracting (e.g., encouraging the patient to distract from the pain)

Research has shown that overly solicitous behaviors or punitive responses from family members or friends are generally not helpful. Research with patients with cancer pain and their families reveals that misconceptions about cancer and pain control on the part of the family have an adverse effect on patient care and outcome.[18]

Those with pain may not be able to fulfill role behavior they perceive as important to their definition of themselves as fathers, mothers, or members of a family or friendship network. For example, a father may not be able to participate in athletic activities with his children and may define this ability as an important part of his role as a father. Families may need assistance changing roles and learning to interact with a person with chronic pain on a long-term basis.

Social and Occupational Functioning

The nature and extent of some chronic pain conditions impact the ability to work and interact in social settings. The stress that accompanies the loss of work involves the loss of a sense of purpose, as well as loss of financial compensation.

Work-related injuries are particularly difficult for workers who believed they were valued employees who became relegated to a "disabled" status after their injury. The process of workers' compensation is complex and sometimes adversarial. Patients might experience the following:

- Be required to participate in independent medical examinations by nontreating physicians to review the appropriateness of treatment
- Be followed by private investigators who routinely investigate claims for fraud
- Be disregarded by coworkers because the pain cannot be seen and the patient "looks good"
- Be sent back to work prematurely
- Be asked to interview for other positions
- Be treated differently by physicians because of their litigation status
- Be denied treatment the treating physician has recommended
- Be financially stressed because of the loss of full-time salary or wages

Patients sometimes feel disbelieved and may feel accused of faking an injury or illness for the purpose of personal gain (e.g., obtaining time off) or malingering. Of course, this process is made difficult for physicians and patients because a few patients are malingerers. Malingering involves the intentional production of false or grossly exaggerated physical or psychological symptoms for the purpose of tangible external incentives, such as obtaining financial compensation, evading criminal prosecution, avoiding work or military duty, and obtaining drugs.[19]

The presence of workers' compensation or litigation status does not mean the patient does not want to improve and return to work or is demonstrating malingering, although these factors may complicate recovery. Evaluating the obstacles to recovery or rehabilitation (e.g., the patient does not want to return to a former job or employer) and addressing these obstacles during treatment (e.g., with vocational counseling) are important components of treating patients with chronic pain.

Psychiatric Disorders and Pain

Painful conditions, like all medical conditions, affect patients with psychiatric disorders. Selected psychiatric disorders are found in greater prevalence in medical settings and in persons with chronic illnesses. Persons with chronic pain are most often diagnosed with depression, anxiety, and substance-use disorders.[20] Consider the following statistics for individuals meeting criteria for major depressive disorder:

- 2% of people in the community[21]
- 5–9% in ambulatory care[21]
- 15–20% of medical inpatients[21]
- 0–58% of persons with cancer[22]
- 43% with nondisabling pain and depression in primary care[23]
- 66% with disabling pain and depression in primary care[23]

A Word about Somatization Disorder

Some psychiatric disorders have as a primary characteristic the existence of abnormal illness behavior and are therefore more likely to present in medical settings. For example, somatization disorder is characterized by the following:

- A pattern of multiple physical complaints
- Significant social and occupational impairment
- Symptoms that occur before age 30
- Symptoms that last for a period of years
- Pervasive complaints unaccounted for by a general medical condition, including the following:
  - Four different pain symptoms
  - Two gastrointestinal symptoms
  - One sexual symptom and
  - One pseudoneurologic symptom[19]

Although the presence of unexplained somatic symptoms is common, somatization disorder is rare.[21]

The diagnosis of undifferentiated somatoform disorder is less restrictive than somatization disorder, requiring one or more physical complaints that cannot be explained by a general medical condition and that cause significant social or occupational distress. Care should be taken before labeling patients with somatoform disorder or as "somatizers" because of current limitations of diagnostic testing and disease criteria.[21]

Pilowsky[24] suggests that a hallmark of abnormal illness behavior is extreme difficulty accepting advice from a physician if it doesn't fit the patient's appraisal of his or her health status. Avoidance of dualism in pain (i.e., the pain is either in the body or the mind) is key in assessing and treating individuals with pain conditions and is especially pertinent when treating individuals with psychiatric illnesses.

■ **Table 4.**
Summary: General Clinical Questions to Ask to Assess Psychosocial Aspects of Pain

Psychosocial Aspects of Pain	Clinical Questions to Ask
Global question	How is the pain affecting your life?
Emotional reactions	What's your mood generally like?
Suicidal thoughts	Do you ever feel like giving up?
	Do you have suicidal thoughts?
Cognitions, coping, beliefs about pain	How do you cope with the pain?
Behavioral reactions	What do you do when you have a flare up of pain?
Family functioning	How do your family members/supportive others respond when you have pain?
Social and occupational functioning	How are work and social activities going?

REFERENCES

1. Hadjistavropoulos HD, Clark J. Using outcome evaluations to assess interdisciplinary acute and chronic pain programs. *The Joint Commission Journal on Quality Improvement.* July 2001; 27(7). Available at: http://www.jcrinc.com/1249/. Accessed on July 26, 2007.

2. Loeser JD. Medical evaluation of patient with pain. In Loeser JD, Butler SH, Chapman CR, Turk DC, eds. *Bonica's Management of Pain (3rd ed).* Philadelphia: Lippincott Williams & Wilkins, 2001:267–278.

3. Jacox AK, Carr DB, Payne R, et al. *Management of Cancer Pain, Clinical Practice Guidelines.* No. 9. Rockville, MD: U. S. Department of Health and Human Services, Public Health Service, Agency for Health Care Policy and Research (AHCPR Publication No. 94-0592), 1994.

4. Galer BS, Dworkin, RH. *A Clinical Guide to Neuropathic Pain.* New York: McGraw Hill Healthcare Information Programs, 2000.

5. Stolov WC. Electrodiagnostic evaluation of acute and chronic pain syndromes. In Loeser JD, Butler SH, Chapman CR, Turk CD, eds. *Bonica's Management of Pain (3rd ed).* Philadelphia: Lippincott Williams & Wilkins, 2001:279–296.

6. Jensen, MP, Karoly, P. Self-report scales and procedures for assessing pain in adults. In Turk DC, Melzack R, eds. *Handbook of Pain Assessment.* New York: Guilford; 2001:15–34.

7. Cork I, Elsharydah S, Zavisca A. A comparison of the verbal rating scale and the visual analog scale for pain assessment. *The Internet Journal of Anesthesiology* 2004;8(1).

8. Clark ME, Gironda RJ, Young RW. Development and validation of the Pain Outcomes Questionnaire-VA. *Journal of Rehabilitation Research & Development.* September/October 2003; 40(5):381–396. Available at: http://www.rehab.research.va.gov/jour/03/40/5/clark.html. Accessed on July 26, 2007.

9. Fishman B, Pasternak S, Wallenstein SL, et al. The Memorial Pain Assessment Card. A valid instrument for the evaluation of cancer pain. *Cancer* 1987;60:1151–1158.

10. Tang NK, Crane C. Suicidality in chronic pain: a review of the prevalence, risk factors and psychological links. *Psychol Med* 2006;36:575–586.

11. Edwards RR, Bingham CO 3rd, Bathon J, Haythornthwaite JA. Catastrophizing and pain in arthritis, fibromyalgia, and other rheumatic diseases. *Arthritis Rheum* 2006;55:325–332.

12. Bishop SR, Warr D. Coping, catastrophizing and chronic pain in breast cancer. *J Behav Med* 2003;26:265–281.

13. Lackner JM, Gurtman MB. Pain catastrophizing and interpersonal problems: a circumplex analysis of the communal coping model. *Pain* 2004;110:597–604.

14. Seminowicz DA, Davis KD. Cortical responses to pain in healthy individuals depends on pain catastrophizing. *Pain* 2006;120:297–306.

15. Turk DC, Winter F. *The Pain Survival Guide: How to Reclaim Your Life.* Washington, DC: American Psychological Association; 2005.

16. Turner JA, Roman JM. Psychological and psychosocial evaluation. In Loeser JD, Butler SH, Chapman CR, Turk DC, eds. *Bonica's Management of Pain (3rd ed).* Philadelphia: Lippincott Williams & Wilkins, 2001. pp. 329–341.

17. Kerns RD, Turk DC, Rudy, TE. The West Haven-Yale Multidimensional Pain Inventory (WHYMPI). *Pain* 1985;23:245–356.

18. Miakowski C, Zimmer EF, Barrett KM, et al. Differences in patients' and family caregivers' perceptions of the pain experience influence patient and caregiver outcomes. *Pain* 1997;72:217–226.

19. *Diagnostic and Statistical Manual of Mental Disorders.* 4th ed text-rev. Washington, DC: American Psychiatric Association; 2000:739.

20. Dersh J, Polatin P, Gatchel R. Chronic pain and psychopathology: Research findings and theoretical considerations. *Psychosom Med* 2002;64:773–786.

21. Sullivan MD, Turk DC. Psychiatric illness, depression, and psychogenic pain. In Loeser JD, Butler SH, Chapman CR, Turk DC, eds. *Bonica's Management of Pain (3rd ed).* Philadelphia: Lippincott Williams & Wilkins, 2001.

22. Massie MJ. Prevalence of depression in patients with cancer. *J Natl Cancer Inst Monogr* 2004;32:57–71.

23. Arnow BA, Hunkeler EM, Blasey CM, et al. Comorbid depression, chronic pain, and disability in primary care. *Psychosom Med* 2006;68:262–268.

24. Pilowsky I. The diagnosis of abnormal illness behavior. *Aust N Z J Psychiatry* 1971;5:136–141.

V.

Types of Pain

ACUTE PAIN

Postoperative Pain

Postoperative pain is arguably the most commonly occurring model of an acute pain condition. Despite its high prevalence, postoperative pain continues to be a challenging condition to treat, even in the face of continuing advances in pain management. The Joint Commission on Accreditation of Healthcare Organizations has developed guidelines for pain management specifically to try to improve consistency and effectiveness of pain care. These guidelines make clear recommendations on not only the importance of treatment of pain in hospitalized patients, but also continued assessment and reassessment of patients to uphold quality of pain management. Yet, a 2003 national survey revealed that 80% of adults surveyed who had undergone major surgery reported pain that was moderate to severe despite treatment with analgesics.[1]

Acute postoperative pain is likely managed by the pain service, anesthesiologist, or surgeon. Specific types of postoperative pain and their individual treatments fall beyond the scope of this manual.

In the event that the responsibility of postoperative pain management falls on the shoulders of the primary care practitioner, some basic steps and considerations should be kept in mind that can improve the likelihood of effective treatment:

- Preoperative discussion should take place with the patient (if possible) to increase awareness of expectations of pain and its management and minimize stress.
- Detailed knowledge of use of analgesics before surgery if applicable is important to estimate analgesic needs.

- Preemptive therapy may actually decrease postprocedure requirements for analgesics:
  - Nonsteroidal antiinflammatory drugs
  - Cyclooxygenase-2 (COX-2) inhibitors (highly used for preemptive therapy in the past are now only valuable in selected patients where the benefit is clear and the patients are appropriate candidates)
  - Local anesthetics by direct injection
  - Opioids
- Multimodal analgesic techniques listed above using more than one method of pain management at the same time can reduce the amount of medications necessary to relieve pain and can minimize uncomfortable side effects of any given medication.

Adequate postoperative pain management is an integral part of medical care in the postoperative period. Benefits of good postoperative pain management include the following:

- Improved patient comfort
- Improved patient satisfaction
- Decreased time to ambulation
- Decreased rates of surgical complications
  - Bowel motility
  - Thrombophlebitic episodes
  - Improved blood flow and wound healing
  - Improved lung mechanics and severity of atelectasis
- Decreased length of hospital stay (nonambulatory patients)
- Decreased return to hospital rates (ambulatory patients)
- Decreased cost of care

CHRONIC PAIN

Back and Neck Pain

The structural framework of the neck and back consist of the vertebrae, musculature, and ligaments. As already stated, the likelihood is that four out of five people will experience some type of back pain in their lives.[2] The epidemiology of neck and back pain is vast. Back pain is also one of the most common forms of chronic pain in patients at all age ranges.[3] Low back pain (LBP) is well-distributed across sex, race, and marital status,[4] and it is among the top 10 complaints of patients older than 16 years of age who present to the primary care practitioner,[5] with a prevalence of up to 20%.[6] Although neck pain often receives less publicity than LBP, millions of people still experience neck pain and/or related arm pain at some point in their lives.

The economic and social magnitude of the impact of neck and back pain—most frequently chronic LBP—is enormous. Although it is difficult to calculate exactly how much back pain costs in the United States, the statistics show that backaches result in the loss of approximately 175 million work days and in a $20 billion loss in productivity. Two percent of the U.S. work force suffers from chronic back pain, costing the U.S. economy a total of $50 billion annually. Backaches are the second most common reason Americans go to the doctor (headaches are the first) and among the most common reasons for surgery (National Institutes of Health data on file).[7]

Temporal Classification of Back and Neck Pain

Acute back or neck pain generally arises spontaneously and usually lasts from a few days to a few months. Such pain may or may not have radicular symptoms associated with it. Treatment for acute back and neck pain is usually symptomatic and typically includes activity as tolerated and some form of analgesia. Bed rest for more than 2 days has now been shown conclusively to worsen prognosis. In fact, the debunking of the myth that rest is helpful, with the consequent reduction of iatrogenic disability, is probably the major advance in the treatment of back pain in the modern era.[8] The reader is referred to Chapter IV for detailed discussion of treatment options for back and neck pain.

Persistent, or *chronic*, back or neck pain may be defined as pain that lasts 3–6 months or longer and does not improve over time. In cases of chronic back pain, there is a high correlation with spondylotic disease. Patients with persistent pain often undergo surgical intervention,[9] although results are inconsistent. It has been recently appreciated that many patients have neither acute back pain nor chronic persistent back pain, but instead have recurrent back pain, or constant back trouble that occasionally becomes severe and disabling. These patients may experience long-term difficulties, including psychological and medical comorbidities. Some common psychological problems include depression, anxiety, and sleep disturbance. Multidisciplinary interventions, emphasizing rehabilitation, are commonly required.

Common pathologic causes of back and neck pain include the following:

- Disc herniation
- Sciatica
- Torticollis
- Spinal stenosis
- Spondylosis
- Spondylolisthesis
- Cauda equina syndrome
- Cancer
  - Primary tumor
  - Metastatic lesion
- Osteomyelitis of the spine
- Injury (e.g., fracture, compression)
  - As a direct result of trauma
  - As a result of osteoporotic disease

Making the diagnosis in cases of chronic back and neck pain can be challenging for primary caregivers and experts alike. Although diagnostic procedures have continued to improve in their accuracy and reliability, up to 85% of chronic cases may end up with no definitive diagnosis.[10] Sometimes the identifiable causes are muscular, but in the face of accompanying neurologic deficit, there may indeed be some degree of neurologic etiology. Although sometimes episodes of back and neck pain have no identifiable anatomic cause, there are many cases where this pain can be linked to a known cause, such as the following:

- Overuse, strenuous activity, or improper use such as repetitive or heavy lifting
- Muscle injury
  - Strain
  - Torticollis
- Whiplash (sudden force injury)
- Concurrent diagnosis of cancer
- Trauma
  - Injury/contusion
  - Fracture
- Degeneration of vertebrae, often caused by stresses on the muscles and ligaments that support the spine or the effects of aging
- Infection
- Abnormal growth, such as a tumor or bone spur
- Obesity with the result of increased weight on the spine and pressure on the disks
- Poor muscle tone
- Muscle tension or spasm
- Ligament or muscle tears
- Joint problems such as arthritis
- Protruding or herniated disk and/or nerve impingement
- Osteoporosis and compression fractures
- Congenital/developmental abnormalities of the vertebrae and bones (i.e., scoliosis)

Evaluation of Low Back Pain

Assessment of LBP should begin with a detailed history of the pain, including the patient's perception of its cause and the location and duration of the pain. A careful history is necessary to formulate diagnostic impressions and determine what the cause of the pain is. The most important goal in assessing the patient with LBP is to rule out "diagnostic imperatives,"—that is, serious illnesses that can present with LBP. These include dissecting aortic aneurysm, cancer or infections involving the spine, inflammatory spondylitis, and referred pain from the abdominal or pelvic viscera. Factors that suggest the need to rule out such disorders include new-onset back pain in an older patient, systemic symptoms (e.g., fever, sweats, and weight loss), history of cancer, and abdominal or pelvic pain.

During the physical examination, observe the patient's gait and overall posture. Scoliosis may point to underlying muscle spasm or neurogenic involvement. The examiner should also test the patient's spinal range of motion. Although the reliability of provocative maneuvers is not high, reproduction of pain on lumbar flexion tends to indicate disk pathology; pain on extension suggests facet joint pathology. The examiner should also palpate the spine for point tenderness, which could help determine the site of pathology. Palpation of the abdomen and pelvis and examination for signs of systemic illness are imperative in the evaluation of all patients with acute or subacute LBP, especially with the risk factors noted above.

Suspicion of lumbosacral radiculopathy, suggested by radiating pain or by accompanying neurologic symptoms, can be confirmed with provocative maneuvers. In the straight leg raise test, pain radiating below the knee when the leg is raised between 30 and 60 degrees suggests nerve root irritation. The straight-leg raise test is used as a test for sciatica, the lay term for *lumbosacral radiculopathy*. The crossed straight leg raise test, which tests/assesses for pain radiating down the contralateral leg when the ipsilateral leg is raised, is a less sensitive, but highly specific test for lumbosacral radiculopathy.[11] A focused neurologic examination should be performed. More details can be found in Chapter IV. Reflexes (knee and ankle) and motor and sensory testing should also be conducted to determine the presence of a neurologic deficit, which could indicate lumbosacral radiculopathy, cauda equina syndrome, or even spinal cord involvement.

Laboratory tests are not usually needed during an initial evaluation of LBP. However, if risk factors suggest tumor or infection, appropriate blood work and imaging studies must be obtained.

▪ Table 5.
Treatment of Back and Neck Pain

Once the diagnostic imperatives have been ruled out, treatment is symptomatic and is directed toward providing pain relief and restoring function.

- ▪ Most patients benefit from **maintenance of activity as tolerated, keeping as active as they can**.
- ▪ This process is often best directed by a physical therapist.

Nonsteroidal antiinflammatory drugs are helpful for acute low back pain, given the potential risks outlined in Chapter IV.

A short course of **opioid analgesics** is often required, although it is easy to overestimate their efficacy.

- ▪ A patient who cannot stand up due to acute low back pain may not stand much better while taking opioids. However, opioids can facilitate more comfortable rest periods and can facilitate reintroduction of activity and exercise.

Muscle relaxants are frequently prescribed for acute low back pain and probably have analgesic efficacy, although they do not have any primary effect on muscles. Although physicians attempting to avoid opioid use often prescribe muscle relaxants, little is accomplished for the patient by this approach because the muscle relaxants share most of the liabilities of the opioids.

The benefits of **nonpharmacologic approaches** should not be underestimated—a well-constructed comparative trial has now shown that a heating pad provided more analgesia than a nonsteroidal antiinflammatory drug.[10]

Many practitioners perform **epidural steroid injections** on patients with acute sciatica to reduce nerve inflammation and prevent chronicity, although this approach has never been validated.

- ▪ **Oral steroids are generally** *not* **indicated** for the treatment of back and neck pain.

Antidepressants have been widely used for both depressed and nondepressed patients with chronic low back problems. The extent to which these medications are used in treating patients with acute low back problems is unknown. Some researchers have hypothesized that the medications may possibly have a pain-relieving effect in addition to antidepressant properties. If so, the medications could help some patients who have chronic pain whether or not the patients are also depressed. The therapeutic objective of using antidepressant medications for low back problems is to reduce pain (See more discussion of antidepressants in Chapter VI.)

(continued)

■ Table 5.
Treatment of Back and Neck Pain (Continued)

> Because the progression of low back pain from acute to chronic is a major problem, it is worth keeping in mind strategies for prevention of this progression. The major risks for chronicity are psychosocial: comorbid psychiatric disorders, previous disabling episodes, poor job satisfaction, and so forth. It is advisable to perform a psychosocial assessment screening on patients with acute low back pain so that high risk patients can be promptly referred for multidisciplinary rehabilitative management, with vocational rehabilitation if needed.

Headache

The most common of all pain syndromes is headache. As stated previously, studies show that the large majority of adults experience headaches and that headache pain is the single largest factor in work absenteeism as well as total expenditures for health care costs.

Headaches are usually characterized by attacks that are separated by symptom-free intervals, but sometimes may become chronic. Headaches can be caused by structural abnormalities, sinus disease, increased intracranial pressure, or even referred pain from the cervical spine.

The following are three major hypotheses concerning the various origins of headache:

1. Neurogenic or vascular abnormalities in the brain
2. Myofascial or skeletal mechanisms from the cervical spine
3. A variety of diseases involving the face

The ability to make a rapid and accurate diagnosis is crucial to the successful management of any headache disorder. Because head pain can have many causes, a rational approach facilitates differential diagnosis and may increase the likelihood of a positive therapeutic outcome.

Classification of Headaches

Headaches are commonly classified as either primary or secondary. The *primary headache* disorders—those *not* associated with an underlying pathology—include migraine, tension-type, and cluster headache. *Secondary headache* disorders—those attributed to an underlying pathologic condition—include any head pain of infectious, neoplastic, vascular, drug-induced, or idiopathic origin. The vast majority of patients who present with headache have one of the primary disorders, as serious secondary causes for presentation with head pain are rare.

A number of diagnostic schemata for headache have been proposed. As early as 1962, for example, the Ad Hoc Committee on Classification of Headache listed the features that are typically present during certain types of headache, but it failed to indicate which features or combinations of features were required to establish a diagnosis. By 1988, recognizing the need for improvement in headache classification, the *International Headache Society (IHS)* published a new system, the second edition of the International Headache Classification (ICHD-2).

The following information is based on and adapted from the updated IHS criteria, ICHD-2, which outline the classification, incidence, and prevalence, and specific characteristics necessary to confirm a broad range of headache disorders.[12]

Primary Headache

Migraine Headache. Migraine is a chronic neurologic disorder characterized by episodic attacks of head pain and associated symptoms. Similar epidemiologic studies conducted 10 years apart show that the prevalence and distribution of migraine have remained stable over the last decade in the United States, with approximately 18% of women and 6% of men satisfying diagnostic criteria for the condition. Studies conducted outside the United States are in agreement with these migraine prevalence rates. Even though it is widespread, migraine remains underdiagnosed; only 48% of Americans who satisfy criteria for migraine reported receiving a physician diagnosis of migraine. Many patients never even seek medical advice and treat themselves with over-the-counter medications for this condition. The IHS recognizes six variants of migraine, but the most common types seen in primary care practice are migraine with aura (formerly "classic" migraine), migraine without aura (formerly "common" migraine), and probable migraine (formerly "migrainous headache").

■ **Table 6.**
Adapted International Headache Society Criteria for Migraine

Migraine with Aura	Migraine without Aura* (At Least Any Two Descriptions)	Migraine without Aura* (At Least Any One Symptom)
Visual symptoms	Unilateral nature	Nausea and/or vomiting
Blind spots	Pulsatile quality of pain	
Flashes of light		Photophobia
"Zigzag" light	Moderate to severe intensity	Phonophobia
Other visual distortions		
Motor weakness	Aggravation by, or causing avoidance of routine physical activity	
Sensory symptoms		
Paresthesia		
Aphasia		
Signs of brain stem dysfunction		
Diplopia		
Ataxia		
Vertigo		

*Patients without aura must have five attacks fulfilling the above criteria, with headaches lasting 4–72 hrs and no signs of a secondary headache disorder, to meet criteria.

Migraine with Aura. Providers should suspect migraine with aura whenever a headache is preceded by one of the neurologic symptoms listed in Table 6.

The symptoms of migraine with aura should be reported as fully reversible, developing over 5–20 minutes and lasting less than 60 minutes. It is commonly observed in clinical practice that not all auras are followed by a headache or a headache that is associated with characteristics of migraine. If aura occurs without subsequent headache, then the condition is a typical aura without headache; if a nonmigraine headache follows aura, then it is classified as a typical aura with a nonmigraine headache.

Migraine without Aura. Migraine without aura is the commonest subtype of migraine. It has a higher average attack frequency and is usually more disabling than migraine with aura. Migraine without aura is characterized by headache pain that is virtually indistinguishable from the pain experienced by patients with aura, except no aura precedes the migraine attack.

Migraine without aura often has a strict menstrual relationship. In contrast to the first edition of *The International Classification of Headache Disorders*, the current edition gives criteria for *pure menstrual migraine* and *menstrually related migraine*, but in the appendix because of uncertainty over whether they should be regarded as separate entities. Because of their frequency, and menstrual relationship, they deserve mention. *(Readers are encouraged to visit http://www.PainEDU.org for more detailed information on migraine headaches and their menstrual relationship.)*

Pure Menstrual Migraine. Pure menstrual migraine has the following distinguishing characteristics:

- Attacks in a menstruating woman
- Fulfilling criteria for migraine without aura
- Attacks occur exclusively on day 1±2 (i.e., days −2 to +3) of menstruation in at least two out of three menstrual cycles and at *no other times of the cycle*

Menstrually Related Migraine. Menstrually related migraine has the following distinguishing characteristics:

- Attacks in a menstruating woman
- Fulfilling criteria for migraine without aura
- Attacks occur on day 1±2 (i.e., days −2 to +3) of menstruation in at least two out of three menstrual cycles and *in addition at other times of the cycle*

Because migraine without aura does not have a single distinguishing feature, the IHS criteria for migraine without aura require the presence of a constellation of symptoms (see Table 6).

Despite the existence of specific criteria of both types of migraine, clinicians frequently misdiagnose migraine. One reason for error is the criteria themselves. The IHS criteria do not include all symptoms frequently observed in episodes of migraine. Consequently, migraine associated with muscle or neck pain, a non-IHS migraine diagnostic criterion, is often diagnosed as tension-type headache (TTH), or migraine associated with nasal symptoms such as rhinorrhea and nasal congestion, also not included as IHS diagnostic criteria, is diagnosed as a "sinus" headache. In both cases, research demonstrates that these headaches are usually migraine. Additionally, clinicians often focus on the presence of a single symptom to make a migraine diagnosis. This often results in even experts having different opinions of whether or not a headache is truly a migraine.

An especially significant complicating factor in the diagnosis of migraine may be the existence of comorbid illness. Migraine has been associated with a number of psychiatric and medical-neurologic illnesses. Therefore, providers should not be surprised to find an increased incidence of affective and anxiety disorders among migraine patients. Bipolar psychiatric disturbances and phobias are also noted. The incidence of stroke, epilepsy, essential tremor, mitral valve prolapse, and Raynaud's disease also are increased in migraine patients compared with their nonmigraine counterparts. *(Readers are encouraged to visit http://www.PainEdu.org for more detailed information on migraine headaches.)*

■ **Table 7.**
Treatment of Migraine Headache Pain

1. Treatment should be adapted to the patient's individual needs, in view of his or her medical history and mental health.
2. Migraine treatment strategies are often considered to be one of two approaches:
a. **Abortive treatment** (getting rid of an acute headache)
b. **Prophylactic treatment** (preventing them)
(continued)

■ **Table 7.**
Treatment of Migraine Headache Pain (Continued)

3. First, **precipitating factors should be identified** so that the patient can learn to **avoid them**, if possible. These factors include the following:

   a. Alcohol

   b. Abrupt changes in climate or weather

   c. Diet

   d. Missing meals

   e. Stress

   f. Hormonal changes (including menstruation, ovulation, and menopause)

   g. Lack of sleep

4. **Teaching** the patient coping skills is also helpful.

5. **With regard to acute measures, all of the treatment strategies are more effective when combined with treating coexisting insomnia.**

6. **Nonsteroidal antiinflammatory drugs** or **high doses of aspirin** are effective in treating migraine.[13] However, the gastrointestinal side effects of such medications may require that they be administered through the rectal or parenteral route. Moreover, an antiemetic may be needed to counteract the effects of treatment.

7. **Serotonin (5-HT) agonists** (e.g., triptans such as sumatriptan, rizatriptan, and zolmitriptan) are the most effective drugs for aborting a migraine episode. **Sumatriptan** is the most commonly prescribed triptan; however, it also has many side effects. Triptans are contraindicated for patients with cardiovascular or cerebrovascular disorders because of their vasoconstrictive action.

8. Other options for acute treatment of migraine include **antiemetics** and **intranasal dihydroergotamine**.

9. Although **ergotamine** treatments were commonly used to treat migraines in the past, they are generally used only for headaches that have been resistant to other treatments.[14]

(continued)

■ **Table 7.**
Treatment of Migraine Headache Pain (Continued)

10. Prophylactic treatments of migraine are usually considered in cases where the patient's migraines are frequent and disabling, a common rule being more than three severe headaches per month. Research indicates that the long-term efficacy of prophylactic measures is only about 55%.
    a. Prophylactic treatment may also be beneficial in cases of menstrually related migraines, with drugs such as **frovatriptan**.
    b. Other drugs found effective for preventing migraine that may be considered despite the occurrence of side effects that may make them more or less reasonable for a given patient include the following:
        i. **Beta blockers**
        ii. **Sodium valproate**
        iii. **Gabapentin**
        iv. **Serotonin antagonists**
        v. **Calcium channel blockers**
    c. Nonpharmacologic treatments, including **biofeedback**, **behavioral therapy**, and **acupuncture**, are also effective in preventing migraine headaches.[13,14]

Tension-Type Headache. TTH is the *most common* type of primary headache. In the general population, estimates by the IHS of the prevalence of episodic TTH vary widely, from 30 to 80%. The IHS criteria for TTH, listed in Table 8, outline a range of specific characteristics that distinguish TTH from migraine and show that the symptoms tend to be less severe, bilateral, nonpulsating, and not aggravated by routine physical activity. Symptoms associated with migraine attacks, such as nausea, phonophobia, or photophobia, are rarely present, but there can be symptomatic overlap. Studies have shown that 25% of TTH patients also have migraine, and 62% of migraineurs have TTH. Moreover, epidemiologic research suggests that TTH, when it coexists with migraine, might represent a segment on the continuum of the same disorder.

In the 2004 IHS diagnostic criteria, episodic TTH, as opposed to chronic daily TTH, is a condition without associated symptoms other than photophobia or phonophobia. Although this further sep-

■ **Table 8.**
Adapted International Headache Society Criteria for
Tension-Type Headache*

Description (At Least Any Two Descriptions)	Associated Symptoms (At Least One)
Pressing or tightening	Absence of nausea or vomiting
Mild to moderate intensity	Photophobia *or* phonophobia (not both)
Bilateral location	
No worsening with exertion	

*Must have had more than 10 previous headache episodes and no evidence of a secondary headache disorder.

arates migraine and tension headache, it leaves more headache presentations of a mixed type. Much of the void is filled by a diagnosis of "probable migraine," which represents a headache that lacks one diagnostic criterion for migraine headache.

■ **Table 9.**
Treatment of Tension-Type Headache Pain

1. Research shows that **nonsteroidal antiinflammatory drugs** are the primary treatment of choice for acute tension-type headaches.[14]

2. **Combining analgesics with caffeine or sedatives** may be more effective than analgesics alone.

3. **There is no scientific evidence that muscle relaxants are an effective treatment.**

4. Tricyclic antidepressants are often prescribed as prophylactic treatment for chronic tension-type headaches. **Amitriptyline** is the most frequently prescribed antidepressant, but it has many side effects. When the patient experiences these side effects, some other antidepressants, such as **nortriptyline or desipramine**, can be used.

5. **Cognitive-behavioral strategies** are also effective for reducing stress, and research shows that these strategies are most effective when combined with **biofeedback or relaxation techniques**.

6. Some other nonpharmacologic treatments include **massage, positioning, and heat or cold applications**.

Cluster Headache. Cluster headaches are the third major type of primary headache and are defined as a strictly unilateral headache, usually occurring once or a few times a day at a characteristic time (e.g., 1 a.m.), lasting for 15–180 minutes, occurring in a series which lasts from several weeks to several months, separated by remissions lasting from months to years.

Findings from prevalence studies of cluster headache are controversial. Patients with cluster headaches generally rate the intensity of their pain as among the worst imaginable, and cluster headache may be the *most severe* of the primary headache disorders. Most often, cluster headache occurs once every 24 hours for 6–12 weeks at a time, with remission periods typically lasting 12 months. Typical age of onset for both men and women is 27–31 years. However, *cluster headaches are one of the few headache syndromes that are more frequent in men than in women*. Population studies of cluster headaches find the occurrence is five times more likely in males. Cluster headaches may be related to cigarette smoking, head trauma, and positive family history for cluster headaches.

Cluster attacks have several differentiating features. Most important of these is the presence of transient autonomic symptoms. These features are listed in Table 10.

■ **Table 10.**
Adapted International Headache Society Criteria for Cluster Headache*

Description (All Four Descriptions)	Autonomic Symptoms (Any Two Symptoms)
Severe headache	Rhinorrhea
Unilateral and ipsilateral quality	Lacrimation
Duration of 15–180 mins	Facial sweating
Orbital, periorbital, or temporal location	Miosis
	Eyelid edema
	Conjunctival injection
	Ptosis

*No evidence of a secondary headache disorder.

■ **Table 11.**
Treatment of Cluster Headache Pain

---

1. **In most cases, patients with cluster headaches should be referred to a specialist.**

2. Acute treatment of cluster headaches includes the following:

   a. Inhalation of **100% oxygen**

   b. Intranasal application of **dihydroergotamine**

   c. Subcutaneous injection of **sumatriptan**

3. There is *no consensus as to prophylactic treatment* of cluster headaches. Some methods include prescribing the following:

   a. **Verapamil**

   b. **Lithium carbonate**

   c. **Methysergide**

   d. **Ergotamine**

   e. **Corticosteroids**

Systemic symptoms, such as bradycardia, hypertension, and increased gastric acid production, may also accompany an attack. Another unique feature is that cluster episodes are *always* on the same side, even when long intervals separate headache episodes.

Diagnosis of Primary Headache in Clinical Practice

Because most office-based evaluations of headache occur when patients are asymptomatic, the primary health care provider relies on *impact-based recognition of headache*. On those occasions when a person is being evaluated during a headache, it is best to rely on IHS criteria, summarized in Table 12.[12]

Given the constraints of clinical practice, however, primary headache disorders can be quickly and reliably recognized by inquiring about the following:

■ Interference with daily living

■ Recurrent disabling headaches should be considered migraine until proved otherwise

■ **Table 12.**
Characteristics of Primary Headache Disorders

	Migraine	Tension-Type	Cluster
Location	Unilateral	Bilateral	Strictly unilateral
Intensity	Moderate/ severe	Mild/moderate	Severe
Duration	4–72 hrs	30 mins to 7 days	15–90 mins
Quality	Throbbing	Pressing/tight- ening	Severe
Associated symptoms	Yes	No	Yes, autonomic
Gender	Female > male	Female > male	Male > female

- Frequency
  - The frequency of headaches alerts the clinician to chronic headache disorders and migraine transformation
  - Daily or near-daily headache patterns should alert the provider to the possibility of medication overuse
- Change in headache pattern over prior 6-month period
  - A negative response reassures the caregiver and the patient that serious underlying disease is unlikely
  - An affirmative answer indicates the need for a more in depth evaluation of possible warning signs that a secondary headache disorder may be present
- Change in existing headaches
  - "Worst headache ever"
- Focal neurologic signs or symptoms such as the following:
  - Papilledema
  - Motor weakness
  - Memory loss
  - Papillary abnormalities
  - Sensory loss
- Association with systemic symptoms

- New-onset headache after age 50
- Medication use
  - More than 2 days a week
    - Overuse of any acute headache remedy, prescription or nonprescription, *may promote more frequent headaches*
      - "Medication-induced migraine"

Secondary Headache

As mentioned in "Classification of Headaches," secondary headache disorders are those attributed to an underlying pathologic condition. Obviously, the focus centers around the headache-causing condition when dealing with diagnosis.

The breakdown of conditions that cause secondary headache identified by the IHS are the following:

- Head and/or neck trauma
- Cranial or cervical vascular disorder
- Cranial nonvascular disorder
- A substance or its withdrawal
- Infection
- Homeostasis
- Disorder of the cranium, neck, eyes, ears, nose, sinuses, teeth, mouth, or other facial or cranial structure
- Psychiatric disorder

The following criteria should be used for assistance in diagnosis and distinguishing secondary from primary headache:

- Another disorder known to be able to cause headache has been demonstrated.
- Headache occurs in close temporal relation to the other disorder, and/or there is other evidence of a causal relationship.
- Headache is greatly reduced or resolves within 3 months (possibly shorter for some disorders) after successful treatment or spontaneous remission of the causative disorder.

Arthritis Pain

In 2002, 43 million American adults reported doctor-diagnosed arthritis, making arthritis one of the nation's most common health problems. As a result of this, arthritis is very commonly seen in primary care practices. Obviously, as the U.S. population ages, these numbers are likely to increase dramatically. The number of people who have doctor-diagnosed arthritis is projected to increase to 67 million in 2030.[15]

Arthritis is actually not a single disease, but a constellation consisting of more than 100 different conditions. Among the most common are osteoarthritis (OA) and rheumatoid arthritis (RA). Considering the costs associated with diagnosis, treatment, and lost productivity due to disability, arthritis is one of the most expensive diseases in the United States today.[16,17] Arthritis is actually the nation's leading cause of disability, limiting everyday activities for 16 million Americans in 2002. Work limitations attributable to arthritis affect more than 5% of the general population and nearly 30% of people with arthritis. Each year, arthritis results in 750,000 hospitalizations and 36 million outpatient visits. Direct medical costs for arthritis were more than $51 billion in 1997. Arthritis is not just an old person's disease. Nearly two-thirds of people with arthritis are younger than age 65.[17]

Osteoarthritis

OA is the most common arthritic condition, affecting from 16 million to 23 million Americans usually 60 years of age or older.[17,18] OA is primarily a disease of the cartilage that produces local tissue response, mechanical change, and ultimately, failure of function.

The joints most commonly involved in presentation of OA typically include the following:

- Cervical spine
- Distal interphalangeal joints
- Feet and ankles
- First carpometacarpal joints
- Hips
- Knees

- Lower spine
- Proximal interphalangeal joints

Patients usually present with symptoms of *morning stiffness lasting no longer than 20–30 minutes*. Presence of stiffness that persists longer should generate inquiry about other possible diagnoses. In the absence of injury, involvement of the shoulders, wrists, and elbows is uncommon.

Diagnosis of OA is assisted by attention to the following:

- Clinical presentation
  - History and physical findings
- Radiographic evaluation
  - Joint-space narrowing of large, weight-bearing joints
  - Increased subchondral bony sclerosis
  - Osteophytes
  - Small synovial effusions with noninflammatory pathology findings
  - Laboratory tests are usually *not* useful and often normal

Rheumatoid Arthritis

RA is the second most common form of arthritis. It is a debilitating and destructive disease and, unlike OA, a systemic inflammatory condition. Women are affected more than men (5:1). Incidence is highest between ages 20 and 50, with a prevalence of 1–2% of adults, ranging from 0.3% in patients younger than 35 to approximately 10% of those older than 65 years old.[18]

RA is a chronic autoimmune disease; patients present with findings including the following:

- Symmetric involvement of small and large joints with the following:
  - Pain
  - Swelling
  - Warmth
  - Tenderness
  - Synovitis

■ **Table 13.**
Quick Comparison of Osteoarthritis vs. Rheumatoid Arthritis

Osteoarthritis	Rheumatoid Arthritis
Usually occurs in patients 60 years or older	Highest incidence between ages 20 and 50
Asymmetric joint involvement	Symmetric joint involvement
Distal and proximal interphalangeal joints	Small and large joints
	Large joint effusion
Lumbar and cervical spine	Inflammatory
Weight-bearing joints	Stiffness lasts hours to full day
Small joint effusion	Laboratory tests useful
Not inflammatory	Elevated erythrocyte sedimentation rate
Morning stiffness lasts 20–30 mins	
Laboratory tests not useful	Elevated C-reactive protein
Radiographic evidence	Anemia of chronic disease
Joint space narrowing of large, weight-bearing joints	Rheumatoid factor present in 90% of patients
Increased subchondral bony sclerosis	Radiographic evidence
	Variable

- ■ Occurs in patients typically younger than OA patients
- ■ Morning stiffness lasts several hours to entire day
- ■ Fever
- ■ Weight loss

Diagnosis of RA is assisted by attention to the following clinical presentation:

- ■ History and physical findings
  - ■ Chronic progressive system inflammation
    - ♦ Joint swelling
    - ♦ Synovitis
- ■ Large joint effusions

- Pathology positive for the following:
    - Elevated white blood cell count (20,000–50,000) with 50–70% polymorphonuclear leukocyte cells
- Laboratory tests
    - Elevated erythrocyte sedimentation rate
    - Elevated C-reactive protein
    - Anemia of chronic disease
    - Rheumatoid factor present in 90% of patients
- Radiographic studies
    - Juxtaarticular osteoporosis may be present
    - Symmetric affectation

In addition to arthritis' structural and mechanical consequences, pain is a significant stress for people with arthritis. People with OA and RA experience both acute and chronic pain, depending on the progression of their condition. A major consideration in dealing with arthritis patients is the patient's level of function, as it is often the criterion by which treatment successes are measured. This functionality is influenced by physical as well as psychosocial factors.

Because patients with arthritis will live the remainder of their lives with some degree of their condition, this, indeed, could be one of the most common chronic painful conditions faced in primary care practices today and in the future. Although they are quite different conditions, treatment strategies of OA and RA are similar. These strategies include those listed in Tables 14 and 15.

■ **Table 14.**
  Treatment of Arthritis Pain

1. Patient education
a. Weight reduction
b. Physical exercise
c. Cognitive-behavioral therapy
Self-help techniques
d. Good nutritional habits
(continued)

■ **Table 14.**
  Treatment of Arthritis Pain (Continued)

2. Assistive devices

3. It is clear that altering the progression of disease in rheumatoid arthritis (RA) has importance in controlling pain. In RA, these drugs are often the first line of therapy. Disease-modifying medications commonly used to achieve this goal include the following:

   a. Methotrexate

   b. Leflunomide

   c. Tumor necrosis factor (TNF-α inhibitors)

   d. Sulfasalazine

4. Topical agents may be beneficial in helping to abate arthritis-related pain.

   a. Capsaicin

   b. Lidocaine 5% patch

5. Hyaluronic acid viscosupplementation may be useful in treating osteoarthritis (OA) and is Food and Drug Administration–approved for OA of the knee.

6. Analgesics

   a. Acetaminophen (in the absence of signs of inflammation)

   b. Nonsteroidal antiinflammatory drugs

      i. Nonspecific nonsteroidal antiinflammatory drugs (Consider coadministration of proton pump inhibitor for gastric protection.)

      ii. Cyclooxygenase-2–selective nonsteroidal antiinflammatory drugs (only in appropriate patients)

   c. Intraarticular injection of glucocorticoids in patients with OA with significant inflammation

   d. Systemic glucocorticoids should be avoided in treatment of OA but may be useful in low doses and short-term use in treatment of RA.

      i. Should be combined with osteoporosis prophylaxis:

         ■ Bisphosphonates

         ■ Calcium supplementation

         ■ Vitamin D supplementation

(continued)

■ **Table 14.**
Treatment of Arthritis Pain (Continued)

7. Opioids should be used in patients with OA or RA when other medications or nonpharmacologic approaches provide inadequate pain relief and affect the patient's quality of life. These include but are not limited to the following:

    a. Morphine

    b. Oxycodone

    c. Oxymorphone

    d. Hydrocodone

8. Tramadol, like opioids, may be effective in treating pain in OA and RA that has been refractory to other treatments.

    Opioids and tramadol may be used in combination with other medications and approaches to minimize the dosage of opioid required and therefore minimize adverse effects of these drugs.

■ **Table 15.**
Surgical Intervention

Procedures	Reasons for Surgery
Procedures such as synovectomy, arthroscopic débridement, and joint replacement surgery often have improved success rates before the development of tendon rupture, contracture, or advanced joint disease. Commonly, the decision to treat with surgical intervention is made on an individual basis with consideration of the following factors.	Pain Function Deformity Stiffness Medical risk factors Patient goals and preferences Prior treatments and successes Radiographic evidence Age Patient quality of life

Gout

Gout is one of the most painful forms of arthritis. Gout typically is an example of an acutely painful arthritic condition, as compared to OA and RA. Gout accounts for approximately 5% of all cases of arthritis. In the United States, it occurs in approximately 840 out of every 100,000 people. Gout is nine times more common in men than women. Gout often affects men in their 40s and 50s, although gout attacks can occur after puberty, which sees an increase in uric acid levels. Gout attacks are more common in women after the menopause.

Gout is thought to occur from buildup of uric acid in the body, resulting in the following:

- Sharp uric acid crystal deposits in the joints, typically the big toe
- Tophi, deposits of uric acid under the skin, appearing as hard lumps
- Uric acid renal calculi

Although the first attack of gout often occurs in the big toe, it can also occur in other locations, such as in the following:

- Ankles
- Elbows
- Fingers
- Heels
- Instep
- Knees
- Wrist

Commonly, gouty "attacks" can be brought on by stress, alcohol consumption, an acute illness, or even medications. The attacks can last from 3 to 10 days and may be separated from each other by months or even years. Presentation of a gouty attack is usually characteristic, with patients presenting with the following symptoms:

- Exquisite tenderness and pain in the big toe
  - Often awaking the patient from sleep at the time of the attack
- Redness
- Swelling

■ **Table 16.**
  Treatment of Gout Pain

1. Traditionally, treatment for acute gout has consisted of **colchicine,** which can be effective if given early in the attack (best if used in the first 12 hours of acute attack).

2. **Nonsteroidal antiinflammatory drugs** can decrease inflammation as well as pain in joints and other tissues. Nonsteroidal antiinflammatory drugs have become the treatment choice for most acute attacks of gout.

3. **Corticosteroids** are important options in patients who cannot take nonsteroidal antiinflammatory drugs or colchicine. Given orally or by injection directly into the joint or intramuscularly, they can be very effective in treating gout attacks.

4. **Resting the affected joint** and applying cold compresses to the area also may help alleviate pain.

■ Warmth of the affected area
■ Stiffness

In addition to signs and symptoms, the clinician can test to confirm or exclude the diagnosis of gout:

■ History of present illness
  ■ Sudden onset of 1 day of arthritic-like symptoms with redness and swelling
  ■ Presence in one single joint
■ Determination of serum uric acid level
■ Examination of joint aspirate for presence of uric acid crystals

Neuropathic Pain

Until recently, the mechanisms of neuropathic pain have been unknown. It is currently thought to be due to injury to or dysfunction of the nervous system. There are likely multiple mechanisms of neuropathic pain.[19] Possibilities include the following:

■ Genetic predisposition to develop pain after nerve injury

- Alteration of the input from peripheral nerves to the dorsal horn of the spinal cord
- Aberrant growth of sympathetic fibers
- Peripheral or central sensitization
- An abnormal inflammatory response. Peripheral nerves, the spinal cord, and the brain react to the environment and change structure and function, emphasizing the plasticity of the nervous system.

Some common causes of neuropathic pain include the following:

- Alcoholism
- Amputation
- Back, leg, and hip problems
- Cancer chemotherapy
- Diabetes
- Facial nerve problems
- Human immunodeficiency virus infection or acquired immunodeficiency syndrome
- Multiple sclerosis
- Shingles [postherpetic neuralgia (PHN)]
- Spine surgery

Assessment of the patient with neuropathic pain involves the standard assessment for pain discussed in Chapter IV. The sensory qualities of neuropathic pain can also be assessed by specific self-report paper and pencil measures. Two instruments that are commonly used are the McGill Pain Questionnaire,[20] an instrument with a long history of research, and the newer, Neuropathic Pain Scale.[21] The *Neuropathic Pain Scale* is a reliable and valid measure of self-reported pain intensity, especially designed with attention to common aspects of neuropathic pain. A difference between the McGill Pain Questionnaire and the Neuropathic Pain Scale is the manner in which they are scored; the McGill Pain Questionnaire results in a composite score of sensory items and the Neuropathic Pain Scale results in 10 separate scores.

A focused neurologic examination should determine the presence of the following[19]:

- Allodynia (the sensation of pain after a stimulus that does not normally evoke pain; allodynia may be experienced by air blowing over the affected area, or light touch, such as the sensation of sheets or clothing)
  - Testing for the presence of dynamic allodynia is accomplished by lightly rubbing the area (e.g., with fingertip or a cotton swab)
  - Static allodynia is found by applying perpendicular pressure (e.g., with a pencil eraser or a cotton swab)
  - Thermal allodynia by applying warm or cold stimuli (e.g., with a test tube or tuning fork)
- Hyperalgesia (abnormally increased pain reactions elicited by stimuli that would normally *not* be painful)
  - Single and multiple pinpricks can be used to test for hyperalgesia
- Myofascial pain
  - Tightening muscles, ligaments, and tendons
- Motor deficiencies
  - Weakness
  - Ataxia
  - Decreased endurance

Laboratory tests in neuropathic pain, such as neuroradiologic tests and electrophysiologic studies, can sometimes be helpful in establishing the diagnosis but are not helpful in determining the presence or severity of pain.

Neuropathic pain can occur in many syndromes, including diabetic peripheral neuropathy (DPN), PHN, polyneuropathy, central pain syndromes (e.g., poststroke pain, phantom pain), and complex regional pain syndrome (CRPS) (types I and II). Some neuropathic pain states are associated with cancer and include those induced by chemotherapy, impingement of tumor on nerves, radiation, and postsurgical neuropathic pain syndromes (e.g., postmastectomy pain).[18] Painful polyneuropathies are often described as "burning and shooting" with "tingling and pins and needles." They generally occur in a stocking-and-glove distribution.

Treatment algorithms for neuropathic pain based on efficacy, tolerability, safety, and the results of published controlled clinical trials have been suggested by Galer and Dworkin[19] and generally include the following:

- Topical analgesics
- Tricyclic antidepressants
- Anticonvulsants
- Opioids
- Other medications (e.g., tizanidine, tramadol) and selected invasive interventions

Diabetic Peripheral Neuropathy

DPN is an often undiagnosed and tragic complication of diabetes. DPN is thought to occur as a result of microvascular insufficiency, a common complication of diabetes. Twenty-five to fifty percent of diabetic patients develop DPN in their lifetime.[22] Although it occurs so commonly, a recent survey by the American Diabetes Association indicated that for most of the respondents who experienced pain, 75% had not been diagnosed. Additionally, in 2005, 56% of symptomatic respondents were not even familiar with the term "diabetic neuropathy."[23]

DPN can have several deleterious effects on patients, not unlike other chronic painful conditions, including the following:

- Depression
- Anxiety
- Insomnia
- Decreased quality of life
  - Inability to perform activities of daily living
  - Increased disability
  - Inability to perceive dangerous conditions
    - Heat
    - Cold
    - Tissue damage

The most common form of DPN is distal symmetrical polyneuropathy of the lower extremities, manifesting itself with pain having the following qualities:

- Shooting
- Burning
- Stabbing pain in the feet or lower legs

A position statement in 2006 by the American Diabetes Association recommends screening of patients for DPN at the time of diagnosis of type 2 diabetes and 5 years after diagnosis of type 1 diabetes.[24] Screening for DPN includes examination of ankle reflexes and sensory function in the feet. Investigation should be performed to inquire about neuropathic symptoms in the feet and lower extremities, as well as physical examination for ulcers, sores, or other forms of tissue damage.

The early recognition and appropriate management of neuropathy in the patient with diabetes are important for a number of reasons:

- Nondiabetic neuropathies may be present in patients with diabetes and may be treatable.
- A number of treatment options exist for symptomatic diabetic neuropathy.
- Up to 50% of DPN may be asymptomatic, and patients are at risk of insensate injury to their feet.
- Autonomic neuropathy may involve every system in the body.
  - Cardiovascular autonomic neuropathy causes substantial morbidity and mortality.

Specific treatment for the underlying nerve damage is currently not available, other than improved glycemic control, which may slow progression but rarely reverses neuronal loss. Effective symptomatic treatments are available for the manifestations of DPN and autonomic neuropathy. Once the diagnosis of DPN is established, special foot care is appropriate for insensate feet to decrease the risk of amputation.[24]

■ **Table 17.**
Treatment of Diabetic Peripheral Neuropathy

Treatment of diabetic peripheral neuropathy (DPN) pain is similar to that of other types of neuropathic pain with some special treatments as well, including the following:

1. **Glycemic control** (paramount importance in DPN)
2. **Antidepressants**
   a. **Tricyclics**, such as amitriptyline, nortriptyline, desipramine, doxepin, imipramine, maprotine, and clomipramine
   b. **Selective serotonin reuptake inhibitors**, such as fluoxetine, paroxitene, sertraline, citalopram, and fluvoxamine
   c. **Selective norepinephrine and serotonin reuptake inhibitors**, such as venlafaxine
   d. **Others**, such as bupropion, trazodone, nefazodone, and mirtazapine
3. **Anticonvulsants**
   a. **Gabapentin** is often considered to be the first-line oral agent for the treatment of neuropathic pain
   b. **Pregabalin** (recent U.S. Food and Drug Administration approval for treatment of DPN). Its presumed pain-relieving effect at the α_2-δ subunit of the presynaptic calcium channel
   c. Others include phenytoin, carbamazepine, topiramate, and valproic acid
4. **Opioids**
5. **Topical analgesics**
   a. **Lidocaine patch 5%** (for postherpetic neuralgia)
   b. **Topical capsaicin**
6. **Duloxetine** (recent U.S. Food and Drug Administration approval for treatment of DPN). Its presumed pain-relieving effect by 5-hydroxytryptamine and norepinephrine reuptake inhibition
7. **Use of well-fitting and cushioned shoes, or athletic shoes**

Postherpetic Neuralgia

PHN is a painful condition caused by the varicella zoster virus in a dermatomal distribution (the area governed by a particular sensory nerve) after an attack of herpes zoster, usually manifesting after the vesicles have crusted over and begun to heal. Each year, approximately 1 million individuals in the United States develop shingles, or herpes zoster. Approximately 20% of these shingles patients, or 200,000 individuals, go on to suffer from PHN.

PHN is thought to result after nerve fibers are damaged during a case of herpes zoster. Damaged fibers cannot transmit electrical signals from the skin to the brain as they normally do and these signals may be erratic or even exaggerated, causing chronic, often excruciating pain that may persist or recur for months—or even years—in the area where shingles first occurred. Some research suggests that this condition is three times more frequent in the cancer patient population due to immunocompromise.[25]

Pain and temperature detection systems are hypersensitive to light mechanical stimulation, which causes severe pain even from gentle touch or pressure (allodynia). Allodynia may be related to formation of new connections involving central pain transmission neurons. Other patients with PHN may have severe, spontaneous pain without allodynia, possibly secondary to increased spontaneous activity in deafferented central neurons or reorganization of central connections. An imbalance involving loss of large inhibitory fibers and an intact or increased number of small excitatory fibers has been suggested. This input on an abnormal dorsal horn containing deafferented hypersensitive neurons supports the clinical observation that both central and peripheral areas are involved in the production of pain.

Treatments are primarily pharmacologic, as noted in "Neuropathic Pain." In addition to other modalities for treatment of neuropathic pain, the lidocaine 5% patch is a topical patch approved by the U.S. Food and Drug Administration for the treatment of PHN. It is effective and extremely well-tolerated and can be safely used in conjunction with other pharmacotherapies because there is no clinically significant absorption of lidocaine. Antiviral agents (e.g., famciclovir) may also be used, the logic being that an antiviral may shorten the clinical course, prevent complications, prevent the development of latency and/or subsequent recurrences, decrease transmission, and eliminate established latency.

Painful Polyneuropathy

Peripheral neuropathy is an umbrella term for a number of patterns of nerve involvement that include mononeuropathy, mononeuropathy multiplex, plexopathy, radiculopathy, and peripheral polyneuropathy. Polyneuropathy can be recognized by classic stocking-and-glove distribution of sensory and motor findings, which in a subgroup of patients is accompanied by pain. The most common causes of peripheral polyneuropathy are diabetes, alcohol use, vitamin deficiencies, hypothyroidism, toxins including medications, and vasculitis. Cryptogenic polyneuropathy (i.e., unknown diagnosis) is a large category; recent evidence suggests that many patients with cryptogenic polyneuropathy have impaired glucose tolerance.

Diabetes may cause a number of different types of neuropathy; peripheral polyneuropathy (discussed on pg. 72) is the most common, but other types include the following:

- Diabetic amyotrophy
- Thoracic radiculopathy
- Autonomic neuropathy
- Third cranial neuropathy

The most important goal in a patient presenting with a peripheral neuropathy is to make the diagnosis because many of the neuropathies can be resolved or stabilized with primary treatment. It is of critical importance to make a diagnosis because disorders that require prompt recognition sometimes masquerade as a "benign" peripheral polyneuropathy. Once the diagnosis is established, or concurrently with diagnostic efforts, the pain must be managed.

Management is basically pharmacologic, analogous to the approach to neuropathic pain in general. Because the area of pain is often widespread in patients with peripheral polyneuropathy, the topical agents may be less practical than in focal neuropathies; in fact, they are increasingly used and may be helpful. The oral medication approach is analogous to other types of neuropathic pain.

Complex Regional Pain Syndrome

CRPS (*type I*), formerly referred to as *reflex sympathetic dystrophy*, is a painful condition that usually develops after minor trauma, such as a sprain, strain, or contusion. CRPS type I may also follow bony fracture, surgery, or relatively benign soft tissue injury. CRPS (*type II*), formerly referred to as *causalgia*, develops after injury to a large nerve (e.g., a gunshot wound to nerve or plexus). CRPS most commonly occurs near or at the site of injury (e.g., in one hand or foot) but can be found in other body parts and may spread from the original site. The spread of pain in CRPS can be related to myofascial dysfunction in proximal muscles or may represent a centralization of the pain process, including a somatoform process.

CRPS is usually described by patients presenting with the following complaints:

- Pain
  - Burning
  - Deep aching
  - Lancinating
- Allodynia
- Edema
- Skin color changes (e.g., mottled, red, blotchy)
- Skin temperature changes (hot or cold compared with the contralateral side of the body)
- Motor weakness
- Sweating (increased or decreased compared to the contralateral side)
- Brittle nails
- Other nonspecific skin changes (e.g., shiny or extremely dry)
- Various movement disorders affecting the involved limb

The allodynia that patients present with is a characteristic feature that often interferes with the patient's ability to tolerate clothing, air conditioning, or any type of touch in the affected area. CRPS is a clinical diagnosis, and the International Association for the Study of Pain has provided diagnostic guidelines.[26]

Treatment for CRPS involves a variety of modalities, including diagnostic and therapeutic nerve blocks, medications, and physiotherapy. Pharmacologic interventions include the following:

- Lidocaine patch (5%)
- Gabapentin or pregabalin
- Intravenous lidocaine
- Mexiletine
- Opioids
- Tricyclic antidepressants
- Tizanidine[18]

Spinal cord stimulation has been efficacious for selected individuals but is only recommended when other more conservative treatments have failed. Finally, patients with true cases of CRPS almost always require psychological treatments designed to increase their pain-coping skills, decrease negative affect (e.g., depression and anxiety), and provide support through a course of rehabilitation that is often difficult.

Pain Syndromes from Peripheral Nerve Injury

Pain syndromes as a result of direct peripheral nerve injury include the following:

- Postthoracotomy pain
  - Affects the intercostal nerves and is often described as an "aching" sensation in the distribution of the incision
- Postmastectomy pain
- Postnephrectomy pain
  - Associated with nerves in the superficial flank and is described as numbness, fullness, or heaviness in the flank

- Various pain syndromes after amputation
  - The most common types of pain after amputation are phantom pain and stump pain, which are distinguished by the location of the pain being either in the "phantom" of the amputated limb or in its stump, respectively
  - May be manifested by the following:
    - Burning dysesthesia
    - Cramping
    - Feelings of distorted posturing of the nonexistent limb

The treatment of focal neuropathic pain syndromes in general follows the World Health Organization (WHO) algorithm with a focus on neuropathic pain syndromes. Although not well-studied, interventional procedures such as scar injections with steroids or neurolytic agents (e.g., phenol or alcohol), neurolytic blocks (e.g., subarachnoid alcohol), or epidural or intrathecal analgesia, can be quite useful.

Plexopathy

Plexopathy is a major cause of pain in cancer patients. It is produced by tumor invasion or compression of the cervical, brachial, or lumbosacral plexuses or as a consequence of radiation therapy. Pain is more common in plexopathy due to tumor invasion than in radiation plexopathy, wherein general neurological deficits are more prominent. It should be noted that pain may precede overt neurologic signs in plexopathies. Distinguishing plexopathy due to tumor from plexopathy due to radiation may be difficult; in general, the distinction is based on the clinical picture, imaging studies, and electrophysiologic studies.

Pain related to the cervical plexus is usually experienced in the face or head and is described as lancinating, burning, or aching. Swallowing or head movement can intensify the pain. It is important to distinguish cervical plexopathy from epidural compression, which can be done through magnetic resonance imaging or computed tomographic imaging.

Brachial plexopathy is associated with cancers of the lung or breast, with most cases associated with upper lobe lung cancer.[27] Pain in the lower plexus usually involves pain in the shoulder that extends to the arm and fourth and fifth digits. Pain in the upper plexus, which occurs less frequently, begins in the shoulder, lateral arm, and index finger and thumb. Brachial plexopathy is usually diagnosed by computed tomographic imaging or magnetic resonance imaging. Patients with lumbosacral plexopathy usually experience pain in the pelvis, buttock, and legs. Similar to cervical and brachial plexuses, lumbosacral plexopathy can be assessed by magnetic resonance imaging or computed tomographic imaging.

Treatment of the plexopathies, again, focuses on diagnosis, primary treatment when available, and analgesic treatment, more or less in parallel. Analgesic treatment proceeds according to the WHO ladder, described in "World Health Organization Analgesic Ladder for Cancer Pain," with a focus on neuropathic pain medications. Interventional treatments can be quite effective in plexopathy pain, which is often intractable to medical management. In particular, subarachnoid alcohol neurolysis, which is in experienced hands a relatively simple and safe outpatient procedure, relieves pain reliably for a few months in most patients. Patients may also do well with prolonged epidural or intrathecal analgesic modalities, but these procedures are in general much more difficult than the neurolytic procedures under an experienced operator.

Peripheral Polyneuropathies

Peripheral polyneuropathies can be recognized by the classic stocking-and-glove distribution of symptoms and signs, as discussed previously in the case of the noncancer patient. Peripheral polyneuropathies can be caused by chemotherapy [e.g., vinca alkaloids, paclitaxel, cisplatin (Platinol), docetaxel, and vinorelbine tartrate], nutritional deficiencies, metabolic problems, alcohol consumption, and other causes. Of course, identification and treatment, when possible, of the underlying cause of the neuropathy are the most important initial step.

Symptomatic treatment of these syndromes involves the cascade of medical treatments for neuropathic pain described on pg. 72, which may lead to implantable analgesic infusion pumps or spinal cord stimulators.

Central Pain Syndrome

Central pain syndrome is a neurologic condition caused by damage to or dysfunction of the central nervous system. This syndrome can be caused by the following:

- Cerebrovascular accident
- Brain or spinal cord trauma
- Epilepsy
- Multiple sclerosis
- Parkinson's disease
- Tumor-based causes (e.g., direct pressure, tissue infiltration)

The character of the pain associated with this syndrome varies widely and may affect a large portion of the body or may be more restricted to specific areas, such as hands or feet. The extent of pain is usually related to the cause of the central nervous system injury or damage.[28]

Patients present with the following signs and symptoms and one of the above conditions:

- Pain that is typically constant
  - Moderate to severe in intensity
  - Worsened by touch, movement, emotions, and temperature changes, usually cold temperatures
  - One or more types of pain sensations, the most prominent being burning
    - Mingled with the burning may be sensations of the following:
      - "Pins and needles"
      - Pressing
      - Lacerating or aching pain
      - Brief, intolerable bursts of sharp pain similar to dental nerve pain
- Individuals may have numbness in the areas affected by the pain

Central pain syndrome often begins shortly after the causative injury or damage, but may be delayed by months or even years, especially if it is related to post–cerebrovascular accident pain. Treatment includes conventional agents used in managing neuropathic pain, including tricyclics, anticonvulsants, and stress reduction.

Fibromyalgia

Fibromyalgia has been recognized as a clinical condition only since 1987. It is characterized by pain, stiffness, and tenderness of the muscles, tendons, and joints. Fibromyalgia was formerly known as *fibrositis*. Considered to be one of the rheumatic diseases, its cause is currently unknown. Researchers have found elevated levels of a nerve chemical signal, called substance P, and nerve growth factor in the spinal fluid of fibromyalgia patients. Serotonin is also relatively low in patients with fibromyalgia. Studies of pain in fibromyalgia have suggested that the central nervous system may be somehow supersensitized. The painful muscle tissue involved is *not* accompanied by tissue inflammation. Therefore, despite potentially disabling body pain, patients with fibromyalgia do not develop body damage or deformity.

This very challenging condition is more common in women and tends to develop during early and middle adulthood or during a woman's childbearing years. Those who have another rheumatic disease such as lupus, RA, or ankylosing spondylitis also are at a higher risk for developing fibromyalgia.

Patients typically present with the following:

- Chronic widespread muscular pain
- Fatigue
- Widespread tenderness

Many people with fibromyalgia also experience additional symptoms such as the following:

- Morning stiffness
- Headaches
- Irritable bowel syndrome
- Irritable bladder
- Cognitive and memory problems (often called "fibro fog")
- Symptoms of temporomandibular joint disorder
- Pelvic pain

- Restless legs syndrome
- Sensitivity to noise and temperature
- Anxiety and depression
- Insomnia

Diagnosis is by process of elimination and assisted by the presence of the following:

- Widespread or total musculoskeletal pain lasting more than 3 months
- Absence of other possible conditions responsible for the complaints
- Presence of more than 11 of 18 anatomically specific tender points

A number of clinicians are concerned that patients with fibromyalgia are psychologically disturbed. This is likely due to the large number of varying complaints from these patients. The likelihood is that these patients are suffering from a high incidence of anxiety and depression as a result of their widespread chronic pain.

Treatment is with conventional therapies and usually should include an antidepressant. Investigation is taking place to see if duloxetine and pregabalin, which have both been recently approved by the Food and Drug Administration for treatment of DPN, may also be effective in treating fibromyalgia.

Myofascial Pain

Myofascial pain is defined as a syndrome consisting of pain in a muscle, which is usually in spasm, and contains taut bands and/or trigger points, palpation of which reproduces the patient's pain, often with a radiating component.[29]

Associated symptoms may include heaviness, "numbness" without neurologic signs, swelling, or decreased range of motion. Trigger points are defined as localized palpable mass within a muscle, palpation of which reproduces the patient's pain, including the radiating component.[30] Myofascial pain is a regional disorder, as opposed to fibromyalgia, which by definition is a widespread disorder. Another distinction is that fibromyalgia is characterized by tender points (which are tender, but nothing is palpable), as opposed to the trigger points of myofascial pain. Myofascial pain is a clinical diagnosis. A variety of stress-producing stimuli have been postulated in the etiology and maintenance of myofascial pain, including physical stress (e.g., fatigue), tissue injury (major or microtrauma), physiologic state (e.g., hormonal balance, nutritional status), personality, and genetic factors.[31]

Myofascial syndromes are treated by physical interventions, such as stretching, strengthening, postural reeducation, other forms of physical therapy, and vapocoolant sprays. Cases that do not respond to conservative therapy can be successfully treated with trigger point injections of a local anesthetic, low-dose steroid, or saline. Recent reports have suggested the efficacy of botulinum toxin in the treatment of refractory cases.[32] Complaints of myofascial pain, especially in the setting of headache, LBP, and CRPS type I, are common and can result from disuse of muscles secondary to pain.

Chronic Abdominal Pain

Abdominal pain can be the result of a variety of causes that individually are beyond the scope of this manual. Some examples of causes of abdominal pain are chronic intestinal obstructive processes, which occur frequently in the setting of abdominal and pelvic cancers. Other causes include visceral tumors (primary or metastatic), venous thrombosis, omental metastases, volvulus of the small intestine, and occlusion of blood flow to visceral organs. Because the issue of decreased bowel motility is quite important in this group of patients, adjunctive treatments and medications in addition to opioids to spare the adverse effects are often used. Adjunctive treatments include subcutaneous infusion of octreotide, antispasmodic agents, and antiemetics. Interventional treatments include neurolytic procedures (e.g., celiac or hypogastric plexus block, which are contraindicated in the presence of bowel obstruction) and spinal analgesic infusions.

Cancer Pain

Although research indicates that the majority of patients with cancer experience some form of pain, pain associated with cancer is frequently left undertreated. Notably, untreated cancer pain is a major risk factor for suicide. Even though cancer pain cannot usually be entirely relieved, several treatment strategies exist to help to alleviate much of the pain and therefore improve the patient's quality of life.

Lack of effective treatment is most often due to inadequate screening and assessment. The goals of screening are twofold:

1. To screen patients routinely to determine the presence and extent of pain
2. To make a diagnosis in patients who have pain

Various barriers in the clinician–patient interaction frequently prevent the recognition of pain when it is present, without which diagnosis and treatment can never take place. The purpose of diagnosis is, like in the case of any pain syndrome, to determine whether a primary treatment exists for the underlying cause of the pain. For example, many patients with cancer develop new sources of pain that are due to treatable infections.[33]

The patient's description of the pain leading to its categorization as *somatic*, *visceral*, or *neuropathic*, is a critical guide to treatment. In cancer pain, *somatic pain* can result from tumor invasion (by direct growth or metastasis) of the bone and muscle. *Visceral pain* commonly occurs in the setting of malignancies involving internal organ systems, such as the pancreas, uterus, or liver. *Neuropathic pain* can be caused by malignant invasion and subsequent damage or disruption of peripheral nerves, plexuses, nerve root, spinal cord, or brain. Frequently, the type of cancer pain is of mixed origin. (For further definitions of the types of pain, refer to Chapter I in the manual or the glossary.) Although opioids are helpful in many types of cancer pain, they are not necessarily the most appropriate first-line treatment for certain types of pain (e.g., mild bone pain) and in some cases are minimally effective.

A psychosocial assessment is also important. Consider the effect of the cancer diagnosis on the patient, the patient's coping responses, the patient's knowledge of pain management and concerns about using controlled substances, the economic effect of pain, and changes in mood.

The diagnostic evaluation of the cause of the pain may require blood tests, radiologic studies, or neurophysiologic testing. Finally, assessment of pain at regular intervals should be ongoing.[27]

Two common cancer pain problems include the following:

- Periprocedural pain
  - Generally as a result of biopsy or removal of the cancerous tissue or organ.
  - Treatment resembles that of any other acute source of periprocedural pain.
- Bony metastasis
  - The most common cause of pain in cancer patients and is often associated with cancers of the lung, prostate, and breast. The most common areas in which they form are in the vertebrae, pelvis, femur, and skull. In many cases, patients have multiple areas of bone metastases and therefore have multiple areas of pain. Such pain is usually described as dull and aching.
  - A diagnosis of bony metastasis is confirmed through radiographic testing.
  - Treatment consists of the following:
    - Primary treatment of the cancer
    - Radiation therapy is often widely used for metastatic bone pain and is highly effective and generally well-tolerated.
    - Pharmacologic management
      - Nonsteroidal antiinflammatory drugs may be more effective than opioids, especially for movement-associated pain.
      - Many clinicians prescribed selective COX-2 inhibitors but now recognize risks associated with these drugs. This drug class still represents a viable option in carefully selected patients.
      - Opioids and other pharmacologic treatments should be added if needed, as discussed in the "Pharmacologic Options for the Management of Pain" section in Chapter VI.
      - Patients who do not respond adequately to medical management should be referred for pain management consultation because they may respond well to intrathecal analgesia or other interventional procedures.

Treatment of Cancer Pain

The treatment of cancer pain involves both pharmacologic and nonpharmacologic interventions. In terms of pharmacologic treatment, the WHO has developed an effective guideline for titration of analgesic therapy for cancer pain, which has become known as the *analgesic ladder*.[27]

World Health Organization Analgesic Ladder for Cancer Pain. The WHO in 1990 and 1996 issued guidelines that involve the treatment of cancer pain. The guidelines are presented in a ladder formation and are referred to as the "analgesic ladder." The steps of the WHO ladder are described in Table 18 and Figure 3.

■ Table 18.
World Health Organization Analgesic Ladder for Cancer Pain

Step 1

The first step involves treatment of mild to moderate pain with acetaminophen, aspirin, or another nonsteroidal antiinflammatory drug. Medications should be administered as needed or round-the-clock and should be titrated upward when necessary. Adjuvant analgesics, or medications that are not generally used for pain but can have an enhancing effect on other analgesics, may also be used.

Step 2

The second step involves adding an opioid for pain that persists beyond treatment in step 1. An opioid, often codeine or oxycodone, is added to the regimen at this step (the nonsteroidal antiinflammatory drug or acetaminophen should be retained).

Step 3

The third step involves treatment with an opioid on a round-the-clock basis for persistent pain. Morphine is generally the agent of choice. Short-acting opioids are often prescribed as needed for pain as a supplement to a "background dose" of long-acting opioids. This type of dosing is called "rescue" or "breakthrough" and is given for exacerbations of pain that occur beyond the constant, background pain. Whenever possible, the same type of opioid should be given for background and breakthrough treatment.

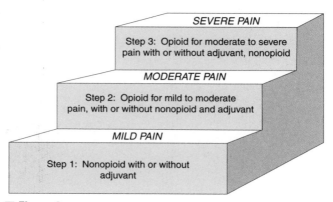

■ **Figure 3.**
World Health Organization Analgesic Ladder for Cancer Pain.

1. **The World Health Organization (WHO) approach to pharmacologic treatment contains five major concepts:**
   a. By the mouth
   b. By the clock
   c. By the ladder
   d. For the individual
   e. With careful documentation

2. In treating patients with cancer, the medication regimen should be individualized. A simple regimen should be developed, and medication should be taken orally unless the patient is unable (e.g., trouble swallowing, obtundation).

3. **Nonsteroidal antiinflammatory drugs** and/or acetaminophen should be prescribed for mild to moderate pain **(step 1 of the WHO ladder)**.

4. With persistent pain or when pain increases, **opioids** should be administered in addition to the nonsteroidal antiinflammatory drugs. The WHO guidelines initially recommended using **"weak" opioids** for initial treatment—for example, codeine, oxycodone, propoxyphene, hydrocodone, and tramadol **(step 2 of the WHO ladder)**.

5. When pain is more severe at the outset or in the case of failure of "weak" opioids, the guidelines recommended using **"strong" opioids**—for example, morphine, hydromorphone, methadone, levorphanol, fentanyl, oxymorphone, and meperidine **(step 3 of the WHO ladder)**.

6. These days, the concepts of "strong" and "weak" opioids have been discredited for most clinical situations, and most clinicians would advocate a modified approach to the WHO ladder:

   a. **Start with nonsteroidal antiinflammatory drugs (cyclooxygenase-2 inhibitors might be a choice in selected patients).**

   b. **Add a short-acting opioid on an as-needed basis if needed.**

   c. **Then add a long-acting opioid on a round-the-clock basis if needed.**

   d. **Adjuvant medications should be added whenever indicated.**

7. Medications should be administered on a regular basis, plus on an as-needed basis, which helps build a constant level of the medication in the body, but also addresses exacerbations of pain, which may be provoked by increased activity during treatment.

8. It is worth emphasizing that patients should enter the rung of the ladder appropriate for their presentation. For example, patients presenting with severe and continuous pain should usually be treated with "strong" opioids at the beginning, which may be most effectively administered intravenously in the acute setting. Patients can then be transitioned, once pain is under control, to a regimen consisting of an nonsteroidal anti-inflammatory drug, a sustained-release opioid, plus a short-acting opioid for breakthrough pain.

9. Long-term opioid use may be associated with tolerance and physical dependence; however, neither tolerance nor physical dependence generally reflects aberrant (drug-abusing) behavior. Finally, because of the potential for serious side effects, patients should be monitored and evaluated regularly.

End-of-Life Considerations

Palliative care is the "active, total care offered to a patient with a progressive disease and their family when it is recognized that the illness is no longer curable, in order to concentrate on the quality of life and the alleviation of distressing symptoms within the framework of a coordinated service."

Pain is experienced by the vast majority of cancer patients at the end of life, but it is only one of many symptoms that dying patients may face.[34] Therefore, the need for the availability of comprehensive palliative care and appropriate pain management in a hospital or home hospice cannot be underestimated.

The WHO defines palliative care as "an approach [that] improves the quality of life of patients and their families facing life-threatening illness, through the prevention, assessment, and treatment of pain and other physical, psychosocial, and spiritual problems."

The WHO underscores the principles that palliative care should strive to achieve the following goals:

- Provide relief from pain and other distressing symptoms
- Affirm life and regard dying as a part of the life cycle
- Intend neither to hasten nor postpone death
- Offer a support system to help patients live as actively as possible until death
- Offer a support system to help family members cope during the patient's illness and during their own bereavement, including supporting the needs of children
- Use a team approach to address the needs of patients and their families, including bereavement counseling if indicated
- Enhance the quality of life and may also positively influence the course of a patient's illness

Development of U.S. palliative care consensus guidelines was discussed during a national leadership conference coordinated by the Center to Advance Palliative Care (*http://www.capc.org*) that was held in December 2001 at the New York Academy of Medicine. The end result of this meeting was National Consensus Project, and ultimately

Clinical Practice Guidelines for Quality Palliative Care.[35] In 2003, the American Cancer Society and the National Comprehensive Cancer Network collaborated to produce *Advanced and Palliative Care Guidelines for Patients*.[36] The purpose of these and other guidelines is to build a framework for standardized approaches to patients with end-of-life care that is thoughtful and comprehensive. Ultimately, this led to the development of *Cancer Pain Treatment Guidelines for Patients*,[36] developed in 2005 by the same collaboration (*http://www.cancer.org*).

Patients dying of cancer or other illnesses often experience fear of impending death. Moreover, patients worry about dependents, losing physical control, dying in pain, and physical decline. Clinicians should directly explore patients' fears, ask what their thoughts are about death, support positive coping, address psychosocial and spiritual concerns, and treat ameliorable problems. Treatment for patients dying of cancer may include supportive therapy and, in some cases, pastoral or faith-based counseling. As cancer progresses, patients are often unable to participate in therapy due to limitations in cognition and speech. Thus, it can be helpful for the patient to discuss preferences for treatment early, particularly if there is conflict among family members. Moreover, it may be helpful to encourage patients to plan practical arrangements (e.g., funeral, wills, advance directives).

Patients and their family members may have fears about becoming addicted to pain medications in the end-of-life setting. In addition, some treatment providers may question opioid doses, especially as they are increased and other medications are added. The polypharmacy generally required to treat patients at the end of life increases the probability of drug interactions, particularly in the presence of borderline cognition, cachexia, low intravascular volume, and reduced glomerular filtration.[34] Therefore, patients and their families need education about pain management and reassurance that their loved one will not become addicted. Patients should also be encouraged to express their wishes about future care, including pain medication and possible trade-offs with wakefulness.

Regulatory and legal concerns about prescribing pain medication are present for some physicians in the end-of-life setting. These fears can be a major barrier to providing appropriate pain management. Fears of sanctions are generally exaggerated. In fact, the opposite problem has occurred multiple times in recent years: successful litigation against a physician for failing to control pain at the end of life. A physician prescribing opioids appropriately for cancer pain is almost never investigated, although due to variability across communities in the United States, local prescribing guidelines should be checked. Documentation of diagnosis and treatment, including the outcomes of opioid treatment, are essential and provide protection in the event of regulatory scrutiny. Read more about regulatory and legal concerns in the "Pharmacologic Options for the Management of Pain" section in Chapter VI.

Delirium is the most common neuropsychiatric complication at the end of life.[34] A clinical approach to treating delirium may begin with screening with the Mini-Mental State Questionnaire to establish the presence of delirium. Delirium is a syndrome with a long differential diagnosis and many treatable causes. Common causes include medications, dehydration, infections, metabolic disorders (e.g., hypercalcemia, hypoglycemia), and brain metastases. The aggressiveness of diagnostic efforts must be appropriate to the clinical situation; clearly, in the setting of impending death, management is symptomatic, as opposed to the more stable situation where quality of life is usually maximized by identifying and treating the cause. Symptomatic treatment of delirium usually consists of high-potency neuroleptics—for example, haloperidol. Although benzodiazepines can be used, they usually worsen the problem in the long-term. Consideration should be given to opioid rotation because accumulation of opioid metabolites can cause delirium. Counseling and education for the patient, family, and staff should also be accomplished.[34]

Preventing toxicity of adjuvant drugs in palliative care is another common challenge in the end-of-life setting. One adjuvant drug at a time should be prescribed in effective, often high, doses. Treatment outcome should be defined before starting treatment, and the adjuvant should be discontinued if deemed ineffective. Sedation and cognition should always be monitored. Finally, opioids should be used first for pain and should have reached dose-limiting toxicity before prescribing adjuvant medications in the terminal setting.[34]

REFERENCES

1. Apfelbaum, Chen, Mehta, Gan, Post-operative pain experience results from a national survey suggest post-operative pain continues to be undermanaged. *Anesth Analg* 2003;97:534–540.

2. Long DM. *Contemporary Diagnosis and Management of Pain.* Newton, PA: Handbooks in Health Care; 2001.

3. *Americans Living With Pain Survey.* Rocklin, CA: American Chronic Pain Association; 2004. Available at: http://www.theacpa.org/documents/FINAL%20PAIN%20SURVEY%20RESULTS%20REPORT.pdf. Accessed July 27, 2007.

4. Cooper JK, Kohlmann T. Factors associated with health status of older Americans. *Age Ageing* 2001;30(6):495–501.

5. Blount BW, Hart G, Ehreth JL. Description of the content of Army family practice. *J Am Board Fam Pract* 1993;6:143–152.

6. Carey TS, Garrett JM, Jackman AM. Beyond the good prognosis. Examination of an inception cohort of patients with chronic low back pain. *Spine* 2000; 25(1):115–120.

7. *Low Back Pain Fact Sheet.* National Institute of Neurological Disorders and Stroke. Bethesda, MD: National Institutes of Health, July 2003. Available at: http://www.ninds.nih.gov/disorders/backpain/detail_backpain.htm. Accessed July 27, 2007.

8. Koes BW, van Tulder MW, Ostelo R, et al. Clinical guidelines for the management of low back pain in primary care: an international comparison. *Spine* 2001;26(22):2504–2513, discussion 2513–2514.

9. Long DM. Chronic back pain. In Wall PD, Melzack R, eds. *Textbook of Pain.* London: Churchill, 1999:539–558.

10. Deyo RA, Weinstein JN. Low back pain. *N Engl J Med* 2001;344:363–370.

11. Nadler SF, Steiner DJ, Erasala GN, et al. Continuous low-level heat wrap therapy provides more efficacy than ibuprofen and acetaminophen for acute low back pain. *Spine* 2002;27(10):1012–1017.

12. IHS Classification ICHD-II. http://www.ihs-classification.org. Accessed Nov. 1, 2006.

13. Saper JR, Silberstein S, Gordon CD, et al. *Handbook of Headache Management: A Practical Guide to Diagnosis and Treatment of Head, Neck, and Facial Pain.* Philadelphia: Lippincott Williams & Wilkins, 1999.

14. Schoenen J, Sandor PS. Headache. In Wall PD, Melzack R, eds. *Textbook of Pain.* London: Churchill, 1999:761–798.

15. Hootman JM, Helmick CG. Projections of U.S. prevalence of arthritis and associated activity limitations. *Arthritis Rheum* 2006;54(1):226–229.

16. Gabriel SE, Mattson FL. Economic and quality-of-life impact of NSAIDs in rheumatoid arthritis: a conceptual framework and selected literature review. *Pharmacoeconomics* 1995;8(6):479–490.

17. National Institute on Aging, 1996; NIH, 2001a.

18. Harris E, Zorab R. *Rheumatoid Arthritis.* Philadelphia: Saunders, 1997.

19. Galer BS, Dworkin, RH. *A Clinical Guide to Neuropathic Pain.* New York: McGraw Hill Healthcare Information Programs, 2000.

20. Melzack R, Casey KL. Sensory motivational and central control determinants of pain: a new conceptual model. In Kenshalo D, ed. *The Skin Senses.* Springfield: Thomas, 1968:423–443.

21. Galer BS, Jensen MP. Development and preliminary validation of a pain measure specific to neuropathic pain: the Neuropathic Pain Scale. *Neurology* 1997;48:332–338.

22. Dyck PJ, Kratz KM, Karnes JL, et al. The prevalence by staged severity of various types of diabetic neuropathy, retinopathy, and nephropathy in a population-based cohort: the Rochester Diabetic Neuropathy Study. Neurology 1993;43:817–824.

23. American Diabetes Association Diabetic Neuropathy Campaign. http://www.diabetes.org/formedia/2005-press-releases/diabeticneuropathy.jsp. Accessed in 2005.

24. American Diabetes Association, Standards of Medical Care in Diabetes. Diabetes Care. 2006 Jan;29 Suppl 1:S4–42.

25. Cherny NI, Portenoy RK. Cancer pain: principles of assessment and syndromes. In Wall PD, Melzack R, ed. *Textbook of Pain.* London: Churchill, 1999:1017–1064.

26. Bruehl S, Harden RN, Galer BS, et al. External validation of IASP diagnostic criteria for complex regional pain syndrome and proposed research diagnostic criteria. *Pain* 1999;81:147–154.

27. Jacox AK, Carr DB, Payne R, et al. *Management of Cancer Pain, Clinical Practice Guidelines.* No. 9. Rockville, MD: U. S. Department of Health

and Human Services, Public Health Service, Agency for Health Care Policy and Research (AHCPR Publication No. 94-0592), 1994.

28. National Institute of Neurological Disorders and Stroke. Available at: http://www.ninds.nih.gov/disorders/central_pain/central_pain.htm. Accessed on July 27, 2007.

29. Travell J, Simons DG. *Myofascial Pain and Dysfunction: The Trigger Point Manual*. Baltimore: Williams, 1992.

30. Fisher AA. Documentation of myofascial trigger points. *Arch Phys Med Rehabil* 1988;69:286–291.

31. Sola AE, Bonica JJ. Myofascial pain syndromes. In Loeser JD, Butler SH, Chapman CR, Turk DC, eds. *Bonica's Management of Pain (3rd ed)*. Philadelphia: Lippincott Williams & Wilkins, 2001:530–542.

32. Cheshire W, Abashian SW, Mann JD. Botulinum toxin in the treatment of myofascial pain syndrome. *Pain* 1994;59:65–69.

33. Gonzales GR, Elliott KJ, Portenoy RK, Foley KM. The impact of a comprehensive evaluation in the management of cancer pain. *Pain* 1991;47:141–144.

34. Bruera E, Higginson I, Neumann CM. Acupuncture. In Loeser JD, Butler SH, Chapman CR, Turk DC, eds. *Bonica's Management of Pain (3rd ed)*. Philadelphia: Lippincott Williams & Wilkins, 2001:1832–1841.

35. National Consensus Project for Quality Palliative Care (2004). *Clinical practice guidelines for quality palliative care*. http://www.nationalconsensusproject.org. Accessed on July 27, 2007.

36. Cancer Pain Treatment Guidelines for Patients, 2005. Available at: http://www.nccn.org/patients/patient_gls/_english/_pain/contents.asp. Accessed on July 27, 2007.

VI.

Approaches to the Management of Pain

NONPHARMACOLOGIC OPTIONS FOR THE MANAGEMENT OF PAIN

The biopsychosocial model encompasses biologic, psychological, and social aspects of pain. Nonpharmacologic options for the management of pain can be divided into physical, psychological, and psychosocial dimensions.

Physical Modalities

Therapeutic Exercise

Therapeutic exercise includes the following:

- Range-of-motion exercises
- Stretching
- Strength training
- Cardiovascular conditioning

Range-of-motion exercises can be delivered in a passive, assisted-active, or active manner. Multiple exercise techniques in each of these categories can be used to increase physical functioning. Although exercise is generally limited to range of motion during acute pain,[1] patients should be encouraged to adopt an exercise program as early as possible. Exercise mobilizes joints and strengthens muscles, in addition to enhancing balance and coordination.

Cardiovascular conditioning is also important for maintenance of long-term health.[2] Facilitating exercise is a primary goal of analgesic therapy.

Patients can become discouraged when their pain increases due to therapeutic exercise. Many patients terminate their treatment far too early to achieve maximal benefit. Physicians can choose physical therapists who specialize in treating persons with chronic pain and can encourage them to persist with an exercise program.

Because the primary goal of treatment for individuals with chronic pain is to restore overall functioning, and injuries or disease often diminish physical capacities, the importance of evaluation and treatment with physical measures cannot be underestimated.

Application of Heat and Cold

Early interventions for acute injuries can be rest, ice, compression, and elevation, which can be remembered by the popular mnemonic acronym RICE. These interventions are directed at diminishing swelling and inflammation and are most often effective between 24 and 48 hours after an acute injury.[3]

The application of heat can be made via hot packs, hot water bottles, moist compresses, heating pads, chemical and gel packs, and immersion in water.[4] Cold can also be applied to reduce inflammation via ice packs, towels soaked in cold water, or gel packs.

The use of heat and cold therapies is somewhat controversial for cancer pain because of the risk of increasing tumor growth. Superficial heat is not contraindicated in some recent cancer guidelines.[5,6] However, caution should be exercised for application of deep heat, including by short wave, microwave, and ultrasound.[5] Heat is also contraindicated for acute musculoskeletal injuries because it can result in increases in hemorrhage and edema.[7]

Care should be taken for superficial and deep heat and cold delivery for the following:

- Individuals with insensate tissue
- Cognitively impaired individuals
- Arterial insufficiency
- Bleeding diathesis
- Individuals with metastatic tumors

Physical Manipulations

For acute pain, physical manipulations, such as instructions on repositioning and appropriate ways to rise from bed or a chair, are important in helping the patient reduce movement-related pain early in the course of postoperative pain.

Short-term immobilization of joints or restriction of movement is often necessary to manage painful joints and facilitate healing. Immobilization of joints at angles that approximate the angle of their optimal functioning (e.g., wrist joints at 30 degrees of dorsiflexion) increase functioning when the immobilization is no longer necessary.[1]

For chronic pain, although immobilization can be helpful in the short-term, the benefits are generally outweighed by undesired consequences (e.g., contracture, atrophy, and cardiovascular deconditioning) if used on a long-term basis.[8]

Therapeutic Massage. Massage can be delivered by stroking, kneading, pressing, or rhythmic motions or a combination.[8,9] Massage is also considered to be a complementary medicine technique. Therapeutic massage provides the following:

- A sense of relaxation
- Reduction of muscle tension
- Promotion of circulation
- Improvements in sleep
- Decreased pain[9,10]

Transcutaneous Electrical Stimulation

Transcutaneous electrical nerve stimulation (TENS) is a counter-stimulation technique that is thought to stimulate peripheral nerves directly and alter painful sensations. TENS involves applying low-voltage electrical stimulation to large nerve fibers. Patients report that a "tingling" sensation replaces painful sensations. TENS has been shown to provide effective pain relief in some forms of acute pain conditions, including postoperative pain, oral-facial pain, and pain associated with childbearing.[11] However, the results of research for TENS in chronic pain are mixed.

Some manufacturers of electrical TENS units indicate that TENS over a cancer site is contraindicated. Recent cancer guidelines state that TENS may be beneficial for patients with mild cancer pain.[5,6]

Other physical treatments, including acupuncture, are covered in "Complementary and Alternative Medicine Approaches."

A Word about Functional-Capacity Evaluations. Individuals with chronic pain may be required to provide documentation of the extent of the injury or illness for purposes of work continuation, reassignment, or qualification for disability benefits. The American Medical Association has established a rating system that provides guidelines for quantifying the degree of disability present. However, many conceptual and practical issues are involved in classifying persons with chronic pain conditions.[12] Many physicians treating pain require that qualified professionals complete functional-capacity evaluations when asked to make work-related capacity decisions for individuals with chronic nonmalignant pain.

Psychological Treatments

Some of the psychological treatments used for treating chronic pain are discussed in this section. A combination of psychological and medical treatments is usually more effective than unidimensional treatment for an individual's complex chronic pain problems.

Behavioral Therapies

Operant conditioning or contingency management involves changing the environment for the purpose of modifying behaviors. Behaviors are elicited by stimuli in the environment and are influenced by both their antecedents and consequences. Reinforcement increases behaviors and can be used to change behaviors.

An example of the use of contingency management for a person with chronic pain is observing the attention that is given in response to his or her pain behaviors. If family members pay special attention to the individual when he or she groans or lies down during the day, the person with pain may be inadvertently reinforced to display pain behaviors. As such, pain behaviors and disability tend to increase over time. In this instance, the focus of the response to the patient by individuals in the environment could be changed to giving the patient attention for active engagement, such as performing exercises during the day or going to work.[13]

Contingency management requires careful thought and a plan tailored for the individual. Family members or significant others may need to be involved. Contingency management can be used effectively to help patients increase their exercise and activity level.

Psychophysiologic Techniques

Psychophysiologic techniques, such as relaxation and biofeedback, are directed toward helping the patient become aware of his or her ability to exert some control over physiologic processes of which he or she is not normally aware (e.g., muscle tension, skin temperature, respiration). Biofeedback uses feedback from a device or computer to give information to patients about their progress. Electromyography biofeedback is directed toward relaxing the muscles, which is particularly important in chronic pain conditions. Patients with low back or cervical pain tend to tense muscles around the site of their pain condition, bracing against it. This often causes increased pain due to muscle fatigue.

Biofeedback is also used in myofascial pain and temporomandibular joint syndrome. In addition to alleviating pain from reducing muscle tension, biofeedback can be used to increase peripheral skin temperature, causing dilation of vessels. This process can be helpful in the treatment of some types of headaches.

The outcome of biofeedback research is generally positive, especially when combined with relaxation training. Individuals with migraine and/or tension-type headaches show 50–55% success rates.[14] A review of mind–body therapies found that relaxation and thermal biofeedback are helpful in the management of recurrent migraine.[15] Relaxation and electromyography biofeedback are effective for recurrent tension headache or as a stand-alone treatment.[15]

Relaxation Techniques

Relaxation techniques are a form of physiologic self-monitoring. Two popular procedures are progressive muscle relaxation and autogenic relaxation. Progressive muscle relaxation is a procedure that involves alternate tensing and relaxing of various muscle groups in sequence. This form of muscle relaxation is often coupled with diaphragmatic breathing and is helpful for patients who are unaware of their level of muscle tension.

Autogenic techniques involve repeating phrases subvocally (e.g., "My right hand feels heavy, warm, and comfortable.") and focusing the patient in a meditative manner as he or she is reclined or sitting quietly in a chair with eyes closed. Guided imagery can be used to focus the patient on changing reactions to his or her painful sensations or to distract from painful experiences. Relaxation differs from hypnosis in that hypnosis involves a suggestion of pain relief and is generally thought to be a more concentrated form of relaxation. Relaxation and imagery have been found to reduce acute pain and procedural pain in patients with cancer pain.[16] Hypnosis is discussed in "Complementary and Alternative Medicine Approaches."

Cognitive-Behavioral Therapy

Cognitive-behavioral therapy (CBT) combines cognitive techniques with behavioral techniques. Cognitive techniques include changing distorted thoughts, such as "My pain is getting worse and will never get any better." Patients learn to observe their thoughts and how they affect their emotions and subsequent behaviors. Interventions are directed at changing the patient's thoughts to ones that are more realistic and engender positive coping behaviors.

Coping skills training includes identifying the patient's primary ways of coping with pain and changing those skills if they are not in the best interest of the patient's functioning. An example might be changing the patient's wishful thinking (passive coping) to seeking social support, increasing activities, or gaining more information about a problem (active coping).

Behavioral techniques that are commonly used in CBT are the psychophysiologic techniques (e.g., relaxation, imagery) discussed in the previous section and increasing appropriate activity, including pacing, problem solving, and stress management. In addition, maladaptive behaviors are identified and targeted for change.

CBT is an active therapeutic approach in which the therapist helps the patient set goals for treatment and engages the patient in completing homework in between sessions. CBT can help individuals with chronic pain focus and change their reactions to painful sensations, decrease negative emotional responses, and increase functioning. Advantages of CBT include a relatively short time course (usually 6–12 weeks), its evidence-based procedures and demonstrated effectiveness, and its applicability to a variety of pain-related difficulties (e.g., depression, anxiety) encountered by patients with chronic pain conditions. However, because of the active nature of this treatment, it is efficacious only to the extent that patients become active participants.[17]

A review of randomized controlled trials on mind–body therapies for managing pain found multimodal approaches effective. Table 19 includes a summary of some of these studies.

■ **Table 19.**
Randomized controlled evidence for multimodal mind–body approaches for pain.

Type of Pain	Evidence for Efficacy
Chronic low back pain[15]	Multimodal approaches combining stress management, coping skills training, cognitive restructuring, and relaxation therapy
Rheumatoid and osteoarthritis[5,15]	Multimodal approaches
	Cognitive-behavioral therapy, educational/informational approach
Migraine headache[5,15]	Thermal biofeedback, relaxation
Tension headache[5,15]	Electromyography (muscle) biofeedback
Surgical pain (delivered presurgically) [5,15]	Hypnosis, imagery, relaxation
Invasive medical procedure pain[5,15]	Multimodal approaches may be helpful when used as an adjunct
Adult cancer pain[5]	A-level evidence: patient education and hypnosis
	B-level evidence: cognitive-behavioral coping skills (distraction and cognitive restructuring)
	Psychotherapy and structured support

Psychosocial Interventions

Family Therapy and Family Interventions. Chronic pain can affect all family members. Family therapy focuses on the family unit and can change the patterns of behavior that are maladaptive. Family therapy should be considered when one or more family members exhibit behaviors that encourage maladaptive coping of the patient, if the family is overwhelmed by other difficulties, or if the patient is a child.[18]

Educational Interventions for Families. Some educational interventions for families have been shown to be helpful especially for families with patients with cancer. One target of such interventions is the patient and family barriers to adequate pain management described by the National Institutes of Health Consensus Statement.[19] These barriers are the following:

- Belief that pain is inevitable in cancer
- Belief that nothing can be done for cancer pain
- Fear of addiction and dependence on opioids
- Fear that drugs will lose their effectiveness
- Fear that reporting pain will exclude the patient from clinical trials or cancer treatments
- Failure to mention pain to providers
- Lack of adherence to treatment regimens
- High cost of medications and treatments
- Cognitive impairment hindering symptom assessment

Decreased pain has been found for cancer patients when education is directed toward alleviating these barriers, compared with those who received standard pain information.[20] Research shows that incongruence in beliefs about pain and pain experience between patients and caregivers results in the following:

- Poorer psychological functioning
- Poorer interpersonal functioning
- Lower quality of life
- Increased anger
- Increased fatigue
- Higher levels of caregiver strain[21]

Coping Skills Training for Couples. Coping skills training generally involves a combination of education, cognitive-behavioral skills, and relaxation training. Keefe et al.[16] trained partners of people with cancer in how to use cognitive behavioral pain-coping skills to assist their loved one toward the end of life. This line of research is new and quite exciting in that it uses the patient's social milieu to improve pain coping and control.

Couples, Sexuality, and Pain. Couples often experience sexual problems after the onset of pain. Very little research has been conducted in this area. Patients with pain frequently experience the following:

- Decreased libido
- Decreased physical arousal
- Dyspareunia
- Postcoital pain

Pain and physical difficulties because of disability or illness can also impede a couple's usual sexual practices. These problems can affect relationships (e.g., satisfaction, intimacy), as well as identity (e.g., decreased feelings of femininity or masculinity). In addition, some medications used to treat pain or depression can cause sexual dysfunction. Prolonged use of opioids and antidepressants (most notably selective serotonin uptake inhibitors) can cause loss of libido and sexual disturbances in men (e.g., inability to attain or maintain an erection) and women (e.g., infertility, amenorrhea).

In evaluating patients with sexual dysfunction or difficulties, listening and asking questions concerning sexual functioning are significant parts of treatment. Many therapeutic modalities can be used to improve sexual dysfunction, including behavioral therapy, cognitive behavioral therapy, couples therapy, and sex therapy. Importantly, asking about sexual dysfunction can reveal treatable medical causes, such as low testosterone levels in men.

Group Therapy and Support Groups

Different types of therapy can be delivered in groups of 5–10 individuals and can range from coping-skills groups to support groups formed and led by persons with medical conditions. Mental health professionals (psychiatrists, psychologists, or social workers) generally lead therapeutic groups. These groups are usually psychoeducational or cognitive-behavioral in format and have been shown to be efficacious in increasing coping with chronic pain.

Patient-led support groups vary in effectiveness; some organized support groups provide emotional support and practical suggestions for members; others may focus more on limitations due to pain, dissatisfactions with the medical system, or other reinforcements for pain and dysfunction, all of which may perpetuate disability. In addition, a number of listservs and chat rooms are devoted to persons with various types of medical difficulties, including chronic pain conditions. The accuracy of information obtained from these sites varies, and patients should be critical of information they obtain through these methods.

Spiritual/Religious Support

Faith-based practices are important for many patients as a source of coping, support, and comfort in facing difficult situations and terminal illness. Patients with terminal illness may have existential questions and concerns best answered by a leader of their faith practice. Spiritual and religious beliefs often help patients make sense of their situations and serve as a guide for their future behaviors. Supportive members of faith communities may provide needed social support and/or assistance with tasks of daily living (e.g., grocery shopping). Physicians may not understand the practices or beliefs of a particular patient, and patients may be hesitant to discuss how faith-based support is helpful to them. To the extent that religious and spiritual beliefs and practices can increase the patient's positive coping, facilitation of this process should occur.

Although a large body of research has been conducted on prayer and physical and mental health, few studies have been conducted on prayer and chronic pain. One study investigating the religious and spiritual practices of orthopedic patients with chronic pain found the following:

- Poorer physical health was related to private spiritual practices.
- Pain duration was associated with less forgiveness and less support from a religious or spiritual community.
- Poorer mental health was related to lack of forgiveness, feeling punished and abandoned by God, lack of daily spiritual experi-

ences, little support from a religious community, and not being religious or spiritual.

- Pain, and interference due to pain, were not related to higher levels of religion or spirituality.[22]

Complementary and Alternative Medicine Approaches

The National Center for Complementary and Alternative Medicine, a division of the National Institutes of Health, defines *complementary and alternative medicine* (CAM) as a "group of diverse medical and health care systems, practices and products that are not presently considered to be a part of conventional medicine."[23]

Complementary medicine means that the practice is used *with* conventional medicine, such as music therapy used to soothe a patient after surgery. *Alternative medicine* is defined as practices that are used *instead* of conventional medicine, such as using herbal preparations as a treatment for rheumatoid arthritis instead of drugs recommended by a doctor who practices conventional medicine.[23]

CAM interventions are divided into the following categories by the National Center for Complementary and Alternative Medicine:

- Alternative medical systems (e.g., Ayurveda, traditional Chinese medicine)
- Mind–body interventions (e.g., meditation, prayer)
- Biologically based therapies (e.g., herbal products, vitamins)
- Manipulative and body-based methods (e.g., chiropractic or osteopathic manipulation, massage)
- Energy therapies (e.g., use of electromagnetic fields, biofield therapies such as Reiki and therapeutic touch)

Prevalence of Complementary and Alternative Medicine Practices

Americans are using many forms of CAM, and usage is growing. Consider the following statistics from nationally representative random surveys in 1991 and 1997:

- CAM use increased from 33.8% in 1991 to 42.1% in 1997.
- There was a 47% increase in probability of visiting an alternative medicine practitioner from 1991 to 1997.
- Approximately 38% of users inform their doctors they use CAM.
- Out-of-pocket payments remained similar (64% and 58.3%).
- Visits to CAM practitioners exceeded total visits to U.S. primary care physicians.
- Fifteen million adults took prescription medication with herbal remedies or high-dose vitamins.[24]

CAM was most sought for chronic conditions, including back and neck pain, anxiety, depression and headaches.[24] The following CAM therapies were most used for back and neck pain:

- Chiropractic
- Massage
- Relaxation techniques
- Other practices (yoga, imagery, herbs, energy work)

Mind–Body Interventions

The most studied mind–body interventions are relaxation, meditation, imagery, biofeedback, and hypnosis. Some of these are more studied and integrated into allopathic, or "conventional," medicine. A few of the more common interventions used for pain within the mind–body category are hypnosis and meditation. Massage, relaxation, and biofeedback are discussed in "Physical Manipulations" and "Psychological Treatments."

Hypnosis is a state of deep relaxation that involves selective focusing, receptive concentration, and minimal motor functioning.[25] A National Institutes of Health Technology Panel found strong support for the use of hypnosis for the reduction of pain.[26] Hypnosis has also been shown to do the following:

- Reduce chemotherapy-induced nausea and vomiting[27]
- Improve recovery time after surgery when performed preoperatively[15]

■ Improve postsurgical pain[15]
■ Improve pain from oral mucositis after bone marrow transplant[28]

There are a variety of meditative practices, many of which derived from Eastern culture or religious practices. Mindfulness-based stress reduction (MBSR) is a modern variant of meditation that has been applied to stress reduction. MBSR purports to change the experience of negative emotions by cultivation of an acute, moment-to-moment awareness of thoughts and feelings. A nonjudgmental attitude toward these thoughts and feelings is learned. This awareness is taught through regular meditative practice. Unlike many other meditative practices, MBSR has been studied for patients with chronic pain[29,30] and cancer.[31]

MBSR has been shown to improve the following:

■ Chronic pain[29,30]
■ Low back pain[29,30]
■ Coping with pain[29,30]
■ Stress[32]
■ Mood[33]
■ Immune system markers in patients with breast and prostate cancer[31]

Mindfulness-based art therapy, a combination of mindfulness practices and art therapy, has been shown to reduce psychological distress and improve the quality of life for patients with breast cancer.[34,35]

Biologically Based Therapies

Herbal Products. Many herbal products purport to relieve pain. A complete review can be found in the Clinical Tools section of http://www.PainEDU.org. Five of the top 10 herbal remedies in the United States are marketed to relieve pain. They are presented in Table 20.[36]

■ **Table 20.**
Herbs marketed to relieve pain.

Herb	Uses	Safety/Adverse Reactions
St. John's wort (*Hypericum perforatum*)	Used for depression, anxiety, headache, muscle and nerve pain	Adverse effects: insomnia, anxiety, fatigue, headache. Is probably safe when used appropriately May interact with drugs with serotonin, triptans, opioids, human immunodeficiency virus drugs, digoxin, warfarin, oral contraceptives, chemotherapy, albuterol
Echinacea (*Echinacea purpura*)	Used for migraines, dyspepsia, pain, dizziness, respiratory infection, wound healing	Adverse effects: allergic reaction, nausea, stomach pain, diarrhea, dizziness May interact with acetaminophen, immunosuppressive therapy
Feverfew (*Tanacetum parthenium*)	Used for migraine	Adverse effects: headache, ulcers, gastrointestinal upset May interact with anticoagulants
Ginger (*Zingiber officinale*)	Used for nausea, gastrointestinal upset, thermal burns, topical analgesic	Generally safe when used appropriately. Adverse effects: increased bleeding risk May interact with diabetic drugs, heart drugs, reflux and stomach ulcer drugs
Ginseng (*Panax quinquefolius*)	Used for memory, depression, headache, fatigue	Adverse effects: anxiety, insomnia, headache May interact with other drugs: nonsteroidal antiinflammatory drugs, antipsychotic drugs, hormones, monoamine oxidase inhibitors, immunosuppressants, opioids, alcohol

Herbal preparations are not subjected to the regulatory processes of other drugs, and therefore, a paucity of studies that assess their efficacy and safety exists. There are some well-controlled studies that, on the whole, document the limited efficacy of herbal treatments for pain relief.[36] However, physicians should know what their patients are taking and ask about herbal preparations in a nonjudgmental manner.

Manipulative and Body-Based Methods

Acupuncture. Acupuncture began in China approximately 2,500 years ago. Its primary purpose according to Chinese philosophy is to assess and rebalance the life force of the individual. This life force is known as *qi* (pronounced "chee."). Qi is located on meridians of the body. Stimulation of certain points on the meridians with small-gauge needles rebalances qi in the body.

Western physicians have adopted forms of acupuncture, including pressure applied with the finger (acupressure), with low-frequency electrical current (electroacupuncture), or at points on the ear (auricular).[37–39] More than 1 million Americans are treated with acupuncture every year.[40]

The evidence is considered strong for the efficacy of acupuncture in postoperative pain and chemotherapy nausea and vomiting.[40,41] A metaanalysis found evidence that acupuncture is effective for pain relief for low back pain over sham acupuncture and no additional treatment.[42] Two reviews for cancer patients found the following:

- Pain relief
- Increased mobility
- Reduced cancer treatment–related pain
- Reduced muscle and bladder spasms
- Reduced vascular problems[41,43]

Literature reviews on the efficacy of acupuncture for short-term acute and for chronic pain indicate an overall positive therapeutic benefit, with the caveat that well-controlled studies are

rare and long-term studies are lacking. Empiric studies are difficult to accomplish for a number of reasons, including the absence
of standardized treatments for certain conditions. Additionally,
many practitioners of acupuncture do not believe the scientific
methods of Western medicine are appropriate to study the efficacy
of acupuncture.

Drawing on a scientific rationale of trigger point or electrical
stimulation therapy, acupuncture is generally recommended for
conditions that involve somatic pain. Adverse effects of acupuncture are bleeding and pain at the needle site. It is contraindicated
for patients with thrombocytopenia, coagulopathy, or neutrope-
nia.[38] Limitations of acupuncture include the possibility of infection if sterile precautions are not taken. In addition, some
practitioners are overzealous about the effects of acupuncture and
may promise more relief than is generally expected from any one
treatment for acute or chronic pain. Properly practiced, acupuncture is considered safe and is an alternative to conventional symptomatic treatments.[44]

Chiropractic or Osteopathic Manipulative Techniques. Chiropractic or osteopathic manipulation involves movement of the spine.
They are used to reduce muscle tension and/or to place the
patient's spine in proper alignment.

Limited evidence from systematic reviews supports chiropractic
treatment for musculoskeletal conditions.[45] More research needs to
be accomplished before these techniques can be recommended for
the majority of patients with musculoskeletal pain.

Energy Therapies. Energy therapies involve manipulating the
patient's energy to revive the energy flow in the body to enhance
health. Energy is generally manipulated without touching the
patient (e.g., therapeutic touch). Reiki and Qigong are also techniques in this category.

There is not enough evidence about these therapies to recommend
them. However, there are no known risks to these treatments.

PHARMACOLOGIC OPTIONS FOR THE MANAGEMENT OF PAIN

Nonopioid Analgesics

Acetaminophen

Acetaminophen has analgesic and antipyretic properties similar to that of aspirin, without the antiinflammatory effect. Acetaminophen is a common treatment of mild to moderate pain and is often the recommended first-line analgesic therapy for the treatment of osteoarthritic pain.

Its mechanism of action is not well-defined, although it is thought to be associated with the nitric oxide cycle. Acetaminophen *does not* interfere with gastric mucosa protection or platelet aggregation. However, doses in excess of 4 g per day should be avoided in all patients to minimize the risk of rare but potentially serious liver toxicity. Patients with chronic alcoholism and/or severe liver disease can develop hepatotoxicity even at therapeutic doses; therefore, care should be taken when prescribing acetaminophen in these patient populations. Clinicians should also be extremely vigilant when managing warfarin therapy in patients taking acetaminophen, as it can cause potentiation of the anticoagulant effects of warfarin.

Acetylsalicylic Acid

Acetylsalicylic acid, or aspirin, can sometimes be as effective as other nonopioid analgesics in relieving pain. Aspirin is commonly used to treat minor to moderate types of pain, including arthritic conditions, where its antiinflammatory effect (similar to other nonsteroidal antiinflammatories) would be of benefit. Gastrointestinal disturbances (usually upper gastrointestinal) and bleeding due to platelet aggregation inhibition are the most common adverse effects seen with aspirin therapy. Although one of the oldest nonopioid analgesics and considered to be a member of the class of nonsteroidal antiinflammatory medications, the exact mechanism of aspirin is still unknown.

Because of the possible association with Reye's syndrome, aspirin *should be avoided* in children younger than age 12 years with acute viral illness, particularly varicella, or influenza-like conditions. Aspirin should also be avoided by patients with peptic ulcer disease or poor kidney function because this medication can aggravate both conditions. Aspirin is avoided in patients taking blood-thinning medications (anticoagulants) such as warfarin because of an increased risk of bleeding.

Aspirin hypersensitivity may occur and can present with two distinct clinical pictures. In one presentation, the patient develops a respiratory reaction, with rhinitis, asthma, or nasal polyps. In another, smaller subset of patients, anaphylactoid symptoms may occur, such as urticaria, rash, hypotension, and shock within minutes of ingestion.

Nonselective Nonsteroidal Antiinflammatory Drugs

Nonselective nonsteroidal antiinflammatory drugs (NSAIDs) are used primarily for treatment of mild to moderate pain and provide additive analgesia when combined with opioids prescribed for more severe pain conditions or inflammatory pain conditions. NSAIDs work by inhibiting the enzyme cyclooxygenase, which catalyzes the conversion of arachidonic acid to leukotrienes, and prostaglandins, which are known to sensitize nociceptors near the location of the pain.[46] In contrast to opioids, NSAIDs have a distinct ceiling effect for analgesia— that is, increasing the dose beyond a certain threshold does not increase analgesia (but can increase toxicity). NSAIDs do not produce physical or psychological dependence.

NSAIDs are particularly good for bone pain and incident pain, or the type of pain that is provoked by activity (e.g., walking). All types of pain may respond to NSAIDs; however, visceral pain is probably less responsive than somatic pain, and neuropathic pain is often unresponsive.[47]

Although NSAIDs are useful for treating pain, patients should be carefully monitored for adverse effects, including renal impairment, bleeding, gastric ulceration, and hepatic dysfunction. Some less common side effects include confusion, precipitation of cardiac failure, pedal edema, and exacerbation of hypertension.

Extreme caution should be used when prescribing NSAIDs in patients who have any of the following risk factors:

- A history of gastric or duodenal perforation
- Bleeding ulcer
- Concomitant use of anticoagulants (e.g., warfarin, heparin)
- Concomitant use of corticosteroids
- Prior history of long duration of use of NSAID therapy
- Advanced age

The optimal strategy for providing analgesia without gastrointestinal toxicity remains to be determined. Concomitant ulceroprotective treatment—for example, proton pump inhibitors or misoprostol—may be prescribed in high-risk patients. Although nonacetylated salicylates, choline-magnesium-trisalicylate, and salsalate appear not to alter platelet function significantly and are often used in this situation, clinical experience suggests that these medications are not as effective as the NSAIDs at relieving pain.

Cyclooxygenase-2 Inhibitors

Research has shown that there are actually two relevant isoforms of cyclooxygenase, COX-1 and COX-2. COX-1 is present in many tissues, including gastrointestinal tract and platelet, whereas COX-2 is present primarily in inflamed/injured tissue and kidney. Thus, inhibition of COX-2 is likely the primary mechanism of action of NSAIDs, whereas inhibition of COX-1 is the mechanism of some of the major toxicities of NSAIDs: gastrointestinal ulceration and bleeding and platelet dysfunction. Agents that selectively inhibit COX-2 appear to relieve pain and inflammation *without* significant gastrointestinal or platelet disturbance. However, the analgesic efficacy of COX-2 inhibitors has not been proved to be superior to traditional NSAIDs. Indeed, with the current swirl of controversy surrounding cardiovascular risks that exists today with selective COX-2 inhibitors, these drugs should be used in appropriate patients who either are not at increased risk for complications or in whom typical NSAIDs are not indicated due to risk factors such as those mentioned previously.

Opioid Analgesics

Opioid analgesics are considered to be a mainstay in the treatment of moderate to severe pain that does not respond to nonopioids alone because they are effective, are fairly easy to titrate, and have a favorable risk to benefit ratio. They are often combined with non-opioids because this permits using a lower dose (i.e., opioid dose-sparing effect). Opioids are the first-line approach to moderate to severe cancer-related pain.

Opioids can exhibit their analgesic effects by acting on both peripheral and central mu, kappa, and delta opioid receptors, which inhibits the transmission of nociceptive input from the periphery to the spinal cord, activates the inhibitory pathways that modulate transmission, and alters limbic system activity. Recent research expands the traditional view and shows that opioids may also work peripherally in areas of inflammation. Evidence also bears out that because responsiveness varies in individuals, a patient who has failed with one should be treated with another to investigate greater efficacy. Opioid analgesics are typically classified according to the receptors to which they bind, and are categorized as follows:

- Pure agonists
- Agonist-antagonists
  - Partial agonists
  - Mixed agonist/antagonists
- Pure antagonists
- Other
  - Tramadol

They may also be subdivided further into divisions based on their pharmacokinetic properties:

- Short-acting
- Long-acting

Pure agonists include the following:

- Codeine
- Dihydrocodeine
- Fentanyl
- Hydrocodone
- Hydromorphone
- Levorphanol
- Meperidine
- Morphine
- Methadone
- Oxycodone
- Oxymorphone
- Propoxyphene

These opioids are classified as *pure agonists* because they bind to the mu opioid receptor, do not have a ceiling effect for analgesia, and do not interfere with the effects of other opioids in this class when prescribed simultaneously. Side effects of full agonists include constipation, sedation, nausea and vomiting, mental clouding, addiction, myoclonus, pruritus, sweating, urinary retention, and respiratory depression.

Partial agonists (e.g., buprenorphine) bind with only partial efficacy at the opioid receptor. They have a ceiling effect for analgesia (like NSAIDs) and may produce a withdrawal syndrome when administered to physically dependent patients.

Finally, *mixed agonists/antagonists* include butorphanol, nalbuphine, and pentazocine. Unlike full agonists, these opioids block opioid analgesia at the mu opioid receptor or are neutral at this receptor while simultaneously producing analgesia by activating another opioid receptor (kappa). Agonist/antagonists should not be prescribed with full agonists because doing so could lead to symptoms of withdrawal and increased pain.[8] Although the agonist/antagonists were initially thought not to cause addiction, experience has revealed the opposite. The agonist/antagonists thus have a limited role, if any, in pain management.

Pure antagonists such as naloxone and naltrexone are administered for prevention or reversal of opioid effects.

Tramadol is a useful agent that is unique in that it has a dual mechanism of action. Tramadol acts as a weak agonist at the mu opioid receptor but also inhibits reuptake of norepinephrine and serotonin, like a tricyclic antidepressant. Both properties are necessary for its full analgesic activity. Tramadol is typically used for mild to moderate pain and can be used up to 400 mg per day, given as 25–100 mg every 4–8 hours as needed. Tramadol does not appear to produce tolerance, and although it can be addictive, this is much less common than with the other opioids. Tramadol is *not* an NSAID and does not share the NSAID liabilities of antiplatelet effect and gastrointestinal complications. Because of its tricyclic-like properties, tramadol should be used only with great caution in patients already on these agents. Also, tramadol can precipitate seizures, so it should be used with great caution, if at all, in patients with a history of seizures, brain metastases, or other risk factors for seizures.

Short-Acting and Long-Acting Opioid Preparations

Opioids may be classified according to whether they are short-acting or long-acting. *Short-acting opioids* include codeine, hydrocodone, hydromorphone, oxycodone, meperidine, and fentanyl (available for transmucosal use as a lollipop or buccal tablet). Short-acting agents are characterized by a relatively short onset of action (30–60 minutes) and relatively short duration of action (2–4 hours). Short-acting opioids are used generally for patients with mild to moderate pain, intermittent pain, or breakthrough episodes that are superimposed on constant background pain.

Other opioids may be characterized as *long-acting* by virtue of their intrinsic pharmacokinetic properties (e.g., methadone, levorphanol) or by virtue of their incorporation into a slow-release delivery system (e.g., controlled-release morphine; controlled-release oxycodone; transdermal fentanyl). Long-acting opioids are generally characterized by a slower onset of action, but a relatively long duration, and are therefore used on a round-the-clock basis for patients with constant background pain. Most patients with cancer pain end up on a long-acting opioid on a fixed-dose schedule for background pain with a short-acting opioid for breakthrough pain. Maximizing the use of long-acting opioids in this setting enhances adherence and affords patients the advantages of more consistent pain relief, increased sleep, decreased episodes of medication taking, and generally improved satisfaction. Although many clinicians have extended this treatment philosophy to individuals with chronic noncancer pain, the long-term advantages and disadvantages of these various approaches to opioid analgesia have not been systematically studied.

Appropriate Dosing of Opioids

An equianalgesic chart should be used when changing from one opioid to another or from one route of administration to another. It is important to remember that the doses listed on equianalgesic charts are just estimates and can vary; the optimal dose for any individual patient is always determined by careful titration and appropriate monitoring. Equianalgesic charts show the oral and intramuscular (IM) doses of opioids that are equivalent to 10 mg of IM morphine. Because few studies exist regarding comparisons between intravenous (IV) doses of different opioids, the American Pain Society[48] recommends that IV doses be based on two assumptions: (1) that half the IV dose will give the same peak effect as a single IM dose and (2) IV infusions or repeated small boluses and IM total dosage will be equal when calculating the 24-hour requirements because IM doses are eventually absorbed.

When a new drug is considered, the equianalgesic chart shows approximate equivalents between the new and old drug. The total dose of each opioid over 24 hours should be recorded, with separate calculations made for parenteral and oral doses of the same opioid if both forms are used. Each 24-hour total should be divided by the equianalgesic dose for that opioid and route, thereby converting the dose into equianalgesic dose units that are each equivalent to 10 mg of IM morphine. The equianalgesic dose units for all drugs should be added. The dose of the new drug can be found by multiplying the sum of the dose units obtained above by the equianalgesic dose for the new drug and route.[48]

The equianalgesic dose conversion charts are derived mainly from single-dose analgesic studies and may not apply to chronic dosing. The American Pain Society Principles of Analgesic Use[48] indicate that dose changes for patients on high doses of opioids can be accomplished in stages by first implementing a partial conversion to minimize the risks of serious miscalculation (withdrawal, severe pain, overdose). For example, a patient with an infusion being changed to an oral preparation might have his or her infusion decreased by 50%, with the remaining 50% of the opioid requirement provided by an oral formulation. Reassessment of this strategy can be made after 24 hours. The half-life of opioids must also be taken into consideration when changing patients to different opioids. Estimates of doses vary widely depending on the half-life of the initial and replacement opioid, sometimes resulting in doses several times the original dose. In cases where the difference between severe pain from underestimating the conversion dose is coupled with safety concerns about overestimating the conversion dose, hospitalization for dose conversion is appropriate.

Routes of Administration of Opioids

The *oral* route of administration should be used first. This route is most convenient and cost-effective. It is a myth that *parenteral* administration of opioids is more effective at relieving pain than *oral* administration. *Effectiveness* (i.e., how well it works) must be distinguished from *potency* (how many milligrams it takes). *Oral* opioids are less potent than *parenteral* opioids—that is, higher doses of *oral* compared with *parenteral* opioids are required to produce the same degree of pain relief because of the first-pass metabolism of opioids in the liver. This has nothing to do with effectiveness—both routes work equally well at *equianalgesic* doses. However, the *parenteral* route, *intramuscular (IM), intravenous (IV)*, and *subcutaneous (SC)*, may be required when the *oral* route is unavailable, rapid titration of opioid dose for severe pain is required, or the *oral* or *transdermal* opioid dose has become so high that only *parenteral* opioids can be conveniently administered. Because the ratio of *oral* to *parenteral* equianalgesic dosages differs among opioids, conversion charts are generally necessary when transitioning a patient from one opioid regimen to another. Liquid forms of opioids can be used when patients have trouble swallowing. Also, a number of liquid opioid preparations are fairly well-absorbed *sublingually* and come in various potencies (e.g., morphine, methadone), thus obviating the need for *parenteral* doses in patients who cannot swallow (e.g., esophageal cancer).

Fentanyl lozenges can be used *transmucosally* in patients with breakthrough pain who are unable to swallow or absorb medication. These fentanyl lozenges have the most rapid onset of action of any nonparenteral opioid. A new rapid-onset (15 minutes) short-acting (60 minutes) *buccal* preparation of fentanyl has just received approval for the management of breakthrough pain in patients with cancer who are already receiving and who are tolerant to opioid therapy for their underlying persistent cancer pain.

When *oral* opioids cannot be delivered secondary to unavailability of the *oral* route (e.g., nausea and vomiting), *rectal* and *transdermal* forms of administration should be considered. *Rectal* administration of opioids is possible but has a relatively slow onset of action and variable pharmacokinetics.[8] The *transdermal* fentanyl patch appears to be a safe and practical alternative to short-acting analgesics in the treatment of cancer pain. The unique pharmacokinetics of the *transdermal* system, including the prolonged time to peak analgesic effect, long elimination half-life, and skin depot concept, should be kept in mind when prescribing the system. A relatively new patient-controlled *transdermal* fentanyl patch is indicated for the short-term management of acute postoperative pain in adult patients requiring opioid analgesia during hospitalization.

IM injections should be avoided as a route of administration of opioid analgesia because of increases in pain that the injection can cause, unreliable absorption, and complications of *IM* shots (e.g., nerve injury, sterile abscesses).[8] In addition, oversedation can occur because of staircased doses given to achieve rapid analgesia. The *SC* route is a useful and underused mode of delivery of both isolated injections and long-term infusions. *SC* injections can provide rapid relief without the need for *IV* access. *SC* infusions can be used with patient-controlled analgesia pumps for long-term home use; patients can receive a continuous infusion plus boluses as needed. Generally a maximum of 2 ml per hour can be delivered this way; however, both morphine and hydromorphone can be concentrated to as high as 50 mg/ml, which covers nearly all situations. Induration or irritation at the infusion site can be a complication of subcutaneous infusion. *IV* patient-controlled analgesia requires *IV* access but does not have the volume limitations of *subcutaneous* infusions. In addition, opioid analgesia has more rapid onset when given *intravenously* versus *subcutaneously*. When *IV* patient-controlled analgesia is used, approximately 85% of individuals receive good to excellent pain control.[49]

Epidural and intrathecal administration of opioids directly to the spinal axis has gained widespread use because of its efficacy, especially for acute pain that has not responded to less invasive measures. However, side effects, such as pruritus, urinary retention, and delayed respiratory depression, are more common with these routes of administration. Opioids alone do not cause the same degree of hypotension from sympathetic blockade similar to that of local anesthetics because of their action only at opioid receptors, nor do they cause motor blockade that reduces patient mobility.[48] However, opioids are generally used epidurally in combination with local anesthetics, due to the dramatic increase in analgesic efficacy of the combination; also, the combination allows relative reduction of opioid requirements and therefore opioid side effects.

Common Adverse Reactions

Constipation is commonly associated with opioid use, and all patients should receive prophylactic bowel therapy unless contraindicated. Increasing fluids, dietary fiber, exercise, and prophylactic medications may relieve constipation. Prophylaxis for opioid-induced constipation involves stimulants, such as senna derivatives, and stool softeners, such as docusate. It is important to note that dietary changes are rarely sufficient to counteract the effects of opioids. If constipation develops, the cause and severity of the constipation should be assessed. A clinical history should include the time of the last two bowel movements, stool consistency, stool amount, use of laxatives, and other symptoms, such as nausea and distention.[47] The presence of fecal impaction, hemorrhoids, fissures, or an empty rectum should be established on physical examination. A good bowel movement every 3 days is a reasonable goal of treatment, depending on the patient's baseline.

After beginning an opioid analgesic, many patients complain of *sedation*. Although sedation usually abates in a few days, many patients report persistent sedation. To minimize sedation, administer opioids at the suggested starting doses, with lower doses for elderly or compromised patients, and then increase the opioid dose as necessary. When sedation develops, assess for other causes of sedation, including other sedating medications, sleep deprivation, systemic illness (e.g., hepatic or renal dysfunction), metabolic disturbances, and central nervous system pathology. Reduce the dosage of opioid if pain can be managed at a lower dose, although this is rarely useful because the patient likely uptitrated out of necessity for pain control. If the patient is using a significant dose of the opioid at bedtime to help with sleep, try nonopioid hypnotics (preferably ones with no morning carryover effect) to spare the total opioid burden. Administration of a coanalgesic (e.g., an NSAID) may allow opioid reduction. "Opioid rotation," or changing from one opioid to another, may reduce side effects. Opioid rotation may be necessary due to elimination of toxic opioid metabolites or to patients' idiosyncratic responses to different opioids. Psychostimulant medications are a useful symptomatic treatment for opioid-induced sedation and include caffeine, modafinil (Provigil) (200 mg every day to twice a day), dextroamphetamine (2.5–10 mg by mouth every day or twice a day), and methylphenidate (5–10 mg by mouth every day or twice a day).[48] Stimulant medication generally should not be taken beyond 2 P.M. to avoid interruption of sleep.

Opioids are thought to worsen the performance of psychomotor tasks because of their sedating and mental-clouding effects. As a result, some safety regulations restrict the use of opioids when driving or using heavy equipment.

A study was conducted to investigate the psychomotor effects of long-term opioid use in 144 patients with low back pain. All subjects were administered two neuropsychological tests (Digit Symbol Substitution Test and Trail Making Test) before being prescribed opioids for pain (oxycodone with acetaminophen or transdermal fentanyl). Tests were then readministered at 90- and 180-day intervals. Test scores significantly improved while subjects were taking opioids for pain, which suggested that long-term use of short- and long-acting opioids does not significantly impair cognitive ability or psychomotor function. This supports the clinical impression that many patients who take opioids for pain over time adjust to the adverse effects of opioids, especially with regard to impaired cognition.[48]

Nausea and vomiting are other common side effects associated with the use of opioids. Although drug-induced nausea is among the most common causes, other causes are possible (e.g., metabolic difficulties such as hypercalcemia or uremia, irritation of the gastrointestinal tract, pharyngeal lesions, brain metastases) and should be ruled out. New onset of nausea or vomiting in a patient who has been on an opioid for over a few weeks is *not* likely related to the opioid. Nausea and vomiting prophylaxis should be instituted in high-risk patients on initiation of opioid therapy. Treatment of nausea and or vomiting should be aggressive if it occurs. To prevent opioid-induced nausea and vomiting in patients at risk, prescribe antiemetics with each opioid dose, at least until the patient's response seems stable and satisfactory. Some common antiemetics prescribed to treat opioid-induced nausea and vomiting are dopamine-blocking agents (e.g., prochlorperazine, 10 mg; haloperidol, 0.5–1 mg; or metoclopramide, 10 mg, before each opioid dose), or 5-hydroxytryptamine 3 (5-HT$_3$) receptor antagonists (e.g., ondansetron).

Opioids can sometimes cause *dysphoria* or *delirium,* as well as confusion, hallucinations, seizures, restlessness, and bad dreams. Opioid-induced delirium can often be resolved after a reduction of opioid and sometimes switching from one opioid to another. Haloperidol, 0.5–2 mg by mouth every 4–6 hours, or other neuroleptic agents are effective symptomatic treatments.[8] It is useful to distinguish mental clouding caused by sedation from mental clouding caused by delirium. Psychostimulants may improve these symptoms in the former case but will usually worsen them in the latter.

Some patients develop *pruritus*, which can result from mast cell destabilization by the opioid and subsequent histamine release, or more likely, from central opioid effects on brain or spinal cord. In many cases, the pruritus can be treated with a routine administration of long-acting, nonsedating antihistamines while opioid dosing continues. Although nalbuphine (an opioid agonist/antagonist) or naloxone may be effective, these agents should be used with caution to avoid precipitating withdrawal symptoms. Administration of an agonist/antagonist (i.e., butorphanol) has been shown to be very effective in treating opioid-induced pruritus without affecting analgesic efficacy. Sometimes switching opioids is the most pragmatic strategy for persistent opioid-induced pruritus.

Opioids occasionally cause multifocal *myoclonus*, which consists of sudden unexpected repetitive (but nonrhythmic) jerks of unrelated muscle groups throughout the body. This can be confused with "benign nocturnal myoclonus," a normal phenomenon consisting of a sudden jumping of seemingly the whole body during periods of drowsiness. Multifocal myoclonus is a characteristic feature of the opioid metabolite accumulation syndrome and should prompt concern, as it can progress to seizures. The approach consists of opioid rotation if possible; if not, the myoclonus can be suppressed with a number of agents (baclofen, valproic acid, clonazepam, gabapentin). Any medication that causes increased drowsiness can increase "benign nocturnal myoclonus," which should not arouse concern unless it is part of a progressive neurologic picture.

Urinary retention is sometimes caused by opioids but may be a more frequent problem associated with epidurally administered opioids. Urinary retention can be relieved with bethanechol or in the short-term with opioid antagonists (naloxone, naltrexone, or nalbuphine). It may be necessary to repeat doses to make certain that the bladder is completely empty, and sometimes catheterization of the bladder is necessary. Persistent urinary retention that is clearly due to an oral opioid should result in opioid rotation, along with measures to reduce opioid requirements.

Respiratory depression is the most important opioid adverse effect. Opioids typically produce a concentration-dependent shift in the carbon dioxide response curve. When this shift becomes great enough, clinical expression of respiratory depression occurs, usually as a decrease in respiratory rate. Usually with clinically appropriate doses, compensation occurs, and respiratory rate does not decline. Tolerance to the respiratory effects of opioids usually develops quickly, and doses can be increased as necessary without concern. However, in the event of a cardiorespiratory event, a patient's response may be exaggerated due to the presence of opioid concentrations in the bloodstream. The point is that even in the absence of clinical signs, there may still be residual effects on respiratory reserve after tolerance develops, and this must be kept in mind with patients on opioid therapy. In cases where respiration is acutely compromised, the first priorities are, as always, establishing an airway and ventilating the patient. Consider using a dilute solution of naloxone (0.4 mg in 10 mL of saline), administered as 1-mL boluses every minute until the patient is breathing appropriately. Some patients are extremely sensitive to opioid antagonists. There is nothing more distressing to patients, family members, nurses, and physicians than overly aggressive administration of naloxone to a terminal patient resulting in a horrific withdrawal syndrome in the patient's last days or weeks. Patients remember opioid withdrawal forever—it is best avoided. Children and patients who weigh less than 40 kg should have 0.1 mg of naloxone diluted in 10 mL of saline to make a 10 mcg/mL solution, given at 0.5 mcg/kg every 2 minutes.[48a] Naloxone administration should not be given for altered mental status unrelated to opioid overdose.

Prescribing Considerations

Two major considerations are important when prescribing opioids: the *fear of regulatory and legal scrutiny* and the *fear of addiction*, which can ultimately contribute to the undertreatment of pain. Fears of sanctions by regulatory agencies are largely exaggerated. When prescribing guidelines are followed, investigations by regulatory agencies are unlikely.

Fear of Regulatory Scrutiny. The Federation of State Medical Boards of the United States has recognized the need for the use of opioids in pain management and in 1998 published the *Model Guidelines for the Use of Controlled Substances for the Treatment of Pain*, which appears here:

1. Evaluation of the Patient. A complete medical history and physical examination must be conducted and documented in the medical record. The medical record should document the nature and intensity of the pain, current and past treatments for pain, underlying or coexisting diseases or conditions, the effect of the pain on physical and psychological function, and history of substance abuse. The medical record should also document the presence of one or more recognized medical indications for the use of a controlled substance. Many clinicians use **SOAPP®**, (**S**creener and **O**pioid **A**ssessment for **P**atients with **P**ain), a brief paper and pencil tool, to facilitate assessment and planning for chronic pain patients being considered for long-term opioid treatment.[48b] The tool and accompanying scoring information can be downloaded from http://www.PainEDU.org.

2. Treatment Plan. The written treatment plan should state objectives that will be used to determine treatment success, such as pain relief and improved physical and psychosocial function, and should indicate if any further diagnostic evaluations or other treatments are planned. After treatment begins, the physician should adjust drug therapy to the individual medical needs of each patient. Other treatment modalities or a rehabilitation program may be necessary depending on the etiology of the pain and the extent to which the pain is associated with physical and psychosocial impairment.

3. Informed Consent and Agreement for Treatment. The physician should discuss the risks and benefits of the use of controlled substances with the patient, persons designated by the patient, or the patient's surrogate or guardian if the patient is incompetent. The patient should receive prescriptions from one physician and one pharmacy where possible. The patient should agree to take medications only as prescribed. If the patient is determined to be at high risk for medication abuse or has a history of substance abuse, the physician may make use of a written agreement between physician and patient outlining patient responsibilities, including (1) urine/serum medication levels screening when requested, (2) number and frequency of all prescription refills, and (3) reasons for which drug therapy may be discontinued (e.g., violation of agreement).

4. Periodic Review. At reasonable intervals based on the individual circumstance of the patient, the physician should review the course of treatment and any new information about the etiology of the pain. Continuation or modification of therapy should depend on the physician's evaluation of progress toward stated treatment objectives such as improvement in patient's pain intensity and improved physical and/or psychosocial function (e.g., ability to work, need of health care resources, activities of daily living, and quality of social life). If treatment goals are not being achieved despite medication adjustments, the physician should reevaluate the appropriateness of continued treatment. The physician should monitor patient compliance with medication use and related treatment plans.

5. Consultation. The physician should be willing to refer the patient as necessary for additional evaluation and treatment to achieve treatment objectives. Special attention should be given to those pain patients who are at risk for misusing their medications and those whose living arrangement pose a risk for medication misuse or diversion. The management of pain in patients with a history of substance abuse or with a comorbid psychiatric disorder may require extra care, monitoring, documentation, and consultation with or referral to an expert in the management of such patients.

6. Medical Records. The physician should keep accurate and complete records to include the following:

- The medical history and physical examination
- Diagnostic, therapeutic, and laboratory results

- Evaluations and consultations
- Treatment objectives
- Discussion of risks and benefits
- Treatments
- Medications (including date, type, dose, and quantity prescribed)
- Instructions and agreements
- Periodic reviews

Records should remain current and be maintained in an accessible manner and readily available for review.

7. Compliance with Controlled Substances Laws and Regulations. To prescribe, dispense, or administer controlled substances, the physician must be licensed in the state and comply with applicable federal and state regulations. Physicians are referred to the *Physicians Manual of the U.S. Drug Enforcement Administration* and *any relevant documents issued by the state medical board* for specific rules governing controlled substances as well as applicable state regulations.

In addition, the Drug Enforcement Agency, along with a number of other agencies, has issued a statement supporting the importance of opioids in the management of pain. Physicians can check these guidelines, as well as others in their communities.

Documentation of the diagnosis, treatment and treatment outcome, as well as periodic review, is essential when prescribing opioids and serves as protection in the event of investigation. An opioid agreement, outlining the expectations of the patient and provider, can be used to document informed consent and the responsibilities of patient and provider. Such agreements often contain stipulations that the physician be the only person to prescribe opioids and that the patient use one pharmacy. These agreements outline appropriate use of opioids, side effect information, and the type of behavior expected from the patient (e.g., no requests for early refills, no changes in doses are made unless the patient has been physically evaluated). They may also define addictive behaviors and indicate the sanctions if the patient engages in these behaviors. Family members and/or significant others may be involved in these conversations so that they can learn more about the risks and benefits of treatments with opioids. Physicians should review any such agreements with their legal counsel before implementation because such agreements may have legal implications.

Fear of Addiction. Another fear that leads to the undertreatment of pain with opioids is addiction. It is important that the clinician understand, and be able to convey to the patient and family, the distinction between physical dependence, addiction, and pseudoaddiction. *Physical dependence* is a physiologic adaptation that occurs in patients receiving opioid analgesics (as well as other medications, including antiepileptics and certain antihypertensives). Physical dependence is characterized by the development of withdrawal symptoms when a medication is stopped or decreased abruptly and is expected in patients receiving opioid analgesics for more than a few days. Withdrawal can be avoided by tapering the dose when discontinuing treatment.

Addiction, on the other hand, is a chronic neurobiologic disease with genetic, psychosocial, and environmental influences. It is characterized by impaired control over drug use, compulsive use, continued use despite harm, and craving. *Pseudoaddiction* is a term used to describe behavior that appears to be addictive, "drug-seeking" behavior but is actually an effort to obtain pain relief by a nonaddicted patient who is not receiving adequate analgesia. Additional information on treatment of patients with comorbid substance abuse disorder is found in Ch. VII, in the section "Patients with Substance Abuse Problems." Although primary care practitioners often manage opioids for patients with chronic pain and cancer, they should not hesitate to refer patients to psychiatry, psychology, or pain management centers for consultation and/or evaluation and treatment.

Adjuvant Analgesic Agents

Adjuvant analgesic agents are a miscellaneous group of pain-relieving drugs whose primary indication traditionally is not for the treatment of pain. They are used to provide treatment for specific types of pain, and at times, to augment the analgesic effect of opioids and/or reduce the side effects of analgesics. Some of the most commonly used adjuvant drugs include corticosteroids, anticonvulsants, antidepressants, local anesthetics, neuroleptic agents, and hydroxyzine.

Corticosteroids. Corticosteroids are often used in palliative care, where they have a number of beneficial effects, including pain reduction, improved appetite, weight gain, antiemetic action, and mood elevation. Steroids are used in the treatment of neuropathic pain due to cord compression, brachial or lumbosacral plexus invasion, or peripheral nerve infiltration. Additionally, they are helpful in treating headache due to increased intracranial pressure, some types of arthritic pain, and pain after visceral obstruction.[47]

Dexamethasone, 12–24 mg/day, and prednisone, 30–100 mg/day, are the most commonly prescribed chronic regimens. Of course, the lowest dose that maintains benefit should be used; often, the best strategy is high initial doses followed by rapid tapering to the minimum effective dose. Beneficial effects of steroids tend to diminish after 2–3 months, and their use is therefore limited to patients with limited time left to live or as a short-term treatment before the institution of other palliative measures.[47] Chronic use of corticosteroids produces weight gain, Cushing's syndrome, proximal myopathy, mental changes, and increased risk of gastrointestinal bleeding.[48] NSAIDs should not, if possible, be used concomitantly with corticosteroids secondary because of risks of gastrointestinal bleeding. Discontinuation of a corticosteroid should be made gradually to minimize the effects of a steroid withdrawal syndrome which may occur due to adrenal suppression.

Anticonvulsants. Anticonvulsants are used for some neuropathic pain conditions to relieve lancinating or stabbing pain.[48] Anticonvulsants have the ability to suppress discharge in pathologically altered neurons, thus inhibiting neural hyperexcitability, which may be responsible for their usefulness in treatment of neuropathic pain conditions.

Gabapentin is a popular treatment choice because it is generally well-tolerated and serious side effects are extremely rare.[47] Gabapentin is indicated for treatment of postherpetic neuralgia but also has been widely studied in treatment of other types of neuropathic pain. Unlike other anticonvulsants, gabapentin rarely causes hematologic or hepatic side effects. Effectiveness studies of gabapentin have shown wide variability in the dose (e.g., 100–3,600 mg) required to produce beneficial results. Consequently, gabapentin should be prescribed in low dosages initially, with titration as needed, and as tolerated.[47] Positive results are usually seen within 2 days, and therefore, upward titration may begin every other day, as needed.[47] Gabapentin is associated with the typical side effects of all central nervous system–acting drugs, including sedation, dizziness, and confusion.

Pregabalin is another anticonvulsant used to treat neuropathic pain. It was approved in 2004 for treatment of diabetic peripheral neuropathy and postherpetic neuralgia.

Other anticonvulsants used to treat pain include carbamazepine and phenytoin; however, the hematologic and hepatic side effects of these drugs have made them less popular than newer agents. Some studies have shown lamotrigine and topiramate useful in the treatment of neuropathic pain, but their higher side effect burden and requirement for prolonged titration have caused them to be a second choice for treatment. Finally, it should be highlighted that opioids are the main treatment choice for cancer pain, even neuropathic cancer pain, unless the pain can be controlled with adjuvants alone.

Antidepressants. Tricyclic antidepressants (TCAs), such as amitriptyline, imipramine, nortriptyline, and desipramine, are useful agents for neuropathic pain, cancer pain, and nonneuropathic pain with certain symptoms (e.g., insomnia, depression, or visceral spasm). Evidence suggests that tricyclic antidepressants suppress pain-signaling through local anesthetic-like effects at sodium channels in neural membranes. They also inhibit reuptake of norepinephrine, serotonin, and dopamine at synapses, which may increase their analgesic effects, as well as improve mood favorably.

Analgesic efficacy is best demonstrated for tricyclic antidepressants such as amitriptyline and nortriptyline, and duloxetine has recently been approved for the treatment of diabetic peripheral neuropathy, although it is not recommended in patients with a history of hepatic disease.

Common side effects include dry mouth, sedation, urinary retention, constipation, and orthostasis. They may also be associated with cardiovascular side effects, such as increased blood pressure, and conduction blockade. They may also lower seizure threshold. Given that the efficacy of these agents is similar, choice of agent depends on the occurrence of side effects. Dosages for these agents are also comparable and should begin with 10–25 mg by mouth before bedtime and titrate upward as needed.[47] The usual beneficial dose for pain is 50–75 mg before bedtime; however, some patients may require 150 mg/day or more.[47] Although serum levels are not clinically useful for adjusting dosages, they are valuable for monitoring toxicity. It takes 2–4 weeks for analgesic effects to begin.

Topical Analgesics. Topical analgesics are targeted toward a specific area of pain. Typically, topical analgesics (e.g., lidocaine patch, capsaicin) are applied directly onto the painful area. They act locally, so serum drug concentration is insignificant and systemic side effects are unlikely. Titration is not needed, and there are no drug interactions. Topical analgesics are used for both neuropathic and musculoskeletal pain. Capsaicin, derived from the active ingredient in chili peppers, is available over the counter and is widely used. Capsaicin depletes substance P from nerve terminals and is thought through this mechanism to decrease peripheral pain transmission. Clinical trials have reported efficacy in neuropathic pain and focal arthritis and musculoskeletal conditions. These trials could not be adequately blinded (capsaicin stings), however, and the effect sizes seen were similar to those seen in unblinded trials.

NSAIDs are used topically around the world for localized pain; such use is less common in the United States, where these preparations must be custom compounded. However, many positive clinical trials and metaanalyses have confirmed the usefulness and safety of these preparations, apparently with a fraction of the systemic exposure of systemic NSAID treatment. Examples of such preparations include ibuprofen 5% and ketoprofen 20% cream.

Topical formulations should be differentiated from transdermal formulations, for which the application site is different from the painful region, and systemic effects, including serum drug concentration and possible side effects, can be found. Titration is needed, and drug interactions should be monitored for transdermal formulations.[50]

Several topical local anesthetics are available for use in pain treatment. EMLA® cream is a eutectic mixture of lidocaine and prilocaine and is used to prevent acute procedure-related pain such as that from venipuncture, circumcision, and skin biopsy. EMLA® is available as a cream and as a stick-on anesthetic disk. Although EMLA® is effective at reducing procedural pain, it must be left on for 30–60 minutes under an occlusive dressing before the procedure, which may be inconvenient. ELA-Max® (4% liposomal lidocaine) is another option for topical anesthesia to prevent acute procedural pain. The advantages of ELA-Max® are that it seems to provide clinically relevant anesthesia at 60 minutes, comparable to that produced by EMLA® at 90 minutes, and without requiring an occlusive dressing. These comparisons are based on a small number of generally poorly designed studies.

Once the barrier of intact skin is not an issue, there are a number of topical anesthetic options. Dentists have used benzocaine and other agents effectively for oral anesthesia for generations. Lidocaine 2% jelly is available for coating instruments that are used for urethral or endotracheal intubation and for the topical treatment of urethritis-related pain.

Lidocaine patch 5% is the only topical analgesic approved by the Food and Drug Administration for postherpetic neuralgia. Unlike the topical anesthetics described previously, the lidocaine patch does not produce anesthesia of the affected skin. With chronic use, systemic absorption also seems to be insignificant. The lidocaine patch should be applied directly to the most painful areas. Up to three patches may be used at a time, and they may be trimmed to conform to the affected area. The recommended dose is to use the patch for 12 hours on and 12 hours off; however, pharmacokinetic data suggest that applying four patches at a time for 18 hours a day was safe. The only significant side effect of the lidocaine patch in some cases has been local skin irritation in some patients.

Neuroleptic Agents. Neuroleptic agents have been used as adjuvant analgesics for many decades; however, their role in the treatment of chronic pain is limited at present. Methotrimeprazine is the only neuroleptic with definite analgesic properties and is occasionally used for patients with opioid tolerance or side effects.[47] Common side effects of neuroleptics include sedation and hypotension. Prolonged use of phenothiazines is associated with tardive dyskinesia.[48] Furthermore, extrapyramidal symptoms can occur, usually in younger patients, and can be treated with diphenhydramine.[48] Other neuroleptics are used for the treatment of anxiety, psychosis, hallucinations, intractable insomnia, nausea, and vomiting.

Anxiolytic/Hypnotic. Hydroxyzine is an antihistamine with anticholinergic (drying) and sedative properties that is used to treat allergic reactions. In addition to its antihistamine effects, hydroxyzine has mild analgesic, antiemetic, anxiolytic, and sedative effects.

Hydroxyzine is usually prescribed at 25–50 mg by mouth or IM every 4–6 hours as needed (0.5–1 mg/kg for children).[48] Although analgesic relief has been demonstrated after IM administration, it is not clear that oral administration produces any analgesic effects.[48] As such, oral administration of hydroxyzine is mainly prescribed to relieve nausea or anxiety.

Adjuvants for Bone Pain. Strontium (a radioisotope) and bisphosphonates are analgesic adjuvants used for metastatic bone pain. Radioisotopes work by delivering radiation to the bone. For example, one study demonstrated that a 10 m curie IV dosage of strontium was an effective adjuvant to local radiotherapy.[48] Although they are effective for the pain of widespread bony metastases, they are complicated by bone marrow suppression.

Bisphosphonates are a class of agents originally used to treat hypercalcemia of malignancy that work by suppressing the process of bone resorption, which seems to be accelerated by malignancy. The most common bisphosphonate used for this indication is pamidronate, which has been shown to reduce skeletal events and pain in patients with metastatic breast cancer and other diseases associated with lytic lesions. Pamidronate is generally well-tolerated and is administered as 90 mg IV in 2 hours every 4 weeks.[48] Another recently introduced agent is zoledronic acid, which has been shown to be effective not only in osteolytic lesions (e.g., breast cancer), but also osteoblastic lesions (e.g.,prostate cancer). The relative roles of these different agents remain to be determined; treatment guidelines are available from the American Society of Clinical Oncology.

RATIONAL POLYPHARMACY AND PAIN MANAGEMENT

The American Society of Anesthesiologists Task Force published the following guidelines in *Anesthesiology* in 2004: "Acute pain management practice guidelines for acute pain management in the perioperative setting: an updated report by the American Society of Anesthesiologists Task Force on Acute Pain Management."

Part of these guidelines mentions the idea that *"Whenever possible, anesthesiologists should use multimodal pain management therapy. Unless contraindicated, all patients should receive an around-the-clock regimen of nonsteroidal antiinflammatory drugs (NSAIDs), cyclooxygenase-2 inhibitors (COXIBs), or acetaminophen. Dosing regimens should be administered to optimize efficacy while minimizing the risk of adverse events. The choice of medication, dose, route, and duration of therapy should be individualized."*

Analgesics exert their activity at various sites along the pain pathway. Thus, in theory, multimodal analgesia [i.e., the use of two or more agents with differing mechanisms or multiple modes of analgesia (e.g., local anesthetics and opioids)] increases the likelihood that pain signals will be interrupted and pain relieved. Research has shown that analgesics with differing mechanisms of action can have additive or synergistic effects through a variety of cellular mechanisms, allowing the use of lower doses of each agent than would be used during monotherapy. A multimodal approach to pain management has long been proposed for treatment of both acute and chronic pain. The World Health Organization, the Agency for Healthcare Research and Quality (formerly the Agency for Health Care Policy and Research), and clinicians endorse the use of more than one agent with different mechanisms of action for the treatment of pain. The goal of multimodal therapy is to increase the efficacy of pain relief with enhanced safety and tolerability.

Below is a diagram by Gottschalk et al. depicting the different sites of action of many of the previously mentioned analgesics, portraying the idea that a multifocal approach could be beneficial.[51]

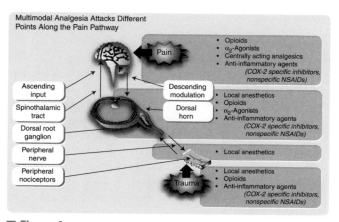

■ **Figure 4.**
Multimodal analgesia attacks different points along the pain pathway. Gottschalk A, Smith D. New concepts in acute pain therapy: preemptive analgesia. *Am Fam Phys* 2001;63:1979–1984.

The idea that multimodal therapy, or rational polypharmacy, should be applied toward effective pain management is actually not new. The logic is that to most successfully treat pain, two strategies are beneficial:

1. Attempt to "attack" pain at as many points along the pathway as possible.
2. Minimize the dose of medications with high adverse effect profiles in concert with other medications. This should likely minimize the incidence of adverse effects.

As stated in the previous guidelines for acute pain management, when treating pain, all decisions should be made with respect to the individualized treatment for the patient.

For more information, please refer to the appendixes medication names and dosing information.

INTERVENTIONAL OPTIONS FOR THE MANAGEMENT OF CHRONIC PAIN

The history of the application of interventional techniques in pain management dates back to 1901, when epidural injections for lumbar nerve root compression were reported.[52] Since then, substantial advances have been made in the administration of epidural injections, and many other interventional techniques have been described. Interventional techniques have been distinguished as the favored, and at times decisive, intervention in both the diagnostic and therapeutic management of chronic painful conditions.

Diagnostic and Therapeutic Blocks

Regional anesthesia refers to regional neural blockade for the purpose of blocking or modifying afferent or efferent neural conduction. *Diagnostic*, or *differential*, *nerve blocks* have been used to determine the source of the pain, differentiate local from central processes, identify nociceptive pathways, and differentiate between local and referred pain,[53] although there are important limitations to these approaches. For example, a sympathetic nerve block can determine whether the pain is sympathetically maintained, which would guide treatment decisions, but with a high false-positive rate. Diagnostic blocks are sometimes used to decide whether a neuroablative block would be effective, but their predictive value in this regard remains to be demonstrated. Local anesthetics and other agents can be infused via an indwelling catheter in the epidural space or along peripheral nerves to provide analgesia for days to weeks. Local anesthetics with or without steroids can be injected into various structures to provide antiinflammatory effects and pain relief. These techniques are useful in treating pain from joints, bursae, and spinal nerves.

Facet Joint Blocks

The facet joints of the spine can be anesthetized by fluoroscopically guided injections of local anesthetic, either into the target joint or onto the medial branches of the dorsal rami that supply them. The rationale for facet joint blocks is based on the observation that if a particular joint is determined to be the source of pain generation, long-term relief can be sought by directing therapeutic interventions at that joint. In managing low back pain, local anesthetic injection into the facet joints or interruption of the nerve supply to the facet joints has been accepted as the standard for diagnosis of facet joint mediated pain.

Trigger Point Injections

Trigger point injections are probably the most extensively used modality of treatment, not only by interventional pain physicians, but by all providers managing pain. Myofascial pain syndrome is a regional muscle pain disorder accompanied by trigger points. It has been described as a common phenomenon in multiple regions, including the spine. Myofascial trigger points are small, circumscribed, hyperirritable foci in muscles and fascia, often found within a firm or taut band of skeletal muscle. In contrast, nonmyofascial trigger points may also occur in ligaments, tendons, joint capsule, skin, and periosteum. Trigger points assist in the proper diagnosis of myofascial pain syndrome.

Neurolysis

Neurolytic agents (alcohol, phenol, and glycerol) injected around the nerve produces destructive changes in the nerve to decrease pain transmission. Other techniques to alter functioning of nerves include cryotherapy (cold) and radiofrequency (heat) lesions. Although these techniques can result in significant pain relief, complete destruction of the nerve can be accomplished only with surgical resection.[54] Neurolysis of the visceral ganglia can be used for visceral pain associated with cancer. Neurolytic techniques are also used to treat neuropathic pain. Neurolytic nerve blocks are generally reserved for intractable pain in the cancer setting, due to their inherent risks and the high rate of pain recurrence. Extreme consideration must be made when selecting patients for this technique, as it is ablative in nature and irreversible.

Interventional Techniques

Sympathetic blocks using regional anesthetic techniques and radiofrequency thermoneurolysis or neuromodulation with spinal cord stimulation or peripheral nerve stimulation are often management options for reflex sympathetic dystrophy, and causalgia, also known as *complex regional pain syndrome* (CRPS) types I and II. Radiofrequency neurolysis is really an extension of a continuous regional sympathetic block or neurolytic block, providing long-term relief with added safety. Consideration of sympathetic blocks is to facilitate management of complex regional pain syndrome with analgesia commensurate with a program of functional restoration and sympatholysis to provide unequivocal evidence of sympathetically maintained pain. Once it is established that sympatholysis is effective, it is important to repeat the procedure to determine whether an increasing duration of effect can be expected in any particular patient. If this is the case, these individual blocks may be all that are necessary to enable a patient to regain function. When sympatholysis completely relieves the symptoms and facilitates exercise therapy but is limited to its duration of effect, it is appropriate to consider a prolonged block using radiofrequency neurolysis. Radiofrequency has been described for lesioning of the cervical sympathetic chain, thoracic sympathetic chain, and lumbar sympathetic chain; in cases of complex regional pain syndrome I and II; as well as for neuropathic pain.

Implantable Technologies

Spinal cord stimulation and peripheral nerve stimulation are techniques that involve electrical stimulation of the spinal cord or peripheral nerves via an implanted pulse generator that delivers electrical signals to these structures. In the United States, the primary indications for spinal cord stimulation are failed back surgery syndrome. Patients experience a "buzzing" feeling that is associated with reduced pain intensity. These signals are thought to stimulate large afferent fibers and inhibit the noxious signals mediated by A delta and C-fibers.[55] Spinal cord or peripheral nerve stimulation appears to be most effective for individuals with chronic neuropathic pain, peripheral vascular disease, or chronic angina.

Implantable intrathecal pumps can deliver a continuous infusion of analgesic medications (e.g., morphine) directly to the spinal cord. Implantable pumps can be useful in the management of cancer pain or intractable chronic pain of noncancer origin. For a few patients, they may be used when the side effects of oral opioids are intolerable. Proper patient selection, as with all forms of pain management strategies, is critical for the success of implantable technologies.

REFERENCES

1. Lee MHM, Itah M, Yang GW, Eason AL. Physical therapy and rehabilitation medicine. In Bonica JJ, ed. *The Management of Pain*. Philadelphia: Lippincott, 1990:1769–1788.

2. Vasudevan S, Hegmann K, Moore A, Cerletty S. Physical methods of pain management. In Raj PP, ed. *Practical Management of Pain*. Baltimore: Mosby, 1992:669–679.

3. Moskal MJ, Matsen FA III. Orthopedic management of pain. In Loeser JD, Butler SH, Chapman CR, Turk DC, eds. *Bonica's Management of Pain (3rd ed)*. Philadelphia: Lippincott Williams & Wilkins, 2001:1807–1814.

4. McCaffery M, Wolff M. Pain relief using cutaneous modalities, positioning, and movement. *Hosp J* 1992;8:121.

5. Miaskowski C, Cleary J, Burney R, et al. *Guideline for the Management of Cancer Pain in Adults and Children. APS Clinical Practice Guidelines Series, No. 3*. Glenview, IL: American Pain Society, 2005.

6. National Comprehensive Cancer Network. NCCN Clinical Practice Guidelines in Oncology: Adult Cancer Pain 2007. Available at http://www.nccn.org/professionals/physician_gls/PDF/pain.pdf. Accessed August 2, 2007.

7. Willick SE, Herring SA, Press JM. Basic concepts in biomechanics and musculoskeletal rehabilitation. In Loeser JD, Butler SH, Chapman CR, Turk DC, eds. *Bonica's Management of Pain (3rd ed)*. Philadelphia: Lippincott Williams & Wilkins, 2001:1807–1814.

8. Jacox AK, Carr DB, Payne R, et al. *Management of Cancer Pain, Clinical Practice Guidelines*. No. 9. Rockville, MD: U. S. Department of Health and Human Services, Public Health Service, Agency for Health Care Policy and Research (AHCPR Publication No. 94-0592), 1994.

9. Field TM. Massage therapy effects. *Am Psychol* 1998;53:1270–1281.

10. Wilke DJ, Kampbell J, Cutshall S, et al. Effects of massage on pain intensity, analgesics and quality of life in patients with cancer pain: a pilot study of a randomized clinical trial conducted within hospice care delivery. *Hosp J* 2000;15(3):31–53.

11. Chabel C. Transcutaneous electrical nerve stimulation. In Loeser JD, Butler SH, Chapman CR, Turk DC, eds. *Bonica's Management of Pain (3rd ed)*. Philadelphia: Lippincott Williams & Wilkins, 2001:1842–1848.

12. Robinson JP. Evaluation of function and disability. In Loeser JD, Butler SH, Chapman CR, Turk DC, eds. *Bonica's Management of Pain (3rd ed)*. Philadelphia: Lippincott Williams & Wilkins, 2001:342–362.

13. Fordyce, W. Operant or contingency therapies. In Loeser JD, Butler SH, Chapman CR, Turk DC, eds. *Bonica's Management of Pain (3rd ed)*. Philadelphia: Lippincott Williams & Wilkins, 2001:1745–1750.

14. Arena, JG, Blanchard E. Biofeedback therapy for chronic pain. In Loeser JD, Butler SH, Chapman CR, Turk DC, eds. *Bonica's Management of Pain (3rd ed)*. Philadelphia: Lippincott Williams & Wilkins, 2001:1759–1767.

15. Astin JA. Mind–body therapies for the management of pain. *Clin J Pain* 2004;20(1):27–32.

16. Keefe FJ, Abernethy AP, Campbell LC. Psychological approaches to understanding and treating disease-related pain. *Ann Rev Psychol* 2005;56:601–630.

17. Turner JA, Romano JM, Psychological and psychosocial evaluation. In Loeser JD, Butler SH, Chapman CR, Turk DC, eds. *Bonica's Management of Pain (3rd ed)*. Philadelphia: Lippincott Williams & Wilkins, 2001:329–341.

18. Tunks ER, Merskey H. Psychotherapy in the management of chronic pain. In Loeser JD, Butler SH, Chapman CR, Turk DC, eds. *Bonica's Management of Pain (3rd ed)*. Philadelphia: Lippincott Williams & Wilkins, 2001:1857.

19. National Institutes of Health (NIH). Consensus Development Program: Symptom Management in Cancer: Pain, Depression and Fatigue. http://consensus.nih.gov/2002/2002CancerPainDepressionFatiguesos022html.htm. Accessed Nov. 1, 2006.

20. Oliver JW, Kravitz RL, Kaplan SH, Meyers FJ. Individualized patient education and coaching to improve pain control among cancer outpatients. *J Clin Oncol* 2001;19(8):2206–2212.

21. Miakowski C, Zimmer EF, Barrett KM, et al. Differences in patients' and family caregivers' perceptions of the pain experience influence patient and caregiver outcomes. *Pain* 1997;72(1–2):217–226.

22. Rippentrop EA, Altmaier EM, Chen JJ, et al. The relationship between religion/spirituality and physical health, mental health and pain in a chronic pain population. *Pain* 2005;116(3):311–321.

23. National Center for Complementary and Alternative Medicine, National Institutes of Health. What is complementary and alternative medicine? May 2002. NCCAM Publication No: D156. http://nccam.nih.gov/health/whatiscam/. Accessed Dec. 15, 2006.

24. Eisenberg DM, Davis RG, Ettner SL, et al. Trends in alternative medicine use in the United States, 1990–1997: results of a follow-up national survey. *JAMA* 1998;280(18):1569–1575.

25. Melchart D, Weidenhammer W, Streng A, et al. Prospective investigation of adverse effects of acupuncture in 97,733 patients. *Arch Intern Med* 2004;164:104–105.

26. NIH Technology Assessment Panel on Integration of Behavioral and Relaxation Approaches into the Treatment of Chronic Pain and Insom-

nia. Integration of behavioral and relaxation approaches into the treatment of chronic pain and insomnia. *JAMA* 1996;276:313–318.

27. Morrow GR, Morrell C. Behavioral treatment for anticipatory nausea and vomiting induced by cancer chemotherapy. *N Engl J Med* 1982;307:1476–1480.

28. Carr DB, Goudas LC, Balk EM, et al. Evidence report on the treatment of pain in cancer patients. *J Natl Cancer Inst Monogr* 2004;32:23–31.

29. Kabat-Zinn J, Lipworth L, Burney R. Four year follow-up of a meditation-based program for the self-regulation of chronic pain: treatment outcomes and compliance. *Clin J Pain* 1987:27:466–475.

30. Kabat-Zinn J, Lipworth L, Burney R. The clinical use of mindfulness meditation for the self-regulation of chronic pain. *J Behav Med* 1985;8:163–190.

31. Carlson LE, Speca M. Mindfulness-based stress reduction in relation to quality of life, mood, symptoms of stress, and immune parameters in breast and prostate cancer outpatients. *Psychosom Med* 2003;65:571–581.

32. Coker KH. Meditation and prostate cancer: integrating a mind/body intervention with traditional therapies. *Semin Urol Oncol* 1999;17:111–118.

33. Carlson LE, Ursuiliak Z, Goodey E, et al. The effects of a mindfulness meditation based stress reduction program on mood and symptoms of stress in cancer patients: 6-month follow-up. *Support Care Cancer* 2001;9:112–123.

34. Monti DA, Peterson C. Mindfulness-based art therapy: results from a two year study. *Psychiatry Times* 2004;21:63–66.

35. Monti DA, Peterson C, Kunkel EJ, et al. A randomized controlled trial of mindfulness-based art therapy (MBAT) for women with cancer. *Psychooncology* 2006;15(5):363–373.

36. Wirth JH, Hudgins JC, Paice JA. Use of herbal therapies to relieve pain: a review of efficacy and adverse effects. *Pain Manage Nurs* 2005;6(4):145–167.

37. Monti DA, Yang J. Complementary medicine in chronic cancer care. *Semin Oncol* 2005;255–231.

38. Deng G, Cassileth BR, Yeung KS. Complementary therapies for cancer-related symptoms. *J Support Oncol* 2004;2(5):419–429.

39. Filshie J, Thompson JW. Acupuncture. In Doyle D, Hanks NC, Calman K, eds. *Oxford Textbook of Palliative Medicine (3rd ed)*. New York: Oxford University Press, 2004:410–424.

40. National Institutes of Health Consensus Conference. Acupuncture. *JAMA* 1998;280:1518–1524.

41. Filshie J, Redman D. Acupuncture and malignant pain problems. *Eur J Surg Oncol* 1985;11:389–394.

42. Manheimer E, White A, Berman B, et al. Meta-analysis: acupuncture for low back pain. *Ann Intern Med* 2005;142:651–663.

43. Filshie J. Acupuncture for malignant pain. *Acupunct Med* 1990;8(2):38–39.

44. Butler SH, Chapman CR. Acupuncture. In Loeser JD, Butler SH, Chapman CR, Turk DC, eds. *Bonica's Management of Pain (3rd ed)*. Philadelphia: Lippincott Williams & Wilkins, 2001:1831–1841.

45. Ernst E. Manual therapies for pain control: chiropractic and massage. *Clin J Pain* 2004;20:8–12.

46. Miyoshi HR. Systemic nonopioid analgesics. In Loeser JD, Butler SH, Chapman CR, Turk DC, eds. *Bonica's Management of Pain (3rd ed)*. Philadelphia: Lippincott Williams & Wilkins, 2001:1667–1709.

47. Katz NP. Pain and symptom management. In Kantoff P, Carroll P, D'Amico A, et al., eds. *Prostate Cancer: Principles and Practice*. Philadelphia: Lippincott Williams & Wilkins, 2002:561–594.

48a. American Pain Society. *American Pain Society Principles of Analgesic Use in the Treatment of Acute Pain and Cancer Pain*. Glenview, IL: American Pain Society; 1999.

48b. Butler SF, Budman SH, Fernandez K, et al. Validation of a screener and opioid assessment measure for patients with chronic pain. *Pain*. 2004;112:65–75.

49. Ashburn MA, Ready LB. Postoperative pain. In Loeser JD, Butler SH, Chapman CR, Turk DC, eds. *Bonica's Management of Pain (3rd ed)*. Philadelphia: Lippincott Williams & Wilkins, 2001:765–779.

50. Jamison RN, Schein JR, Vallow R, et al. Neuropsychological effects of long-term opioid use in chronic pain patients. *J Pain Sympt Manage* 2003;26:913–921.

51. Galer BS, Dworkin, RH. *A Clinical Guide to Neuropathic Pain*. New York: McGraw Hill Healthcare Information Programs, 2000.

52. Gottschalk A, Smith D. New concepts in acute pain therapy: preemptive analgesia. *Am Fam Physician* 2001;63:1979–1984.

53. Cathelin, M. Mode d'action de la cocaine inject dons l'espace epidural par le proceda de canal sacre. *CR Soc Biol* 1901.

54. Buckley FP. Regional anesthesia with local anesthetics. In Loeser JD, Butler SH, Chapman CR, Turk DC, eds. *Bonica's Management of Pain (3rd ed)*. Philadelphia: Lippincott Williams & Wilkins, 2001:1893–1952.

55. Butler SH, Charlton JE. Neurolytic blockade and hypophysectomy. In Loeser JD, Butler SH, Chapman CR, Turk DC, eds. *Bonica's Management of Pain (3rd ed)*. Philadelphia: Lippincott Williams & Wilkins, 2001: 1967–2006.

VII.

Pain Management in Special Patient Populations

INFANTS AND CHILDREN

The myth that pediatric patients do not experience the same degree of pain as adults do was routinely taught to clinicians in training until fairly recently. The foundation of faulty logic was that infants and children had nervous systems that were not yet fully developed, and do not retain memories of their earlier years. Actually, recent animal studies show the opposite is true and that due to a stronger inflammatory response, along with decreased central inhibition, infants and children most likely deal with a higher level of pain than adults do. Indeed, it may be purely the lack of the ability to appropriately communicate the severity of pain that results in undertreatment of pain in this patient population.

Assessment of pain in this special population can be challenging, but *is* possible. Indeed, observational tools as well as physiologic parameters such as heart rate, respiratory rate, and oxygen saturation have been shown to be valid means to assess the degree of pain that a child is feeling.

Tables 21 and 22 are two examples of the commonly used validated observational tools for assessment of pain in infants and children.

■ Table 21.
CRIES Neonatal Postoperative Pain Scale[1]

	0	1	2
Crying	No	High-pitch, consolable	Inconsolable
Required FiO_2 to maintain SaO_2 at least 95%	No	<30%	>30%
Increased heart rate and blood pressure	No	11–20% increased	>20% increased
Expression	Calm	Grimace	Grimace and grunt
Sleepless	No	Frequent awakening	Constantly awake

Scores are added up to an assessment range of a 0–10 pain level.

■ Table 22.
Face, Legs, Activity, Cry, and Consolability Scale[2]

	0	1	2
Face	No particular expression or smile	Occasional grimace or frown, withdrawn, disinterested	Frequent to constant quivering chin, clenched jaw
Legs	Normal position or relaxed	Uneasy, restless, tense	Kicking or legs drawn up
Activity	Lying quietly, normal position, moves easily	Squirming, shifting back and forth, tense	Arched, rigid, or jerking
Cry	No cry (awake or asleep)	Moans or whimpers, occasional complaint	Crying steadily, screams or sobs, frequent complaints

(continued)

■ **Table 22.**
Face, Legs, Activity, Cry, and Consolability Scale[2] (Continued)

	0	1	2
Consol-ability	Content, relaxed	Reassured by occasional touching, hugging or being talked to, distractible	Difficult to console or comfort

Scores are added up to an assessment range of a 0–10 pain level.

Management of pain in the pediatric population should occur within a relationship among the treatment team, the child, and his or her parents or guardians. The parents or guardians usually end up being the single most important and passionate advocate for aggressive pain management in infants and children.

Effective treatment usually combines pharmacologic and non-pharmacologic interventions.

Nonpharmacologic interventions include several psychological techniques such as imagery and relaxation training. Moreover, some practical techniques include minimizing unnecessary procedures and discussing procedures in an age-appropriate manner.

With respect to pharmacologic treatments, the medications used to treat pain in infants and children are similar to those used in adults. However, some special considerations are important. Aspirin and its derivatives should be avoided in patients with pain coexisting with any kind of viral syndrome-like symptoms who are younger than age of 19 unless specifically indicated, due to the incidence of Reye's syndrome. Most analgesics and local anesthetics are metabolized through the liver, and in the first 6 months of life, the liver may be relatively immature and require dosage adjustments of medications to compensate for this immaturity. Newborn infants usually have a decreased glomerular filtration rate in the first week of life. Newborn infants also have a relatively higher percentage of body weight that is water, resulting in an increased volume of distribution.

Treatment interventions for children with cancer pain include analgesics, adjuvants, regional analgesia, chemotherapy, and radiation therapy. It is important to note that most medications have not been tested in children, and therefore, prescribing medications to children should follow the World Health Organization approach. Acetaminophen is relatively safe for relief of mild pain, and can be administered orally or rectally.[3] Nonsteroidal antiinflammatory drugs (NSAIDs) are not recommended for patients with cancer who also suffer from thrombocytopenia. When pain is moderate to severe, opioid analgesics are effective and should be administered orally whenever possible. Children should be administered "rescue" doses, particularly if they are receiving continuous infusion. Regular monitoring of side effects is important given that children are often unable to communicate side effects that they may be experiencing (e.g., pruritus, constipation).

The following table provides a good set of basic principles that should routinely be considered when treating and assessing pain in infants and children.

■ **Table 23.**
Basic Principles of Pain Management in Infants and Children

Neuroanatomic components and neuroendocrine systems are sufficiently developed to allow transmission of painful stimuli in the neonate and child.
Pain in newborns and children is often unrecognized and undertreated. Neonates *do* feel pain, and analgesia should be prescribed when indicated during medical care.
If a procedure is painful in adults, it should be considered painful in newborns, *even if they are preterm.*
Compared with older age groups, infants and children may experience a greater sensitivity to pain and are more susceptible to the long-term effects of painful stimulation.

(continued)

■ **Table 23.**
  Basic Principles of Pain Management in
  Infants and Children (Continued)

Adequate treatment of pain may be associated with decreased clinical complications and decreased mortality.

Sedation does not provide pain relief and may mask the child's response to pain.

A lack of behavioral responses (including crying and movement) does not necessarily indicate a lack of pain.

Severity of pain and the effects of analgesia can be assessed in the pediatric patient. Health care professionals have the responsibility for providing a systematic approach to pain management, including assessment, prevention, and treatment of pain in this patient population.

Treatment should include the appropriate use of environmental, behavioral, and pharmacologic interventions.

Environment should be as conducive as possible to the well-being of the child and family.

Education and validation of competency in pain assessment and management for all clinicians are a professional responsibility and very important when it comes to caring for pediatric and adult patients.

Adapted from The National Pain Management Guideline. Agency for Health Care Policy and Research. *Management of postoperative and procedural pain in infants, children, and adolescents.* 1992. Publication No. 92-0032. Available at http://www.ncbi.nlm.nih.gov/books/bv.fcgi?rid=hstat6.chapter8991. Accessed August 2, 2007.

ELDERLY PATIENTS

Elderly patients with pain are another group of patients who are often understudied and undertreated. Despite the fact that the prevalence of pain increases with age, the use of analgesic medication declines.[4] The reasons for the undertreatment are due to human error. Some include the following:

- Underreporting of pain by patients due to accepting it as a consequence of aging
- Sensory impairments might hinder the patient's ability to communicate the degree and source of pain
- Public and clinician attitudes about aging and pain influence tendencies to treat
- Long-term care facilities consist of staff that may be less educated about pain management than those working in acute care facilities
- Cognitive impairment can interfere with the elderly patients' ability to complete pain assessment instruments and adhere to a prescribed treatment regimen
- Reluctance to prescribe opioids due to adverse effects, such as confusion or delirium

All elderly patients should be considered at increased risk for undertreatment of pain. Assessment of function is critical in assessing pain in elderly patients. The ability to perform activities of daily living is of paramount importance in elderly patients, as they may be solely responsible for their own care or the care of a spouse. Because depression and signs of chronic pain may frequently coexist, elderly patients may exhibit decreased socialization, which may go unrecognized, and they may further suffer from the inability to care for themselves.

The likelihood is that pain in elderly patients stems from one of three causes. First, there is the likelihood that it is as a result of a coexisting medical illness. Second is the likelihood of a result of aging, such as spinal stenosis or osteoarthritis. Finally, there is the likelihood that it is a part of a neuropsychiatric disorder. Of course, there may be overlap, but this categorization usually helps to establish the best course of treatment. The treatment must obviously try to address the specifics of the causes.

Treatments for elderly patients with mild to moderate pain include acetaminophen and NSAIDs. Acetaminophen is considered effective and safe. NSAIDs can cause increased risk of gastric and renal toxicity, cognitive impairment, constipation, and headache.

Opioids are often used to treat pain in elderly patients. Although opioids have been traditionally viewed as more risky than nonopioid "adjuvant" analgesics, such as tricyclic antidepressants or anticonvulsants, the truth may actually be exactly the opposite. Addiction and tolerance with opioids seem, from clinical experience, to be significantly less of a problem in the elderly, whereas the risks of the adjuvant agents, such as mental status changes and falling, appear to be greater. Thus, the risk to benefit ratio may favor opioids over other agents in the elderly. Of course, this remains a controversial issue. Due to differences in metabolism, some older patients appear to be more likely to experience opioid side effects such as cognitive and neuropsychiatric dysfunction than younger patients. Therefore, a slow titration schedule beginning with minimal doses might be preferable to more aggressive titration as in a younger patient.

Similarly, interventional treatment, such as spinal cord stimulation and intrathecal analgesia, although often perceived as invasive and risky, may actually be safer than long-term pharmacologic approaches for some elderly patients. Other treatment options include cognitive-behavioral therapy, physical therapy, and multidisciplinary treatment. Aggressive rehabilitation is particularly important in the elderly, who are particularly prone to rapid deconditioning and whose ability to function depends on fine degrees of conditioning. Clinicians should be careful not to undertreat pain in the elderly; approach the treatment of pain in this population with patience and balance.

PREGNANT AND LACTATING PATIENTS

When possible, the use of nonpharmacologic treatments should be maximized for noncancer pain in pregnancy. These include judicious rest, pacing, various harnesses designed for pregnancy, ice and heat, and other physical therapy modalities. In general, NSAIDs are avoided. Acetaminophen is generally considered safe in clinical practice. Despite a dearth of data, opioids are widely used for severe pain during pregnancy and are considered relatively safe.

It is important to consider consulting with the obstetrician-gynecologist of record before administering pain medications to pregnant or lactating patients when questions exist with regard to safety.

The Food and Drug Administration has created a categorization of drugs based on empirical findings and safety for use in pregnancy[5]:

Category A

Adequate, well-controlled studies in pregnant women have not shown an increased risk of fetal abnormalities.

Category B

Animal studies have revealed no harm to the fetus; however, there are no adequate and well-controlled studies in pregnant women.

Or

Animal studies have shown an adverse effect, but adequate and well-controlled studies in pregnant women have failed to demonstrate risk to the fetus.

Or

No animal studies have been conducted, and there are no adequate and well-controlled studies in pregnant women.

Category C

Animal studies have shown an adverse effect, and there are no adequate and well-controlled studies in pregnant women.

Category D

Studies in animals or pregnant women have demonstrated a risk to the fetus. However, the benefits of therapy may outweigh the potential risk.

Category X

Studies in animals or pregnant women have demonstrated positive evidence of fetal abnormalities. The use of the product is contraindicated in women who are or may become pregnant.

There are many problems with the current system of drug labeling and categories in pregnancy, however. There are very few drugs in category A and very few drugs in category X. In fact, 70% of drugs are category C, but not all category C drugs have the same level of risk. New pregnancy labeling soon to be implemented by the Food and Drug Administration will include summary of risk assessment, clinical considerations, and data, and, it is hoped, provide more detailed guidelines for safe use of medications in this special patient population.

TERMINALLY ILL PATIENTS

Please refer to Chap. V for information about end-of-life care and palliative care guidelines.

COGNITIVELY IMPAIRED PATIENTS

As mentioned previously, pain is a common phenomenon in the elderly patient population because the likelihood of these patients suffering from conditions such as cancer and arthritis problems is increased. Cognitive impairment is another condition with increased incidence in this patient population. Undertreatment of pain in this patient population is only compounded by the coexistence of cognitive impairment. Indeed, cognitive impairment may be responsible for preventing one of the single most important signs needed to treat pain—the ability to communicate suffering. This can make the accurate assessment of pain in those with severe cognitive impairment one of the most significant challenges in the field of pain management.[6] This also makes information available from family and caregivers invaluable.

Pain management in the absence of a detailed history can prove quite challenging. Although caregiver information is critical, it may be incomplete due to the lack of exhibition of normal pain behavior. Sometimes, the signs that cognitively impaired patients exhibit are not discrete or obvious, but may be the only clues available, including the following:

- Changes in body posture
- Grimacing
- Decreased willingness to participate in activities that would normally be engaging
- Somnolence due to exhaustion
- Increased nonspecific vocalization
- Agitation
- Crying
- Resistance to physical contact
- Resistance to ambulation

To successfully approach pain assessment and management in the cognitively impaired patient, the practitioner should realize that the most accurate data for assessing pain are obtained in the following order:

1. Patient's report of pain
2. Reports of patient's pain by family or friends or other caregiver
3. Patient's behaviors
4. Physiologic parameters (most useful in acute pain)[7]

A possible recent event that is the cause of the pain (e.g., recent fall) should be included in the investigation.

Clinicians should avoid relying on their own subjective judgment to estimate the degree of a patient's pain. Efforts should be directed toward seeing if a patient can use some form of self-report. This requires that the patient be able to communicate the existence of pain through vocal or nonvocal communication and to rate the intensity of the pain. Several studies have demonstrated that elderly patients with mild to moderate cognitive impairment can respond fairly reliably to measures of pain intensity.[8–10]

The following steps recommended by the *Consensus Statement from the Veteran's Health Administration National Pain Management Strategy*

Coordinating Committee are quite valuable in helping to try to assess and treat pain in the cognitively impaired patient:

- Observation of behaviors to assess pain
  - When a patient is unable to use a self-report method despite efforts toward education, assessment must rely on observation of behaviors. Family members or consistent caregivers can provide valuable insight into the patient's usual behaviors and changes in behaviors that might indicate the presence of pain.[11]
  - Some common pain behaviors in cognitively impaired older persons have been identified.[11,12] These include signs mentioned previously. However, some patients with cognitive impairment exhibit little or no specific behaviors associated with pain. These pain behaviors have not been systematically evaluated in younger patients with cognitive impairments.
  - Pain behaviors should be observed and assessed both at rest and during movement.[9,13–15] Weiner and Herr[6] and others have noted that it is important to consider other causes of behaviors when relying on observation to assess pain. It is important to consider these other potential causes of distress behavior so that analgesic treatment does not mask problems such as infections, constipation, bladder problems, and primary mood disorders.

- Empirical trials of analgesics
  - Empirical trials of analgesic medication can be used as part of a pain assessment. This should be done in conjunction with other methods of assessment to evaluate the hypothesis that the behaviors are indicative of significant pain.[16,17] This should not be a first-line method of assessment. There are no tested protocols for this practice. It is very important to consider other potential causes of distress behaviors or agitation that could be masked or worsened by analgesics. Many analgesics can negatively alter cognitive status, and this should be considered during the course of a trial.

Changes in function and activity as well as other pain behaviors should always be assessed in the context of an analgesic trial.

- Tools for assessment of pain in cognitively impaired patients
  - A number of devices and protocols have been developed to aid in the assessment of patients who have impaired communication due to failures in cognition. These devices are based on observation of behaviors. Most of the available instruments have been developed for use with elderly patients. All the tools currently available suffer from a lack of studies to determine adequate reliability and validity. Clinicians should be very cautious about using an instrument that does not have established reliability and validity even if it appears to have face value.[11]

A comprehensive review of currently published tools for assessing pain in nonverbal persons with dementia is available at The City of Hope Web site (http://www.cityofhope.org),[18] as listed below:

- Abbey Pain Scale[19]
- Assessment of Discomfort in Dementia[20]
- Checklist of Nonverbal Pain Indicators[13]
- Discomfort Scale-Dementia of the Alzheimer's Type[21]
- Doloplus 2[22]
- Face, Legs, Activity, Cry, and Consolability Pain Assessment Tool
- Nursing Assistant-Administered Instrument to Assess Pain in Demented Individuals[23]
- Pain Assessment in Advanced Dementia Scale[24]
- Pain Assessment for the Dementing Elderly[25]
- Pain Assessment Scale for Seniors with Severe Dementia[26]

Although successful treatment of pain in the cognitively impaired patient remains challenging, it is the clinician's responsibility to use all possible means available to successfully manage this difficult condition.

PATIENTS WITH SUBSTANCE-ABUSE PROBLEMS

The risk of inadequately managing pain increases with patients with addictive disorders or substance abuse problems. It can be helpful to use objective screening and management tools such as the **SOAPP**®[27] (**S**creener and **O**pioid **A**ssessment for **P**atients with **P**ain) and **COMM**™[28] (**C**urrent **O**pioid **M**isuse **M**easure), which can be downloaded from http://www.PainEDU.org.

Many factors are responsible for this undertreatment:

- Inadequate clinician training in pain management and addiction medicine
- Lack of acknowledged differences between dependence, addiction, and tolerance
- Fear of contributing to addictive behavior by using opioids
- Societal prejudices on patients with addictive disorders
- Fear of regulatory penalization.

Challenges in treating pain in this patient population are compounded by the patient's perception that the pain they experience is a major cause of their addictive behavior and also an obstacle to withdrawal of the offending agent. Patients with addictive disorders sometimes have problems managing opioids by themselves, and this may indeed lead them to be deprived of a potentially valuable component of their pain treatment.

A joint statement from 21 health organizations and the Drug Enforcement Administration released in 2001 titled Promoting Pain Relief and Preventing Abuse of Pain Medications: A Critical Balancing Act *states the following important points with respect to pain management in patients with substance abuse problems:*

> "As representatives of the health care community and law enforcement, we are working together to prevent abuse of prescription pain medications while ensuring that they remain available for patients in need.
>
> Both health care professionals, and law enforcement and regulatory personnel, share a responsibility for

ensuring that prescription pain medications are available to the patients who need them and for preventing these drugs from becoming a source of harm or abuse. We all must ensure that accurate information about both the legitimate use and the abuse of prescription pain medications is made available. The roles of both health professionals and law enforcement personnel in maintaining this essential balance between patient care and diversion prevention are critical.

Preventing drug abuse is an important societal goal, but there is consensus, by law enforcement agencies, health care practitioners, and patient advocates alike, that it should not hinder patients' ability to receive the care they need and deserve."

This consensus statement is necessary based on the following facts:

- Undertreatment of pain is a serious problem in the United States, including pain among patients with chronic conditions and those who are critically ill or near death. Effective pain management is an integral and important aspect of quality medical care, and pain should be treated aggressively.

- For many patients, opioid analgesics, when used as recommended by established pain management guidelines, are the most effective way to treat their pain and often the only treatment option that provides significant relief.

- Because opioids are one of several types of controlled substances that have potential for abuse, they are carefully regulated by the Drug Enforcement Administration and other state agencies. For example, a physician must be licensed by state medical authorities and registered with the Drug Enforcement Administration before prescribing a controlled substance.

- In spite of regulatory controls, drug abusers obtain these and other prescription medications by diverting them from legitimate channels in several ways, including fraud, theft, and forged prescriptions and via unscrupulous health professionals.

- Drug abuse is a serious problem. Those who legally manufacture, distribute, prescribe, and dispense controlled substances must be mindful of and have respect for their inherent abuse potential. Focusing only on the abuse potential of a drug, however, could erroneously lead to the conclusion that these medications should be avoided when medically indicated, generating a sense of fear rather than respect for their legitimate properties.

- Helping doctors, nurses, pharmacists, other health care professionals, law enforcement personnel, and the general public become more aware of both the use and abuse of pain medications enable all clinicians to make proper and wise decisions regarding the treatment of pain.

Below is a table with some basic principles and strategies for using opioids in the patient with a known substance abuse problem. Never forget that consultation with a specialist in pain management may always be a valuable choice in management of difficult patient populations.

■ Table 24.
Strategies of Opioid Use in the Patient with Known History of Substance Abuse

Support the individual to help achieve and sustain recovery from addiction.
Provide medications in manageable amounts to patients.
Use schedules and dosages that are less likely to cause euphoric effects, but retain efficacy.
Require a written agreement between you and the patient with respect to abuse of prescribed medications.
Communicate as appropriately necessary with significant others.
See patient frequently to assess for signs and symptoms of abuse.
If there are signs of medication abuse, obtain frequent urine screens, schedule frequent clinic visits, and encourage substance abuse counseling.
If safety concerns outweigh the potential of treatment, discontinue opioid therapy, and use nonopioid approaches.

REFERENCES

1. Krechel SW, Bildner J. CRIES: a new neonatal postoperative pain measurement score. Initial testing and reliability. *Paediatric Aneasthesia* 1995; 5(1):53–61.

2. Merkel SI, Shayefitz JR, Lewis TV, Malwiya S. The FLACC: a behavioral scale for scoring postoperative pain in young children. *Pediatr Nurs* 1997;23(3):293–297.

3. Jacox AK, Carr DB, Payne R, et al. *Management of Cancer Pain, Clinical Practice Guidelines.* No. 9. Rockville, MD: U. S. Department of Health and Human Services, Public Health Service, Agency for Health Care Policy and Research (AHCPR Publication No. 94-0592), 1994.

4. Sorkin BA, Rudy TE, Hanlon RB, Turk DC. Chronic pain in older and. young patients: differences appear less important than similarities. *J Gerontol* 1990;45(2):64–68.

5. United States Food and Drug Administration. Current Categories for Drug Use in Pregnancy. Available at http://www.fda.gov/fdac/features/ 2001/301_preg.html#categories. Accessed August 2, 2007.

6. Weiner DK, Herr K. Comprehensive interdisciplinary assessment and treatment planning: an integrated. overview. In Weiner DK, Herr K, Rudy TE, eds. *Persistent Pain in Older Adults: An Interdisciplinary Guide for Treatment.* New York: Springer, 2002:18–57.

7. Assessing Pain in the Patient with Impaired Communication: A Consensus Statement from the VHA National Pain Management Strategy Coordinating Committee, October 2004. Available at http://www1.va.gov/ pain_management/docs/Cognitivelyimpairedconsensusstatement.doc. Accessed August 2, 2007.

8. Chibnall J, Tait R. Pain assessment in cognitively impaired and unimpaired older adults: a comparison of four scales. *Pain* 2001;92:173–186.

9. Weiner MF, Koss E, Patterson M, et al. A comparison of the Cohen-Mansfield agitation inventory with the CERAD behavioral rating scale for dementia in community-dwelling persons with Alzheimer's disease. *J Psychiatr Res* 1998;32(6):347–351.

10. Ferrell BA, Ferrell BR, Rivera L. Pain in cognitively impaired nursing home patients. *J Pain Symptom Manage* 1995;10(8):591–598.

11. Herr K, Garand L, American Geriatric Society Panel on Persistent Pain in Older Persons 2002. The management of persistent pain in older persons. *J Am Geriatr Soc* 2001;50:5205–5224.

12. Asplund K, Norberg A, Adolfsson R, Waxman HM. Facial expressions in severely demented patients: a stimulus-response study of four patients with dementia of the Alzheimer's type. *Int J Geriatr Psychiatry* 1991;6: 599–606.

13. Feldt KS. The checklist of nonverbal pain indicators. *Pain Manag Nurs* 2000;1:13–21.

14. Feldt KS, Ryden M, Miles S. Treatment of pain in cognitively impaired compared with cognitively intact older patients with hip fractures. *J Am Geriatr Soc* 1998;46(9):1079–1085.

15. Weiner D, Pieper C, McConnell E, et al. Pain measurement in elders with chronic low back pain: traditional and alternative approaches. *Pain* 1996;67(2–3):461–467.

16. Baker A, Bowring L, Brignell A, Kafford D. Chronic pain management in cognitively impaired patients: a preliminary research project. *Perspectives* 1996;20:4–8.

17. Kovach CR, Weissman DE, Griffie J, et al. Assessment and treatment of discomfort for people with late-stage dementia. *J Pain Symptom Manage* 1999;18:412–419.

18. Berkman Research Institute. Special Populations, Pain in the Elderly. Available at http://www.cityofhope.org/prc/elderly.asp. Accessed August 2, 2007.

19. Abbey J, Piller N, De Bellis A, et al. The Abbey Pain Scale: a 1-minute numerical indicator for people with end-stage dementia. *Int J Palliat Nurs* 2004;10(1):6–13.

20. Kovach CR, Noonan PE, Griffie J, et al. Use of the assessment of discomfort in dementia protocol. *Appl Nurs Res* 2001;14(4):193–200.

21. Hurley AC, Volicer B, Hanrahan PA, et al. Assessment of discomfort in advanced Alzheimer patients. *Res Nurs Health* 1992;15(5):369–377.

22. Wary B. Doloplus-2, une echelle pour evaluer la douleur. *Soins Gerontol* 1999;19:25–27.

23. Snow AL, O'Malley K, Kunik M, et al. A conceptual model of pain assessment for non-communicative persons with dementia. *Gerontologist* 2004;44:807–817.

24. Joint Statement from 21 Health Organizations and the Drug Enforcement Administration. Promoting Pain Relief and Preventing Abuse of Pain Medications: A Critical Balancing Act. 2001. Available at http://www.ampainsoc.org/advocacy/promoting.htm. Accessed August 2, 2007.

25. Pain Assesment for the Dementing Elderly, City of Hope. Available at http://www.cityofhope.org/prc/Review%20of%20Tools%20for%20 Pain%20Assessment/PADE%20Text.htm. Accessed August 2, 2007.

26. Pain Assessment Scale for Seniors with Severe Dementia. City of Hope. Available at http://www.cityofhope.org/prc/Review%20of%20Tools %20for%20Pain %20Assessment/PACSLAC%20Text.htm

27. Butler SF, Budman SH, Fernandez K, et al. Validation of a screener and opioid assessment measure for patients with chronic pain. *Pain.* 2004;112:65–75.

28. Butler SF, Budman, SH, Fernandez K, et al. Development and validation of the Current Opioid Misuse Measure. *Pain.* 2007;130:144–156.

VIII.

Patient Level Opioid Risk Management

RISKS OF OPIOID THERAPY

Chronic pain is a major public health problem in the United States, and opioids, for better or worse, remain an essential tool in the armamentarium against acute and chronic pain. Owing to substantial efforts to improve awareness and treatment of chronic pain, the availability of opioids has increased dramatically in the past several decades. Although much more remains to be done to ensure appropriate access to opioids, opioid prescribing is currently at the highest level in decades, allowing patients with cancer and noncancer pain unprecedented access to these analgesics.

Opioids, like all medications, are associated with risks, and the prevalence of negative consequences of opioid use has risen concomitantly with their increased use. The risks of greatest concern have been *abuse* and *addiction*. Prescription opioid abuse is rising faster than any other type of drug abuse and is now second only to marijuana in terms of prevalence of abuse and addiction, and ahead of cocaine and heroin by many measures. Current projections suggest that approximately 1.5 million Americans meet criteria for abuse or addiction to prescription opioids, which is nearly 1% of the population. Although some clinicians have been comforted by a mythology that addiction does not occur in "legitimate" pain patients, the reality is that there is significant overlap between patients with pain and those with addictive disorders; because the prevalence of chronic pain and of addiction is so high, no clinician is free from treating patients with comorbid pain and addiction. This becomes clear when one considers that the background rate of active substance abuse is approximately 10% in the general U.S. population; that substance abuse increases the risk for certain types of pain; that 20–40% of pain patients on opioids have substance abuse problems; and that pain is the number one reason patients see doctors. The presence of comorbid addiction significantly complicates the treatment of pain, and the presence of comorbid pain significantly complicates the treatment of addiction.

A unique feature of prescription drug abuse as a complication of medical prescribing is that the problem occurs not only in patients, but also in their families and the community. Because one of the major sources of abused prescription opioids is the prescriptions of friends and family, it is clear that many of the patients to whom clinicians prescribe are the source of medications that put their family and the community at risk, either from intentional diversion by the patient or by theft or other unintentional pathways to diversion. The prescriber therefore has unique obligations to prescribe opioids in a manner that minimizes potential harm to nonpatient collaterals.

Side effects, such as nausea, vomiting, dizziness, sweating, and constipation, are commonly experienced risks of opioid therapy that can to a great extent be prevented or treated. Another risk of opioid therapy, which has not been widely publicized although observed for centuries, is endocrine disturbance, particularly testosterone deficiency.

REGULATION OF OPIOIDS

The use of opioid analgesics in the United States is governed by a combination of policies at federal and state levels. The Food and Drug Administration approves medications as safe and effective for medical use. After a drug has been approved, a licensed physician can prescribe the medication for any purpose he or she sees fit, whether or not it is described in the product label, as long as it is consistent with community standards of good medical practice. Opioid analgesics are also subject to laws governed by the Controlled Substances Act of 1970 and enforced by the Drug Enforcement Administration. According to the legislation, drugs with abuse potential are assigned to one of five categories, with progressively higher categories associated with increased abuse liability. Schedule I includes drugs with no officially recognized medicinal value in the United States, such as lysergic acid diethylamide (LSD) and marijuana. Most opioid analgesics fall into the Schedule II [e.g., oxycodone (Oxycontin), oxycodone and acetaminophen (Percocet), fentanyl] or Schedule III [e.g., hydrocodone (Vicodin), codeine with acetaminophen, buprenorphine] category.

All clinicians must be familiar with the rules regarding controlled-substance prescribing in their states. Such regulations control activities such as calling in prescriptions, writing refills, calling in emergency supplies, and so forth. Prescribing opioids to patients with pain in the course of usual medical practice, and in the context of a legitimate doctor–patient relationship, is permitted. Moreover, the courts increasingly expect clinicians to attend to patients' pain issues, including if this requires the use of opioid analgesics. It is rare for physicians acting in the context of appropriate medical practice, and maintaining adequate records, to be censured for prescribing opioids to patients with pain.

One common source of confusion is whether physicians can prescribe to patients with addiction. The simple answer is that physicians with current licenses and Drug Enforcement Administration registrations can prescribe opioids, including methadone or buprenorphine, to patients with pain, whether or not the patient has an addictive disorder (although this may not always be advisable). To prescribe for the "maintenance treatment" of addiction, a physician must have a special license or waiver to prescribe maintenance treatment, whether or not the patient has pain. Of course, in the patient with comorbid pain and addiction, it may not be clear under which regulation the medication is prescribed to treat pain or the addiction. Nonetheless, physicians must be mindful of the applicable regulations. Unless specially licensed, physicians must be prescribing for pain, not addiction, even in patients with comorbid addictive disorders, and the medical chart must reflect this practice.

OPIOID RISK MINIMIZATION IN CLINICAL PRACTICE

Although there are no validated guidelines for the use of opioids in chronic pain, the following are a reasonable set of considerations and recommendations consistent with current thinking in the field.

The prescribing of opioids for the treatment of pain is no different than the prescribing of any medication for any disorder. As in the example of insulin treatment for diabetes, all therapies have complications, which are more likely to occur (by definition) in high-risk patients. Therefore, patients should be screened for risk level on initiation of therapy and reassessed periodically. **SOAPP**® (**S**creener and **O**pioid **A**ssessment for **P**atients with **P**ain), to be used when considering initiating opioid treatment, and **COMM™** (**C**urrent **O**pioid **M**isuse **M**easure) a follow-up tool for patients who are prescribed opioids, can be downloaded from http://www.PainEDU.org.

If indicated, opioid therapy can be initiated on a trial basis, and the trial can continue for as long as the patient is on treatment. In general, a trial period of 3 months can be recommended. At each follow-up visit, with a tool such as COMM™, the patient goes through a semistructured assessment that assesses key outcome variables, but that need not be excessively time-consuming if approached systematically. Based on the assessment, there are five options for how to handle the opioid therapy:

1. Continue it without change.
2. Adjust the regimen.
3. Add a long- or short-acting agent.

4. Rotate to another opioid.

5. Discontinue opioid therapy.

Of course, other therapeutics can be implemented as a result of the visit, such as instituting nonopioid analgesic approaches (e.g., acupuncture, physical therapy, psychological therapies, nonopioid analgesics).

Although this chapter is focused on prescribing practices that minimize the risks of opioid therapy, this can be effectively presented in the context of an overall approach to opioid therapy (see figure below). Opportunities to optimize outcome, by maximizing efficacy and minimizing risks, present themselves at every point of the algorithm and are be discussed in more detail below.

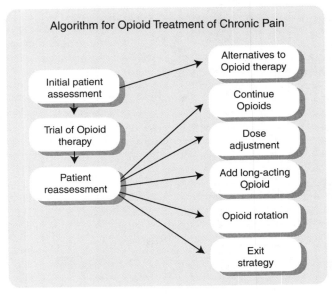

■ Figure 5.

Initial Patient Assessment

As in all other areas of medicine, the initial assessment of the patient with chronic pain has several purposes, including developing a diagnosis, cataloging previous therapies, understanding the patient's status on multiple dimensions (pain, function, psychological, social), setting treatment goals, and creating a treatment plan. With respect to opioid therapy, the purposes of the initial assessment are to determine whether opioid therapy is indicated, assess previous experience with opioid therapy, and determine the risk of opioid abuse. The table below indicates the key elements relevant to opioid therapy that should be added to the routine initial medical evaluation. With these additional elements of the medical history, the clinician can categorize patients into the following risk strata:

Low risk: no history of substance abuse; minimal if any risk factors
    Can be managed by primary care provider

Medium risk: past history of substance abuse (no prescription opioid abuse); significant risk factors
    Comanage with addiction and/or pain specialists

High risk: active substance abuse problem; history of prescription opioid abuse
    Opioids may not be appropriate
    Refer to center specializing in management of patients with comorbid pain and addictive disorders

■ **Table 25.**
Initial Evaluation Guide

History of present illness (pain)	Pain diagnosis
	Previous pain treatments
	Previous experience with opioid therapy
	Effectiveness on pain and function
	Compliance

(continued)

■ **Table 25.**
Initial Evaluation Guide (Continued)

History of present illness (pain) *(continued)*	Subjective experience with opioid therapy (e.g., euphoria)
	Use of opioids for nonprescribed purposes (insomnia, "stress," mood)
Past history	Illnesses relevant to opioid therapy (e.g., respiratory, hepatic, renal disease)
	Medical illnesses suggestive of substance abuse
	Hepatitis
	Human immunodeficiency virus infection
	Tuberculosis
	Cellulitis
	Sexually transmitted diseases
	Elevated liver function tests
	Trauma, burns
Psychiatric history	Current or past mental illness
	History of substance abuse, including alcohol, tobacco
	None
	Past, in remission
	Current
	Which substance(s), routes, prescription drugs
Social history	Arrests
	Motor vehicle accidents, driving under the influence
	Domestic violence
	Fires
	Contact with substance abusers
Family history	Substance abuse
	Family support

Initiating an Opioid Trial

If a patient appears to be an appropriate candidate for opioid therapy, it is appropriate to initiate a trial. In reality, many patients are prescribed opioids without a formal declaration of long-term opioid therapy. This occurs, for example, in a patient with chronic pain who receives a short-term opioid prescription for a pain flare and continues to receive frequent refills before the clinician (and patient) realize that, in fact, the patient is now on long-term opioid therapy. Although in principle these documented steps will be initiated at the time of initiation of opioid therapy, in practice, they are often initiated "when the light bulb goes off."

A written treatment agreement and the expressed informed consent of the patient are highly recommended when managing chronic pain with long-term opioid therapy. The physician should discuss the risks and benefits of the use of controlled substances with the patient, with persons designated by the patient, or with the patient's surrogate or guardian if the patient is incompetent.

The written treatment plan should state objectives and goals as well as expectations regarding behavior, limits, consequences, and stipulations, which may include (1) urine/serum medication levels screening when requested, (2) number and frequency of all prescription refills, and (3) reasons for which drug therapy may be discontinued (e.g., violation of agreement or lack of benefit). The contract should generally stipulate that the patient should receive prescriptions from one physician and one pharmacy. Treatment requires ongoing assessment and modifications of the treatment plan and agreed-on contract as appropriate.

Patients should be advised that opioid therapy is always considered a trial, and the advisability of continued opioid therapy, based on a risk–benefit assessment, is continually revisited for the duration of treatment, no matter how long. The spirit of these discussions is based on fundamental principles of medicine and entered into as a collaboration with the patient to maximize pain relief, functional outcomes, and goal attainment. These goals may be enhanced by opioid therapy or may be undermined by opioid therapy—determining this is the purpose of the opioid trial. If opioids are found not to be helpful to the patient or the patient is unable to comply with therapy, the opioids will be discontinued in an appropriate manner because this is in the best interest of the patient.

An important difference between opioid therapy and nonabusable drug therapies is in the role of patient self-report. As is well known in the addiction community, the patient's self-report in the context of opioid therapy must be taken with a grain of salt because in a number of conditions, patient self-report loses its reliability; this applies to pain intensity, functional improvement, compliance with therapy, and substance abuse–related issues. The physician accustomed to obeying the mantra of "always believe the patient" must learn to modify this approach in the setting of opioid therapy and to consider self-report as one of many sources of information about the patient's status. Again, this is done for the sake of the patient.

A trial of opioid therapy is usually begun with as-needed doses of a short-acting product combining an opioid and a nonopioid analgesic. Common choices include hydrocodone/acetaminophen, oxycodone/acetaminophen, oxycodone/ibuprofen, and codeine/acetaminophen. The nonopioid component maximizes the balance of analgesia and side effects of the regimen. The use of short-acting as-needed doses allows the clinician and patient to assess the opioid requirement.

Short-acting agents are the most widely abused opioids in the United States. Long-acting products, with the exception of extended-release oxycodone products (e.g., OxyContin, due to the ease with which the extended-release formulation can be converted to a high-potency immediate-release formulation), tend to be less abused than short-acting preparations. Also, individuals with addictive disorders tend to be able to comply better with medications that are taken at fixed doses round the clock rather than on an as-needed basis. Therefore, in a patient at risk for substance abuse, an opioid trial at times may be more appropriately initiated with a transdermal opioid (e.g., fentanyl) or an extended-release oral formulation, although these products can certainly be abused as well. The patient's pain profile should be taken into account as well: Patients with a fairly consistent pain profile (pain intensity is more or less the same all the time) are more likely to succeed with a sustained-release-only regimen; patients with intermittent pain may not do well.

A final consideration in the choice of opioid is tramadol. Tramadol is an analgesic that derives part of its pain-relieving properties from an opioid effect (just like morphine), but part from nonopioid effects (inhibition of reuptake of norepinephrine and serotonin, like many antidepressants). Tramadol is far less likely to be abused than other opioid analgesics, although it certainly can be abused. Tramadol is now available in an extended-release formulation as well. Patients with insufficient analgesia on tramadol can always be advanced to other opioid therapies.

No discussion of minimizing the risk of opioid therapies would be complete without discussing the nonabuse risks of opioids, such as constipation, nausea, vomiting, and dizziness. These side effects are very common early in opioid therapy and frequently cause patients to stop taking the prescription. Most guidelines call for implementing a prophylactic bowel regimen in all patients started on opioid therapy, although in patients at low risk for constipation, this can be held in reserve. Patients should be instructed to anticipate these side effects and given instructions on how to deal with them should they occur, potentially including a prescription for an antiemetic.

Follow-Up Visit

It is helpful to follow a structured assessment in following patients on long-term opioid therapy. Follow-up assessment that clinicians can use should be based on the "four A's":

1. Analgesia: What is the patient's average pain intensity?
2. Activities: How has the patient been functioning?
3. Adverse events: Has the patient had side effects?
4. Aberrant behavior: Has there been any evidence of abuse, misuse, or addiction?

Based on capturing the above information, the clinician can develop two more "A's": assessment and action plan.

Analgesia

Patients on opioids for chronic pain rarely enjoy complete pain relief. In fact, many patients live with pain in the "moderate" range—typically 4–7 on a 0–10 numerical rating scale—despite the common perception that opioids are extremely "strong" medications. It is critical to manage patient expectations early so that patients (and clinicians) are not disappointed with the result of partial pain relief and some functional restoration. *In the assessment of analgesia, at least partial pain reduction is necessary evidence for the appropriateness of continuing opioid therapy.* Many clinicians are familiar with the type of patient who, despite ongoing opioid therapy, continues to have reports of severe pain (8–10 out of 10), or even ratings that are "off the scale," but who insist that the opioids are "taking the edge off" the pain. These patients are at high risk for having psychosocial issues amplifying their pain perception and may constitute an exception to the generally useful dictum that in making decisions about analgesic regimens the clinician should rely primarily on the patient's self-report. Patients with persistently high pain intensity ratings and no evidence of functional improvement should have their dose increased (as long as there are not significant side effects), should have nonopioid analgesic approaches added (medical, rehabilitative, or psychosocial), or should be tapered off opioid therapy.

Activities

A judgment that a patient indeed is benefiting from opioid therapy is more convincing if there has been some evidence of functional improvement. Function can be construed broadly and includes activities of daily living, psychological function, social function, sleep, employment, and so forth. Even a slight improvement in pain intensity accompanied by clear evidence of increased function is very persuasive of opioid benefit. On the other hand, a picture of persistently high pain scores and no functional improvement—or actual functional deterioration—generally suggests that an opioid taper is appropriate.

Adverse Events

Patients have many more adverse effects of opioid therapy than they report. Therefore, adverse effects should be elicited prospectively. Often, patients fear that if they report side effects, the medication will be stopped. Although switching opioids is often the most effective solution for opioid-induced side effects, a number of other approaches can be used to address side effects without changing medications, and thereby improve the patient's outcome on opioid therapy.

One underappreciated side effect of long-term opioid therapy is endocrine disturbance. Most men and many women on long-term opioid therapy develop opioid-induced androgen deficiency (OPIAD), a form of central hypogonadism. In men, this is manifested by loss of libido, alteration in hair growth, mood disturbances, alteration of male role, loss of muscle strength and mass, and potentially osteoporosis and fractures. In women, the manifestations have been less well defined but may include alterations in menses and infertility. It is appropriate to measure the following on an annual basis for all patients on long-term opioid therapy: luteinizing hormone, follicle-stimulating hormone, total and free testosterone, sex hormone–binding globulin, and prolactin. It is also appropriate to screen for symptoms of OPIAD. There is no consensus on the management of OPIAD. A reasonable approach would be to switch opioids if feasible (although there is no information on whether one opioid is less likely to cause OPIAD than another); if OPIAD persists, and opioids remain indicated, then it is reasonable to supplement testosterone, preferably under the guidance of an endocrinologist.

Aberrant Behaviors

Many patients use their medication in a way that would not be condoned, or even anticipated by, their clinicians. Noncompliance is ubiquitous in medicine and may be unintentional (e.g., taking the wrong dose by mistake, forgetting a dose), intentional but not related to abuse (e.g., taking an extra Percocet to help sleep, unauthorized dose escalation for a pain flare), or intentional and related to abuse (taking extra to get high, faking pain to get opioids, using the medication in an out-of-control manner). The clinician seeing the patient for pain often does not have the luxury that an addiction specialist in an addiction treatment center may have, whose patients all openly acknowledge their problematic drug use. The pain clinician often sees a confusing and subtle pattern of behaviors and needs to make a judgment as to whether the behaviors represent a pattern potentially indicating abuse, addiction, or criminal behavior, or whether the behaviors can be adequately explained by more benign causes: cognitive or language difficulties, administrative or insurance reasons, comorbid psychological conditions, or pseudoaddiction. Research has shown that most patients engage in a number of aberrant behaviors. The challenge is for the clinician to judge when these aberrant behaviors occur and what actions to take in view of the fact that confirmation can rarely be made with 100% certainty in the pain management setting.

Opioid Management Plan

Continuation of Opioid Therapy

Continuation of opioid therapy is not a default decision—it is a specific action that is justified by the patient assessment. Patients who have been stable with their dosing, who are benefiting in terms of pain reduction and/or improved function, who are tolerating their medication, and who have minimal aberrant behaviors are appropriate for continuation of therapy. Continuing therapy that is patently ineffective (whether or not it "takes the edge off") or that has been associated with functional deterioration (not explained by other factors) cannot be justified, whether or not there are other available management options.

Dose Adjustment

The dose can be too high, too low, or not administered optimally. Opioids need to be dosed on a case-by-case basis based on the response. Patients with persistent unrelieved pain, who are otherwise tolerating their doses, can have their dose increased. Patients with dose-limiting side effects need to have their dose decreased, or their side effects managed another way; the dose cannot be increased. For some patients, the therapeutic index can be improved by altering the mode of administration. For example, patients with side effects at the peak of exposure to a short-acting opioid may do better with smaller, more frequent doses or with a long-acting opioid. In contrast, patients on long-acting opioids with side effects during periods of minimal pain may do better on intermittent doses of a short-acting opioid. Finally, some patients cannot find a dose that allows them to enjoy pain relief without significant side effects. Those patients are candidates for opioid rotation. If a therapeutic index cannot be found with a few opioids for an individual patient, that patient is probably not a candidate for opioid therapy and should be moved to "exit strategy."

Addition of a Long-Acting Opioid

There is little if any evidence that long-acting opioids are better in general than short-acting opioids for patients with chronic pain. However, there are particular types of patients for whom the addition of a long-acting opioid to a short-acting one, or even the substitution of long-acting for short-acting, may improve clinical outcomes. The clearest example is the patient who is taking substantial doses of short-acting opioids multiple times per day. Because tolerance is often first manifested by decreased duration of action, such patients may be forced to take their medication every 3 or even 2 hours. The addition of a long-acting agent may be extremely helpful. Another example is the patient with a compliance problem, due either to cognitive issues or abuse-related problems. Stopping the short-acting medication and substituting a long-acting medication may allow such patients to continue to benefit from opioid therapy in a manner that reduces risk. It is important for clinicians to realize that all currently marketed opioids can be abused, and substituting a long-acting opioid for a short-acting one may reduce risk in some circumstances but does not eliminate the risk completely. Furthermore, some long-acting opioids, such as extended-release oxy-codone, are highly prized by abusers.

Opioid Rotation

It has been observed that individual patients may do poorly on one opioid but better after switching to another. Various explanations have been offered for this phenomenon. One holds that because some opioids are associated with the accumulation of toxic metabolites after prolonged use (e.g., morphine, hydromorphone), switching to another allows for the clearance of metabolites accumulated from the first opioid. Another theory is that different opioids may bind in different patterns to sub-types of the opioid receptor, providing different profiles of efficacy and side effects. Regardless, if a patient cannot seem to find an effective and well-tolerated dose of one opioid, it is reasonable to try one or two more opioids before giving up on opioid therapy or referring to a specialist for further management. It is of critical importance to note that switching patients who are on substantial doses of one opioid to another opioid can be tricky and, if done inappropriately, can lead to underdosing, severe painful flare-ups or withdrawal, or overdose and death, particularly with methadone. Clinicians should have a clear sense of their comfort zone with opioid rotation and should get input as needed.

Exit Strategy

When is it appropriate to stop opioid therapy in an individual patient? Although there has been little guidance on this issue, the following list of criteria is reasonable:

- There has been no convincing benefit from opioid therapy despite reasonable attempts at dose adjustment, management of side effects, and opioid rotation.
- Opioids cannot be tolerated at a dose that provides meaningful analgesia.
- Persistent compliance problems exist despite a patient treatment agreement and efforts at appropriate limit setting.

■ Presence of a comorbid condition can make opioid therapy more likely to harm than help, such as an active substance abuse problem. (Note that the risk–benefit of opioid therapy depends as much on the treatment setting as on the patient and the medicine.)

It is critically important to distinguish between abandoning opioid therapy, abandoning pain management, and abandoning the patient. Exiting a patient from opioid therapy is often difficult for clinicians because of the patient's possible failure to understand that when this decision is made, it is for the welfare of the patient, not for the welfare of the doctor. Approaching the decision to taper off opioid therapy from the perspective of helping the patient in the long run helps avoid many (but not all) awkward confrontations. There are many other approaches to pain management than opioid therapy, and a patient can be tapered off from opioid therapy while alternative pain management approaches are pursued (albeit with reasonable expectations). Also, abandoning opioid therapy does not mean abandoning the patient. Often, the most reasonable course is to offer the patient continued medical guidance (without opioid therapy), even in the case of an addicted patient who pursues comanagement of the addictive disorder.

DOCUMENTATION

As in all cases, but especially when treating high-risk patients and those with substance-use disorders, the physician should keep accurate and complete records. Within the records, the following information should be included:

■ The medical history and physical examination
■ Diagnostic, therapeutic, and laboratory results
■ Evaluations and consultations
■ Treatment objectives
■ Discussion of risks and benefits

- Treatments
- Medications (including date, type, dosage, and quantity prescribed)
- Instructions and agreements
- Periodic reviews

Records should remain current and be maintained in an accessible manner and readily available for review.

REFERENCES

This chapter is a summary of the following:

Katz NP, Inflexxion Inc. Patient Level Opioid Risk Management. 2007. http://www.PainEDU.org/manual.asp. Accessed July 30, 2007.

Glossary

Acute pain. The result of an injury or potential injury to body tissues and activation of nociceptive nerve fibers at the site of local tissue damage. This type of pain is usually time-limited and occurs after trauma, surgery, or a disease process. Acute pain is generally thought to have the biologic functions of alerting the individual to harm and preparing for the "fight-or-flight" response to danger.

Addiction. A primary, chronic, neurobiologic disease with genetic, psychosocial, and environmental factors influencing its development and manifestations. Addiction involves a compulsive desire to use a drug despite continued harm.

Adjuvants. Pain-relieving medications whose primary indication traditionally is not for the treatment of pain. Adjuvants may be used to treat certain types of pain (e.g., neuropathic pain) or may be used to augment the analgesic effect of opioids or to manage their side effects. This term is derived mainly from the cancer pain literature and includes medications such as tricyclic antidepressants and anticonvulsants that were initially prescribed for other indications.

Allodynia. The presence of pain from a stimulus that is not normally painful. For example, pain caused by clothing or bedclothes rubbing over the skin would be considered allodynia.

Anergia. Lack of energy.

Anhedonia. Psychological condition characterized by the inability to derive pleasure from normally enjoyable activities. This is one indication of depression.

Anticonvulsants. Medications used to treat seizures. Due to presumed common mechanisms underlying epilepsy and neuropathic pain, many anticonvulsants are effective in treating neuropathic pain.

Antidepressants. A class of medications used to treat depression that includes tricyclic-type antidepressants, selective serotonin reuptake inhibitors, serotonin-norepinephrine reuptake inhibitors, and monoamine oxidase inhibitors. Some antidepressants, especially tricyclic-type anti-depressants, have been found to have analgesic efficacy. Antidepressants are often used for treating depression associated with chronic pain conditions. See "Selective serotonin reuptake inhibitor" and "Tricyclic antidepressant" for more information. Other antidepressants in a miscellaneous category are bupropion, mirtazapine, nefazodone, and trazodone.

Antiemetic. Medication used for nausea and vomiting. Antiemetics are also used to facilitate treatment in migraine headaches that cause vomiting.

Biofeedback. Feedback from a device or computer to provide information about physiologic processes about which patients are not normally aware (e.g., muscle tension, skin temperature). Biofeedback may help relieve muscle tension caused by bracing muscles due to chronic pain.

Breakthrough pain. An exacerbation of pain that occurs beyond constant, background pain. Short-acting opioids are often prescribed for this purpose. One subcategory of breakthrough pain is "incident pain," which is pain by certain "incidents"—for example, walking.

Cancer pain. Pain associated with cancer that can be the result of cancer itself or treatments for cancer (surgery, radiation, chemotherapy). It can be visceral, somatic, or neuropathic in nature.

Catastrophizing. A cognitive coping style that involves an increasingly downward cycle of negative thoughts that has been associated with depression and negative outcomes in chronic pain.

Central sensitization. Process by which pain is amplified and maintained centrally (in the spinal cord or brain) in addition to the processes in peripheral tissues. This general concept is thought to underlie some types of allodynia or hyperalgesia. It may also explain why surgically removing the "cause of the pain" may not eliminate the pain.

Centralization. This is a loosely defined term of a pain process that begins in the periphery and over time becomes sustained partially or completely by central mechanisms. This concept overlaps with that of central sensitization. Centralization or central sensitization may also underlie evolution of the phenomenology of a chronic pain syndrome, such as the "spread" of reflex sympathetic dystrophy to other limbs.

Chronic pain. Pain that persists beyond the expected healing period. Chronic pain may be associated with levels of underlying pathology that do not explain the presence or extent of pain, and is often associated with affective and behavioral responses to the chronicity of the pain. Sources often define chronic pain as that persisting beyond three or six months after an injury.

Cluster headaches. A strictly unilateral headache, usually occurring once or a few times a day at a characteristic time (e.g., 1 A.M.), lasting for 15–180 minutes, occurring in a series that lasts for weeks to months, separated by remissions lasting from months to years. Cluster headaches are usually episodic but have been known to last up to 14 days. Cluster headaches tend to occur more often in men, usually are one sided, but can shift from side to side in some patients.

Cognitions (thoughts). Cognitions can exert powerful effects on the patient's physical reactions, responses, and interpretations of pain.

Cognitive-behavioral therapy. A form of psychological treatment that combines cognitive psychotherapeutic techniques with behavioral techniques and is used to help patients change their thoughts and behaviors to increase coping with pain, decrease negative affect, and increase functioning.

Constipation. A condition in which bowel movements are infrequent or incomplete.

Complex regional pain syndrome type I (reflex sympathetic dystrophy). Chronic pain that includes clinical findings of regional pain, sensory changes, allodynia, abnormalities of temperature, abnormal pseudomotor activity, edema, and an abnormal skin color that occur after a noxious event.

Complex regional pain syndrome type II (causalgia). Includes all the features of complex regional pain syndrome type I as well as a peripheral nerve lesion.

Delirium. A syndrome characterized by combinations of cognitive deficits, fluctuating levels of consciousness, changes in sleep patterns, psychomotor agitation, hallucinations, delusions, and/or perceptual abnormalities. Causes are multifactorial and can include psychotropic medications, opioids, metabolic changes, cancer treatment, sepsis, or brain tumor or metastases.

Diabetic neuropathy. Damage or dysfunction of the peripheral nervous system due to diabetes mellitus. There are several distinct subtypes of diabetic neuropathy, each with different clinical features, prognosis, and treatment approaches. These include diabetic third cranial nerve palsy, diabetic radiculopathy, diabetic amyotrophy (radiculoplexopathy), and peripheral polyneuropathy (the classic "stocking-and-glove neuropathy"). Also see "Painful peripheral polyneuropathy."

Distraction. A cognitive coping technique that involves turning attention away from painful sensations.

Dyspareunia. Painful or difficult coitus.

Equianalgesic dose. The dose of one opioid that gives the same amount of pain relief as a dose of another opioid or another route of administration. For example, the equianalgesic dose of hydromorphone, for 10 mg of intramuscular morphine, is 1.5 mg intramuscularly. These comparisons are always averages and vary from patient to patient.

Full, or pure, agonists. Class of opioids that produce analgesic effects by binding to the mu opioid receptor. Opioid analgesics do not have a ceiling effect for analgesia and do not interfere with the effects of other opioids in this class when prescribed simultaneously. Examples include morphine, fentanyl, oxycodone, oxymorphone, hydromorphone, meperidine, codeine, and methadone. They are distinguished from the partial agonists, agonist/antagonists, and pure antagonists.

Heat. Refers to the application of heat via hot packs, hot water bottles, moist compresses, heating pads, chemical and gel packs, and immersion in water for the purpose of relief of pain.

Hyperalgesia. The phenomenon whereby stimuli that are normally painful produce exaggerated pain. It can be ascertained by the response to single and multiple pinpricks on neurologic examination.

Hyperpathia. A painful syndrome characterized by increased reaction to a stimulus, especially a repetitive stimulus, as well as increased threshold.

Hypopathia. Refers to decreased responses to stimulation.

Incident pain. Refers to the subset of breakthrough pain that is provoked by specific types of activity (e.g., walking, moving the arm).

Long-acting opioids. An opioid with a relatively long duration of action. By tradition, opioids that last longer than about 6–8 hours are referred to as *long-acting*, but the border between short- and long-acting is not precise. Long-acting opioids, also known as *slow-release* or *controlled-release opioids*, may have a long duration by virtue of their intrinsic pharmacokinetics (e.g., methadone), by having been formulated in a tablet that delivers the medication over a long period of time [e.g., morphine (Kadian), oxycodone (OxyContin)], or by having been formulated in another type of delivery system [e.g., fentanyl (Duragesic) patch]. Several opioids are available in both short- and long-acting forms (e.g., morphine, oxycodone, fentanyl).

Malingering. Intentional production of false or grossly exaggerated physical or psychological symptoms for the purpose of tangible external incentives, such as obtaining financial compensation, evading criminal prosecution, avoiding work or military duty, and obtaining drugs.

Metabolite accumulation syndrome. Several opioids are metabolized to compounds that can accumulate and produce a characteristic syndrome. The features of this syndrome include anxiety, jitteriness, tremor, multifocal myoclonus, encephalopathy, convulsions, and death. This syndrome classically occurs with normeperidine, a metabolite of meperidine (Demerol), but has also been reported with morphine and hydromorphone. Other opioids have been reported to cause delirium and similar symptoms, but not due to metabolite accumulation, and without the other characteristic features noted above.

Mixed agonists/antagonists. Opioids that block opioid analgesia at the mu opioid receptor (mu) or are neutral at this receptor while simultaneously producing analgesia by activating the kappa receptor. Available agonist/antagonists include nalbuphine (Nubain), pentazocine (Talwin), and butorphanol (Stadol).

Modulation. The process of modification of nociceptive signals that takes place in the dorsal horn of the spinal cord and elsewhere with input from ascending and descending pathways.

Morphine conversion guide. A written guideline for the equianalgesic dosing of opioids.

Multimodal treatment. Treatment by more than one modality (e.g., physical therapy, medical, psychological).

Mucositis. Inflammation or sloughing of the oropharyngeal and gastrointestinal mucosae. This occurs stereotypically after bone marrow transplant and its related chemotherapy and is a well-recognized stereotypic severe pain syndrome.

Muscle de-education. Occurs when pain or avoiding pain leads to the failure to activate muscles or the abnormal activation of muscles in movement.

Myofascial pain. Pain localized to a region of muscle or soft tissue, associated with *trigger points* (palpable tender nodules or cords within the muscle). By definition, the pain must be reproduced by palpation of the trigger point, often with a referred component. The pain may be associated with subjective feelings of "numbness," "heaviness," and so forth, but no neurologic deficits. See also "Trigger points."

Neuropathic pain. Pain that is caused by a lesion or dysfunction of the nervous system.

Nociceptive pain. Pain that results from injury to or inflammation of somatic tissues.

Nonpharmacologic treatment. Treatment that does not involve use of drugs (e.g., physical therapy, biofeedback, psychological treatment).

Nonsteroidal antiinflammatory drug (NSAID). An aspirin-like drug used to reduce inflammation caused by injured tissue and pain.

Numerical Rating Scale (NRS). A method of rating pain intensity that involves written or verbal numerical notation of pain [e.g., 11-point scale from 0 ("no pain") to 10 ("pain as bad as it could be")].

Pain. An unpleasant sensory and emotional experience associated with actual or potential tissue damage or described in terms of such damage.

Pain assessment. Evaluation of a variety of aspects of perceived sensations of pain, including intensity, duration, frequency, description, location, and emotional responses.

Pain behaviors. Verbal or nonverbal expressions including behavioral reactions such as grimacing, rubbing the affected part, guarding, or restricting movement and sighing.

Painful peripheral polyneuropathy. A generalized disorder of peripheral nerves, usually affecting the distal fibers, with proximal shading, typically occurring symmetrically. Peripheral polyneuropathies may be classified as axonal or demyelinating and have many causes, particularly metabolic and toxic. Certain types, such as diabetic, alcoholic, vasculitic, and idiopathic, tend to be most painful.

Palliative care. The supportive care of the terminal patient. Such support typically focuses on pain and symptom management, end-of-life psychological and social issues, coordinating care with the family, and preparing the family for grieving before and after the patient's death. Recently the term has been expanded to refer to management of pain and symptoms early in the course of illness before the patient is thought of as terminal.

Partial agonists. Opioid analgesics that produce analgesia by binding to the mu opioid receptor, but with less intrinsic efficacy at that receptor than "full agonists." These agents have a ceiling effect for analgesia and may precipitate withdrawal if administered to a physically dependent patient. Examples of partial agonists include nalbuphine, pentazocine, and butorphanol.

Pathophysiology. The physiology of abnormal states.

Peripheral sensitization. Process by which neurons in peripheral nerves become abnormally responsive to noxious or nonnoxious stimuli, thereby facilitating exaggerated pain perception.

Perception. The final process by which the subject integrates all nociceptive and modulating influences, in the context of psychological and social background and situation information, to form the final experience of pain.

Pharmacological treatment of chronic pain. Treatment of pain with medicine.

Physical dependence. A state of adaptation that is manifested by a drug class–specific withdrawal syndrome that can be produced by abrupt cessation, rapid dose reduction, decreasing blood level of the drug, or administration of an antagonist.

Physical therapy. Physical interventions, including passive modalities (e.g., application of heat and cold) and active modalities (e.g., range of motion, exercise) used to strengthen muscles, increase cardiovascular activity, and restore normal functioning.

Postherpetic neuralgia (PHN). Pain persisting beyond the healing of an acute herpes zoster rash. More recently, postherpetic neuralgia has been redefined by some as zoster-associated pain, recognizing that this is a spectrum of pain that occurs before, during, and for variable times after acute herpes zoster.

Primary afferent nociceptors. Pain receptors (A delta or C fibers) that respond to noxious mechanical, thermal, and chemical stimuli.

Primary headaches. Headaches that are autonomous without a specific lesion or disease process.

Pseudoaddiction. Is a term that is used to describe behavior that appears like addictive, "drug-seeking" behavior but is actually an effort to obtain pain relief. Behaviors from pseudoaddiction are said to be distinguished from addictive behaviors when the behaviors resolve after treatment of pain.

Psychiatric comorbidities. Concomitant psychiatric disorders that occur in individuals with a medical condition such as chronic pain.

Quantitative sensory testing (QST). Testing of sensations with calibrated stimuli such that both stimulus and response can be quantitated. In common usage, **quantitative sensory testing** refers to the use of devices that apply calibrated thermal (hot or cold) stimuli to the skin to record the patient's perception of thermal sensory and pain thresholds.

Referred pain. The perception of pain in parts of the body distant from the pathology from which the pain originates. Examples include arm pain during an acute myocardial infarction or eye pain during vertebral artery dissection.

Rest pain. Pain experienced while in an inactive or resting state.

Secondary headaches. Headache associated with primary disease processes, such as brain tumors, head trauma, vascular disorders, and substance use and withdrawal.

Silent nociceptors. Afferent nerves that do not respond to external stimulation unless inflammatory mediators are present.

Serotonin–adrenalin reuptake inhibitor (SNRI). A type of antidepressant that acts on different mechanisms than other types of antidepressants. An example is venlafaxine. Serotonin-norepinephrine reuptake inhibitor–type drugs are generally used to treat depression associated with chronic pain.

Somatoform disorder. Pain that is produced or amplified by psychological processes. Criteria are less restrictive than somatization disorder and require one or more physical complaints that cannot be explained by a general medical condition and cause significant social or occupational distress.

Somatic pain. Pain arising from somatic structures (e.g., skin, bones, muscle, joint). It is typically well-localized ("my left finger") and worsened by palpation or movement of the affected part.

Somatization disorder. Psychological disorder characterized by a pattern of multiple physical complaints (e.g., pain symptoms, gastrointestinal symptoms, sexual problems) present before the age of 30 that causes significant social and occupational impairment.

Selective serotonin reuptake inhibitor (SSRI). A type of antidepressant that is generally used to treat depression. Little evidence exists for the analgesic effects of selective serotonin reuptake inhibitors. Examples of medications in this class are citalopram, fluoxetine, fluvoxamine, paroxetine, and sertraline.

Stress management. Techniques designed to aid in the reduction of physiologic hyperarousal due to stress.

Transcutaneous electrical nerve stimulation (TENS). A pain reduction technique that involves applying low-voltage electrical stimulation to the skin, putatively stimulating large nerve fibers.

Tolerance. The loss of effect of a pharmacologic agent over a prolonged period of use, or the need to escalate the dose of the agent to maintain the same pharmacologic effect.

Topical analgesics. Analgesics that are applied to the skin or mucosa and act locally, presumably with insignificant systemic exposure. Examples include EMLA cream and the lidocaine patch.

Transdermal analgesics. Analgesics that are applied to the skin or mucosa, are systemically absorbed, and produce their therapeutic effects and side effects by systemic actions. Examples include the fentanyl patch and the buprenorphine patch.

Transduction. Process by which noxious stimulation of tissues is translated into neural signals in nociceptive nerve fibers. The deepest understanding of this process relates to the role of endogenous chemicals at afferent nerve endings in translating these stimuli (e.g., a burn) into nociceptive impulses.

Transmission. The process by which nerve signals from the periphery are sent to the dorsal horn of the spinal cord along the nociceptive afferents.

Tricyclic antidepressants. A class of antidepressant that is used clinically for treatment of neuropathic pain and for sleep disturbance, generally in lower doses than required for treating depression. Examples are amitriptyline, doxepin, imipramine, nortriptyline.

Trigger points. Tender nodules or cords within a muscle, palpation of which reproduces localized and/or radiating pain. Trigger points define *myofascial pain*. This phenomenon is distinct from *tender points*, which are tender areas of muscle or soft tissue *not associated* with palpable abnormalities in the texture of the muscle. Tender points occur in fibromyalgia and rheumatic diseases. See also "Myofascial pain."

Visceral pain. Refers to pain arising from pathology of the visceral organs, such as bowel obstruction or pancreatitis. Such pain is typically poorly localized (e.g., "My whole belly hurts") and is associated with visceral symptoms (e.g., nausea, vomiting).

Visual analogue scale (VAS). A method of measuring pain intensity that consists of a 10-cm line with anchors at the ends. Common anchors are "no pain" and "pain as bad as it could be." Patients draw a vertical line through the horizontal line and the result in centimeters is multiplied by 10, yielding a number between 0 and 100.

Windup. A process that has been observed in experimental animals whereby repeated stimulation of a peripheral structure (e.g., the skin) with an electric or other stimulus produces a greater and greater central response (e.g., pain). The mechanism of windup is thought to be sensitization of neurons in the spinal cord that receive nociceptive input, with the result that subsequent stimuli produce greater effects. Windup is an example of central sensitization, which is, in turn, an example of neural plasticity.

World Health Organization (WHO) analgesic ladder. Recommendations from the World Health Organization for titration of therapy for cancer pain, referred to as the "analgesic ladder." The ladder presents a three-step algorithm for using medications initially in the treatment of cancer pain and includes five major treatment concepts: (1) by the mouth, (2) by the clock, (3) by the ladder, (4) for the individual, and (5) with attention to detail.

Index

Page numbers followed by *t* indicate tables; those followed by *f* indicate figures.

A Caribbean
Mystery

Agatha Christie

To my old friend
John Cruickshank Rose
with happy memories of my
visit to the West Indies

CONTENTS

CHAPTER ONE

MAJOR PALGRAVE TELLS A STORY

'TAKE ALL THIS business about Kenya,' said Major Palgrave.

'Lots of chaps gabbing away who know nothing about the place! Now *I* spent fourteen years of my life there. Some of the best years of my life, too –'

Old Miss Marple inclined her head.

It was a gentle gesture of courtesy. Whilst Major Palgrave proceeded with the somewhat uninteresting recollections of a lifetime, Miss Marple peacefully pursued her own thoughts. It was a routine with which she was well acquainted. The locale varied. In the past, it had been predominantly India. Majors, Colonels, Lieutenant-Generals – and a familiar series of words: *Simla. Bearers. Tigers. Chota Hazri – Tiffin. Khitmagars,* and so on. With Major Palgrave the terms were slightly different. *Safari. Kikuyu. Elephants. Swahili.* But the pattern was essentially the same. An elderly man who needed a listener so that he could, in memory, relive days in which he had been happy. Days when his back had been straight, his eyesight keen, his hearing acute. Some of these talkers had been handsome soldierly old boys, some again had been regrettably unattractive; and Major Palgrave, purple of face, with a glass eye, and the general appearance of a stuffed frog, belonged in the latter category.

Miss Marple had bestowed on all of them the same gentle charity. She had sat attentively, inclining her head from time to time in gentle agreement, thinking her own thoughts and enjoying what there was to enjoy: in this case the deep blue of a Caribbean Sea.

So kind of dear Raymond – she was thinking gratefully, so really and truly kind... Why he should take so much trouble about his old aunt, she really did not know. Conscience, perhaps; family feeling? Or possibly he was truly fond of her...

She thought, on the whole, that he *was* fond of her – he always had been – in a slightly exasperated and contemptuous way! Always trying to bring her up to date. Sending her books to read. Modern novels. So difficult – all about such unpleasant people, doing such very odd things and not, apparently, even enjoying them. 'Sex' as a word had not been mentioned in Miss Marple's young days; but there had been plenty of it – not talked about so much – but enjoyed far more than nowadays, or so it seemed to her. Though usually labelled Sin, she couldn't help feeling that that was preferable to what it seemed to be nowadays – a kind of Duty.

Her glance strayed for a moment to the book on her lap lying open at page twenty-three which was as far as she had got (and indeed as far as she felt like getting!).

> '"Do you mean that you've had no sexual experience at ALL?" demanded the young man incredulously. "At *nineteen?* But you *must*. It's vital."
>
> 'The girl hung her head unhappily, her straight greasy hair fell forward over her face.
>
> '"I know," she muttered, "I know."
>
> 'He looked at her, stained old jersey, the bare feet, the dirty toe nails, the smell of rancid fat... He wondered why he found her so maddeningly attractive.'

Miss Marple wondered too! And really! To have sex experience urged on you exactly as though it was an iron tonic! Poor young things...

'My dear Aunt Jane, why must you bury your head in the sand like a very delightful ostrich? All bound up in this idyllic rural life of yours. REAL LIFE – that's what matters.'

Thus Raymond – and his Aunt Jane – had looked properly

abashed – and said 'Yes,' she was afraid she *was* rather old-fashioned.

Though really rural life was far from idyllic. People like Raymond were so ignorant. In the course of her duties in a country parish, Jane Marple had acquired quite a comprehensive knowledge of the facts of rural life. She had no urge to *talk* about them, far less to *write* about them – but she knew them. Plenty of sex, natural and unnatural. Rape, incest, perversion of all kinds. (Some kinds, indeed, that even the clever young men from Oxford who wrote books didn't seem to have heard about.)

Miss Marple came back to the Caribbean and took up the thread of what Major Palgrave was saying...

'A very unusual experience,' she said encouragingly. '*Most* interesting.'

'I could tell you a lot more. Some of the things, of course, not fit for a lady's ears –'

With the ease of long practice, Miss Marple dropped her eyelids in a fluttery fashion, and Major Palgrave continued his bowdlerised version of tribal customs whilst Miss Marple resumed her thoughts of her affectionate nephew.

Raymond West was a very successful novelist and made a large income, and he conscientiously and kindly did all he could to alleviate the life of his elderly aunt. The preceding winter she had had a bad go of pneumonia, and medical opinion had advised sunshine. In lordly fashion Raymond had suggested a trip to the West Indies. Miss Marple had demurred – at the expense, the distance, the difficulties of travel, and at abandoning her house in St Mary Mead. Raymond had dealt with everything. A friend who was writing a book wanted a quiet place in the country. 'He'll look after the house all right. He's very house proud. He's a queer. I mean –'

He had paused, slightly embarrassed – but surely even dear old Aunt Jane must have heard of queers.

He went on to deal with the next points. Travel was nothing nowadays. She would go by air – another friend, Diana Horrocks, was going out to Trinidad and would see Aunt Jane was all right

11

as far as there, and at St Honoré she would stay at the Golden Palm Hotel which was run by the Sandersons. Nicest couple in the world. They'd see she was all right. He'd write to them straight away.

As it happened the Sandersons had returned to England. But their successors, the Kendals, had been very nice and friendly and had assured Raymond that he need have no qualms about his aunt. There was a very good doctor on the island in case of emergency and they themselves would keep an eye on her and see to her comfort.

They had been as good as their word, too. Molly Kendal was an ingenuous blonde of twenty odd, always apparently in good spirits. She had greeted the old lady warmly and did everything to make her comfortable. Tim Kendal, her husband, lean, dark and in his thirties, had also been kindness itself.

So there she was, thought Miss Marple, far from the rigours of the English climate, with a nice bungalow of her own, with friendly smiling West Indian girls to wait on her, Tim Kendal to meet her in the dining-room and crack a joke as he advised her about the day's menu, and an easy path from her bungalow to the sea front and the bathing beach where she could sit in a comfortable basket chair and watch the bathing. There were even a few elderly guests for company. Old Mr Rafiel, Dr Graham, Canon Prescott and his sister, and her present cavalier Major Palgrave.

What more could an elderly lady want?

It is deeply to be regretted, and Miss Marple felt guilty even admitting it to herself, but she was not as satisfied as she ought to be.

Lovely and warm, yes – and *so* good for her rheumatism – and beautiful scenery, though perhaps – a trifle monotonous? So *many* palm trees. Everything the same every day – never anything *happening*. Not like St Mary Mead where something was always happening. Her nephew had once compared life in St Mary Mead to scum on a pond, and she had indignantly pointed out that smeared on a slide under the microscope there would be plenty of life to be observed. Yes, indeed, in St Mary Mead, there was always something going on. Incident after incident flashed through Miss Marple's mind, the mistake in old Mrs Linnett's cough mixture – that very odd behaviour of young Polegate – the time when Georgy Wood's mother had come down to see him – (but *was* she his mother –?) the real cause of the quarrel between Joe Arden and his wife. So many interesting human problems – giving rise to endless pleasurable hours of speculation. If only there were something here that she could – well – get her teeth into.

With a start she realised that Major Palgrave had abandoned Kenya for the North West Frontier and was relating his experiences as a subaltern. Unfortunately he was asking her with great earnestness: 'Now don't you agree?'

Long practice had made Miss Marple quite an adept at dealing with that one.

'I don't really feel that I've got sufficient experience to judge. I'm afraid I've led rather a sheltered life.'

'And so you should, dear lady, so you should,' cried Major Palgrave gallantly.

'You've had such a very varied life,' went on Miss Marple, determined to make amends for her former pleasurable inattention.

'Not bad,' said Major Palgrave, complacently. 'Not bad at all.' He looked round him appreciatively. 'Lovely place, this.'

'Yes, indeed,' said Miss Marple and was then unable to stop herself going on: 'Does anything ever happen here, I wonder?'

Major Palgrave stared.

'Oh rather. Plenty of scandals – eh what? Why, I could tell you –'

But it wasn't really scandals Miss Marple wanted. Nothing to get your teeth into in scandals nowadays. Just men and women changing partners, and calling attention to it, instead of trying decently to hush it up and be properly ashamed of themselves.

'There was even a murder here a couple of years ago. Man called Harry Western. Made a big splash in the papers. Dare say you remember it.'

Miss Marple nodded without enthusiasm. It had not been her kind of murder. It had made a big splash mainly because everyone concerned had been very rich. It had seemed likely enough that Harry Western had shot the Count de Ferrari, his wife's lover, and equally likely that his well-arranged alibi had been bought and paid for. Everyone seemed to have been drunk, and there was a fine scattering of dope addicts. Not really interesting people, thought Miss Marple – although no doubt very spectacular and attractive to *look* at. But definitely not *her* cup of tea.

'And if you ask me, that wasn't the only murder about that time.' He nodded and winked. 'I had my suspicions – oh! – well –'

Miss Marple dropped her ball of wool, and the Major stooped and picked it up for her.

'Talking of murder,' he went on. 'I once came across a very curious case – not exactly personally.'

Miss Marple smiled encouragingly.

'Lot of chaps talking at the club one day, you know, and a chap began telling a story. Medical man he was. One of his cases. Young fellow came and knocked him up in the middle of the night. His wife had hanged herself. They hadn't got a telephone, so after the chap had cut her down and done what he could, he'd got out his car and hared off looking for a doctor. Well, she wasn't dead but pretty far gone. Anyway, she pulled through. Young fellow seemed devoted to her. Cried like a child. He'd noticed that she'd been odd for some time, fits of depression and all that. Well, that was that. Everything seemed all right. But actually, about a month later, the wife took an overdose of sleeping stuff and passed out. Sad case.'

Major Palgrave paused, and nodded his head several times. Since there was obviously more to come Miss Marple waited.

'And that's that, you might say. Nothing there. Neurotic woman, nothing out of the usual. But about a year later, this medical chap was swapping yarns with a fellow medico, and the other chap told him about a woman who'd tried to drown herself, husband got her out, got a doctor, they pulled her round – and then a few weeks later she gassed herself.

'Well, a bit of a coincidence – eh? Same sort of story. My chap said – "I had a case rather like that. Name of Jones (or whatever the name was) – What was your man's name?" "Can't remember. Robinson I think. Certainly not Jones."

'Well, the chaps looked at each other and said it was pretty odd. And then my chap pulled out a snapshot. He showed it to the second chap. "That's the fellow," he said – "I'd gone along the next day to check up on the particulars, and I noticed a magnificent species of hibiscus just by the front door, a variety I'd never seen before in this country. My camera was in the car and I took a photo. Just as I snapped the shutter the husband came out of the front door so I got him as well. Don't think he realised it. I asked him about the hibiscus but he couldn't tell me its name." Second medico looked at the snap. He said: "It's a bit out of focus – But I could swear – at any rate I'm almost sure – *it's the same man.*"

'Don't know if they followed it up. But if so they didn't get anywhere. Expect Mr Jones or Robinson covered his tracks too well. But queer story, isn't it? Wouldn't think things like that could happen.'

'Oh, yes, I would,' said Miss Marple placidly. 'Practically every day.'

'Oh, come, come. That's a bit fantastic.'

'If a man gets a formula that works – he won't stop. He'll go on.'

'Brides in the bath – eh?'

'That kind of thing, yes.'

'Doctor let me have that snap just as a curiosity –'

Major Palgrave began fumbling through an overstuffed wallet murmuring to himself: 'Lots of things in here – don't know why I keep all these things…'

Miss Marple thought she did know. They were part of the Major's stock-in-trade. They illustrated his repertoire of stories. The story he had just told, or so she suspected, had not been originally like that – it had been worked up a good deal in repeated telling.

The Major was still shuffling and muttering – 'Forgotten all about *that* business. Good-looking woman *she* was, you'd never suspect – now *where* – Ah – that takes my mind back – what tusks! I must show you –'

He stopped – sorted out a small photographic print and peered down at it.

'Like to see the picture of a murderer?'

He was about to pass it to her when his movement was suddenly arrested. Looking more like a stuffed frog than ever, Major Palgrave appeared to be staring fixedly over her right shoulder – from whence came the sound of approaching footsteps and voices.

'Well, I'm damned – I mean –' He stuffed everything back into his wallet and crammed it into his pocket.

His face went an even deeper shade of purplish red – He exclaimed in a loud, artificial voice:

'As I was saying – I'd like to have shown you those elephant tusks – Biggest elephant I've ever shot – Ah, hallo!' His voice took on a somewhat spurious hearty note.

'Look who's here! The great quartette – Flora and Fauna – What luck have you had today – Eh?'

The approaching footsteps resolved themselves into four of the hotel guests whom Miss Marple already knew by sight. They consisted of two married couples and though Miss Marple was not as yet acquainted with their surnames, she knew that the big man with the upstanding bush of thick grey hair was addressed as 'Greg', that the golden blonde woman, his wife, was known as Lucky – and that the other married couple, the dark lean man and the handsome but rather weather-beaten woman, were Edward and Evelyn. They were botanists, she understood, and also interested in birds.

'No luck at all,' said Greg – 'At least no luck in getting what we were after.'

'Don't know if you know Miss Marple? Colonel and Mrs Hillingdon and Greg and Lucky Dyson.'

They greeted her pleasantly and Lucky said loudly that she'd die if she didn't have a drink at once or sooner.

Greg hailed Tim Kendal who was sitting a little way away with his wife poring over account books.

'Hi, Tim. Get us some drinks.' He addressed the others. 'Planters Punch?'

They agreed.

'Same for you, Miss Marple?'

Miss Marple said Thank you, but she would prefer fresh lime.

'Fresh lime it is,' said Tim Kendal, 'and five Planters Punches.'

'Join us, Tim?'

'Wish I could. But I've got to fix up these accounts. Can't leave Molly to cope with everything. Steel band tonight, by the way.'

'Good,' cried Lucky. 'Damn it,' she winced, 'I'm all over thorns. Ouch! Edward deliberately rammed me into a thorn bush!'

'Lovely pink flowers,' said Hillingdon.

'And lovely long thorns. Sadistic brute, aren't you, Edward?'

'Not like me,' said Greg, ___ ___. Full of the milk of human kindness.'

Evelyn Hillingdon sat down by Miss Marple and started talking to her in an easy pleasant way.

Miss Marple put her knitting down on her lap. Slowly and with some difficulty, owing to rheumatism in the neck, she turned her head over her right shoulder to look behind her. At some little distance there was the large bungalow occupied by the rich Mr Rafiel. But it showed no sign of life.

She replied suitably to Evelyn's remarks (really, how kind people were to her!) but her eyes scanned thoughtfully the faces of the two men.

Edward Hillingdon looked a nice man. Quiet but with a lot of charm… And Greg – big, boisterous, happy-looking. He and Lucky were Canadian or American, she thought.

She looked at Major Palgrave, still acting a *bonhomie* a little larger than life.

Interesting…

Chapter Two

Miss Marple makes Comparisons

I

IT WAS VERY gay that evening at the Golden Palm Hotel.

Seated at her little corner table, Miss Marple looked round her in an interested fashion. The dining-room was a large room open on three sides to the soft warm scented air of the West Indies. There were small table lamps, all softly coloured. Most of the women were in evening dress: light cotton prints out of which bronzed shoulders and arms emerged. Miss Marple herself had been urged by her nephew's wife, Joan, in the sweetest way possible, to accept 'a small cheque'.

'Because, Aunt Jane, it will be rather hot out there, and I don't expect you have any very thin clothes.'

Jane Marple had thanked her and had accepted the cheque. She came of the age when it was natural for the old to support and finance the young, but also for the middle-aged to look after the old. She could not, however, force herself to buy anything very *thin!* At her age she seldom felt more than pleasantly warm even in the hottest weather, and the temperature of St Honoré was not really what is referred to as 'tropical heat'. This evening she was attired in the best traditions of the provincial gentlewoman of England – grey lace.

Not that she was the only elderly person present. There were representatives of all ages in the room. There were elderly tycoons with young third or fourth wives. There were middle-aged couples from the North of England. There was a gay family from Caracas complete with children. The various countries of South America were well represented, all chattering loudly in Spanish or Portuguese. There was a solid English background of two clergymen, one doctor and one retired judge. There was even a family of Chinese. The dining-room service was mainly done by women, tall black girls of proud carriage, dressed in crisp white; but there was an experienced Italian head waiter in charge, and a French wine waiter, and there was the attentive eye of Tim Kendal watching over everything, pausing here and there to have a social word with people at their tables. His wife seconded him ably. She was a good-looking girl. Her hair was a natural golden blonde and she had a wide generous mouth that laughed easily. It was very seldom that Molly Kendal was out of temper. Her staff worked for her enthusiastically, and she adapted her manner carefully to suit her different guests. With the elderly men she laughed and flirted; she congratulated the younger women on their clothes.

'Oh, what a smashing dress you've got on tonight, Mrs Dyson. I'm so jealous I could tear it off your back.' But she looked very well in her own dress, or so Miss Marple thought: a white sheath, with a pale green embroidered silk shawl thrown over her shoulders. Lucky was fingering the shawl. 'Lovely colour! I'd like one like it.' 'You can get them at the shop here,' Molly told her and passed on. She did not pause by Miss Marple's table. Elderly ladies she usually left to her husband. 'The old dears like a man much better,' she used to say.

Tim Kendal came and bent over Miss Marple.

'Nothing special you want, is there?' he asked. 'Because you've only got to tell me – and I could get it specially cooked for you. Hotel food, and semi-tropical at that, isn't quite what you're used to at home, I expect?'

Miss Marple smiled and said that that was one of the pleasures of coming abroad.

'That's all right, then. But if there *is* anything –'

'Such as?'

'Well –' Tim Kendal looked a little doubtful – 'Bread and butter pudding?' he hazarded.

Miss Marple smiled and said that she thought she could do without bread and butter pudding very nicely for the present.

She picked up her spoon and began to eat her passion fruit sundae with cheerful appreciation.

Then the steel band began to play. The steel bands were one of the main attractions of the islands. Truth to tell, Miss Marple could have done very well without them. She considered that they made a hideous noise, unnecessarily loud. The pleasure that everyone else took in them was undeniable, however, and Miss Marple, in the true spirit of her youth, decided that as they had to be, she must manage somehow to learn to like them. She could hardly request Tim Kendal to conjure up from somewhere the muted strains of the 'Blue Danube'. (So graceful – waltzing.) Most peculiar, the way people danced nowadays. Flinging themselves about, seeming quite *contorted*. Oh well, young people must enjoy – Her thoughts were arrested. Because, now she came to think of it, very few of these people *were* young. Dancing, lights, the music of a band (even a steel band), all that surely was for *youth*. But where was youth? Studying, she supposed, at universities, or doing a job – with a fortnight's holiday a year. A place like this was too far away and too expensive. This gay and carefree life was all for the thirties and the forties – and the old men who were trying to live up (or down) to their young wives. It seemed, somehow, a *pity*.

Miss Marple sighed for youth. There was Mrs Kendal, of course. She wasn't more than twenty-two or three, probably, and she seemed to be enjoying herself – but even so, it was a *job* she was doing.

At a table nearby Canon Prescott and his sister were sitting. They motioned to Miss Marple to join them for coffee and she did so. Miss Prescott was a thin severe-looking woman, the Canon was a round, rubicund man, breathing geniality.

Coffee was brought, and chairs were pushed a little way away from the tables. Miss Prescott opened a work bag and took out some frankly hideous table mats that she was hemming. She told Miss Marple all about the day's events. They had visited a new

Girls' School in the morning. After an afternoon's rest, they had walked through a cane plantation to have tea at a *pension* where some friends of theirs were staying.

Since the Prescotts had been at the Golden Palm longer than Miss Marple, they were able to enlighten her as to some of her fellow guests.

That very old man, Mr Rafiel. He came every year. Fantastically rich! Owned an enormous chain of supermarkets in the North of England. The young woman with him was his secretary, Esther Walters – a widow. (Quite all *right*, of course. Nothing improper. After all, he was nearly eighty!)

Miss Marple accepted the propriety of the relationship with an understanding nod and the Canon remarked:

'A very nice young woman; her mother, I understand, is a widow and lives in Chichester.'

'Mr Rafiel has a valet with him, too. Or rather a kind of Nurse Attendant – he's a qualified masseur, I believe. Jackson, his name is. Poor Mr Rafiel is practically paralysed. So sad – with all that money, too.'

'A generous and cheerful giver,' said Canon Prescott approvingly.

People were regrouping themselves round about, some going farther from the steel band, others crowding up to it. Major Palgrave had joined the Hillingdon-Dyson quartette.

'Now those people –' said Miss Prescott, lowering her voice quite unnecessarily since the steel band easily drowned it.

'Yes, I was going to ask you about them.'

'They were here last year. They spend three months every year in the West Indies, going round the different islands. The tall thin man is Colonel Hillingdon and the dark woman is his wife – they are botanists. The other two, Mr and Mrs Gregory Dyson – they're American. He writes on butterflies, I believe. And all of them are interested in birds.'

'So nice for people to have open-air hobbies,' said Canon Prescott genially.

'I don't think they'd like to hear you call it hobbies, Jeremy,' said his sister. 'They have articles printed in the *National Geographic* and in the *Royal Horticultural Journal*. They take themselves very seriously.'

A loud outburst of laughter came from the table they had been observing. It was loud enough to overcome the steel band. Gregory Dyson was leaning back in his chair and thumping the table, his wife was protesting, and Major Palgrave emptied his glass and seemed to be applauding.

They hardly qualified for the moment as people who took themselves seriously.

'Major Palgrave should not drink so much,' said Miss Prescott acidly. 'He has blood pressure.'

A fresh supply of Planters Punches was brought to the table.

'It's so nice to get people sorted out,' said Miss Marple. 'When I met them this afternoon I wasn't sure which was married to which.'

There was a slight pause. Miss Prescott coughed a small dry cough, and said – 'Well, as to that –'

'Joan,' said the Canon in an admonitory voice. 'Perhaps it would be wise to say no more.'

'Really, Jeremy, I wasn't going to say *anything*. Only that last year, for some reason or other – I really don't know *why* – we got the idea that Mrs Dyson was Mrs Hillingdon until someone told us she wasn't.'

'It's odd how one gets impressions, isn't it?' said Miss Marple innocently. Her eyes met Miss Prescott's for a moment. A flash of womanly understanding passed between them.

A more sensitive man than Canon Prescott might have felt that he was *de trop*.

Another signal passed between the women. It said as clearly as if the words had been spoken: '*Some other time…*'

'Mr Dyson calls his wife "Lucky". Is that her real name or a nickname?' asked Miss Marple.

'It can hardly be her real name, I should think.'

'I happened to ask him,' said the Canon. 'He said he called her Lucky because she was his good-luck piece. If he lost her, he said, he'd lose his luck. Very nicely put, I thought.'

'He's very fond of joking,' said Miss Prescott.

The Canon looked at his sister doubtfully.

The steel band outdid itself with a wild burst of cacophony and a troupe of dancers came racing on to the floor.

Miss Marple and the others turned their chairs to watch. Miss Marple enjoyed the dancing better than the music; she liked the shuffling feet and the rhythmic sway of the bodies. It seemed, she thought, very *real*. It had a kind of power of understatement.

Tonight, for the first time, she began to feel slightly at home in her new environment... Up to now, she had missed what she usually found so easy, points of resemblance in the people she met, to various people known to her personally. She had, possibly, been dazzled by the gay clothes and the exotic colouring; but soon, she felt, she would be able to make some interesting comparisons.

Molly Kendal, for instance, was like that nice girl whose name she couldn't remember, but who was a conductress on the Market Basing bus. Helped you in, and never rang the bus on until she was sure you'd sat down safely. Tim Kendal was just a little like the head waiter at the Royal George in Medchester. Self-confident, and yet, at the same time, worried. (He had had an ulcer, she remembered.) As for Major Palgrave, he was undistinguishable from General Leroy, Captain Flemming, Admiral Wicklow and Commander Richardson. She went on to someone more interesting. Greg for instance? Greg was difficult because he was American. A dash of Sir George Trollope, perhaps, always so full of jokes at the Civil Defence meetings – or perhaps Mr Murdoch the butcher. Mr Murdoch had had rather a bad reputation, but some people said it was just gossip, and that Mr Murdoch himself liked to encourage the rumours! 'Lucky' now? Well, that was easy – Marleen at the Three Crowns. Evelyn Hillingdon? She couldn't fit Evelyn in precisely. In appearance she fitted many roles – tall thin weather-beaten Englishwomen were plentiful. Lady Caroline Wolfe, Peter Wolfe's first wife, who had committed suicide? Or there was

Leslie James – that quiet woman who seldom showed what she felt and who had sold up her house and left without ever telling anyone she was going. Colonel Hillingdon? No immediate clue there. She'd have to get to know him a little first. One of those quiet men with good manners. You never knew what they were thinking about. Sometimes they surprised you. Major Harper, she remembered, had quietly cut his throat one day. Nobody had ever known why. Miss Marple thought that she did know – but she'd never been quite sure…

Her eyes strayed to Mr Rafiel's table. The principal thing known about Mr Rafiel was that he was incredibly rich, he came every year to the West Indies, he was semi-paralysed and looked like a wrinkled old bird of prey. His clothes hung loosely on his shrunken form. He might have been seventy or eighty, or even ninety. His eyes were shrewd and he was frequently rude, but people seldom took offence, partly because he was so rich, and partly because of his overwhelming personality which hypnotised you into feeling that somehow, Mr Rafiel had the right to be rude if he wanted to.

With him sat his secretary, Mrs Walters. She had corn-coloured hair, and a pleasant face. Mr Rafiel was frequently very rude to her, but she never seemed to notice it – She was not so much subservient, as oblivious. She behaved like a well-trained hospital nurse. Possibly, thought Miss Marple, she had been a hospital nurse.

A young man, tall and good-looking, in a white jacket, came to stand by Mr Rafiel's chair. The old man looked up at him, nodded, then motioned him to a chair. The young man sat down as bidden. 'Mr Jackson, I presume,' said Miss Marple to herself – 'His valet-attendant.'

She studied Mr Jackson with some attention.

II

In the bar, Molly Kendal stretched her back, and slipped off her high-heeled shoes. Tim came in from the terrace to join her. They had the bar to themselves for the moment.

'Tired, darling?' he asked.

'Just a bit. I seem to be feeling my feet tonight.'

'Not too much for you, is it? All this? I know it's hard work.' He looked at her anxiously.

She laughed. 'Oh, Tim, don't be ridiculous. I love it here. It's gorgeous. The kind of dream I've always had, come true.'

'Yes, it would be all right – if one was just a guest. But running the show – that's work.'

'Well, you can't have anything for nothing, can you?' said Molly Kendal reasonably.

Tim Kendal frowned.

'You think it's going all right? A success? We're making a go of it?'

'Of course we are.'

'You don't think people are saying, "It's not the same as when the Sandersons were here".'

'Of course *someone* will be saying that – they always do! But only some old stick-in-the-mud. I'm sure that we're far better at the job than they were. We're more glamorous. You charm the old pussies and manage to look as though you'd like to make love to the desperate forties and fifties, and I ogle the old gentlemen and make them feel sexy dogs – or play the sweet little daughter the sentimental ones would love to have had. Oh, we've got it all taped splendidly.'

Tim's frown vanished.

'As long as *you* think so. I get scared. We've risked everything on making a job of this. I chucked my job –'

'And quite right to do so,' Molly put in quickly. 'It was soul-destroying.'

He laughed and kissed the tip of her nose.

'I tell you we've got it taped,' she repeated. 'Why do you always worry?'

'Made that way, I suppose. I'm always thinking – suppose something should go wrong.'

'What sort of thing –'

'Oh, I don't know. Somebody might get drowned.'

'Not they. It's one of the safest of all the beaches. And we've got that hulking Swede always on guard.'

'I'm a fool,' said Tim Kendal. He hesitated – and then said, 'You – haven't had any more of those dreams, have you?'

'That was shellfish,' said Molly, and laughed.

Chapter Three

A Death in the Hotel

Miss Marple had her breakfast brought to her in bed as usual. Tea, a boiled egg, and a slice of paw-paw.

The fruit on the island, thought Miss Marple, was rather disappointing. It seemed always to be paw-paw. If she could have a nice apple now – but apples seemed to be unknown.

Now that she had been here a week, Miss Marple had cured herself of the impulse to ask what the weather was like. The weather was always the same – fine. No interesting variations.

'The many-splendoured weather of an English day,' she murmured to herself and wondered if it was a quotation, or whether she had made it up.

There were, of course, hurricanes, or so she understood. But hurricanes were not weather in Miss Marple's sense of the word. They were more in the nature of an Act of God. There was rain, short violent rainfall that lasted five minutes and stopped abruptly. Everything and everyone was wringing wet, but in another five minutes they were dry again.

The black West Indian girl smiled and said Good Morning as she placed the tray on Miss Marple's knees. Such lovely white teeth and so happy and smiling. Nice natures, all these girls, and a pity they were so averse to getting married. It worried Canon Prescott a good deal. Plenty of christenings, he said, trying to console himself, but no weddings.

Miss Marple ate her breakfast and decided how she would spend her day. It didn't really take much deciding. She would get up at her leisure, moving slowly because it was rather hot and her fingers weren't as nimble as they used to be. Then she would rest for ten minutes or so, and she would take her knitting and walk slowly along towards the hotel and decide where she would settle herself. On the terrace overlooking the sea? Or should she go on to the bathing beach to watch the bathers and the children? Usually it was the latter. In the afternoon, after her rest, she might take a drive. It really didn't matter very much.

Today would be a day like any other day, she said to herself.

Only, of course, it wasn't.

Miss Marple carried out her programme as planned and was slowly making her way along the path towards the hotel when she met Molly Kendal. For once that sunny young woman was not smiling. Her air of distress was so unlike her that Miss Marple said immediately:

'My dear, is anything wrong?'

Molly nodded. She hesitated and then said: 'Well, you'll have to know – everyone will have to know. It's Major Palgrave. He's dead.'

'Dead?'

'Yes. He died in the night.'

'Oh, dear, I *am* sorry.'

'Yes, it's horrid having a death here. It makes everyone depressed. Of course – he *was* quite old.'

'He seemed quite well and cheerful yesterday,' said Miss Marple, slightly resenting this calm assumption that everyone of advanced years was liable to die at any minute.

'He seemed quite healthy,' she added.

'He had high blood pressure,' said Molly.

'But surely there are things one takes nowadays – some kind of pill. Science is so wonderful.'

'Oh yes, but perhaps he forgot to take his pills, or took too many of them. Like insulin, you know.'

Miss Marple did not think that diabetes and high blood pressure were at all the same kind of thing. She asked:

'What does the doctor say?'

'Oh, Dr Graham, who's practically retired now, and lives in the hotel, took a look at him, and the local people came officially, of course, to give a death certificate, but it all seems quite straightforward. This kind of thing is quite liable to happen when you have high blood pressure, especially if you overdo the alcohol, and Major Palgrave was really very naughty that way. Last night, for instance.'

'Yes, I noticed,' said Miss Marple.

'He probably forgot to take his pills. It is bad luck for the old boy – but people can't live for ever, can they? But it's terribly worrying – for me and Tim, I mean. People might suggest it was something in the food.'

'But surely the symptoms of food poisoning and of blood pressure are *quite* different?'

'Yes. But people do *say* things so easily. And if people decided the food was bad – and left – or told their friends –'

'I really don't think you need worry,' said Miss Marple kindly. 'As you say, an elderly man like Major Palgrave – he must have been over seventy – is quite liable to die. To most people it will seem quite an ordinary occurrence – sad, but not out of the way at all.'

'If only,' said Molly unhappily, 'it hadn't been so *sudden.*'

Yes, it had been very sudden, Miss Marple thought as she walked slowly on. There he had been last night, laughing and talking in the best of spirits with the Hillingdons and the Dysons.

The Hillingdons and the Dysons... Miss Marple walked more slowly still... Finally she stopped abruptly. Instead of going to the bathing beach she settled herself in a shady corner of the terrace. She took out her knitting and the needles clicked rapidly as though they were trying to match the speed of her thoughts. *She didn't like it – no, she didn't like it. It came so pat.*

She went over the occurrences of yesterday in her mind.

Major Palgrave and his stories...

That was all as usual and one didn't need to listen very closely... Perhaps, though, it would have been better if she had.

Kenya – he had talked about Kenya and then India – the North West Frontier – and then – for some reason they had got on to murder – And even *then* she hadn't really been listening...

Some famous case that had taken place out here – that had been in the newspapers –

It was after that – when he picked up her ball of wool – that he had begun telling her about a snapshot – *A snapshot of a murderer* – that is what he had said.

Miss Marple closed her eyes and tried to remember just exactly how that story had gone.

It had been rather a confused story – told to the Major in his club – or in somebody else's club – told him by a doctor – who had heard it from another doctor – and one doctor had taken a snapshot of someone coming through a front door – someone who was a murderer –

Yes, that was it – the various details were coming back to her now –

And he had offered to show her that snapshot – He had got out his wallet and begun hunting through its contents – talking all the time…

And then still talking, he had looked up – had looked – not at her – but at something behind her – behind her right shoulder to be accurate. And he had stopped talking, his face had gone purple – and he had started stuffing back everything into his wallet with slightly shaky hands and had begun talking in a loud unnatural voice about elephant tusks!

A moment or two later the Hillingdons and the Dysons had joined them…

It was then that she had turned her head over her right shoulder to look… But there had been nothing and nobody to see. To her left, some distance away, in the direction of the hotel, there had been Tim Kendal and his wife; and beyond them a family group of Venezuelans. But Major Palgrave had not been looking in that direction…

Miss Marple meditated until lunch time.

After lunch she did not go for a drive.

Instead she sent a message to say that she was not feeling very well and to ask if Dr Graham would be kind enough to come and see her.

CHAPTER FOUR

MISS MARPLE SEEKS MEDICAL ATTENTION

DR GRAHAM WAS a kindly elderly man of about sixty-five. He had practised in the West Indies for many years, but was now semi-retired, and left most of his work to his West Indian partners. He greeted Miss Marple pleasantly and asked her what the trouble was. Fortunately at Miss Marple's age, there was always some ailment that could be discussed with slight exaggerations on the patient's part. Miss Marple hesitated between 'her shoulder' and 'her knee', but finally decided upon the knee. Miss Marple's knee, as she would have put it to herself, was always with her.

Dr Graham was exceedingly kindly but he refrained from putting into words the fact that at her time of life such troubles were only to be expected. He prescribed for her one of the brands of useful little pills that form the basis of a doctor's prescriptions. Since he knew by experience that many elderly people could be lonely when they first came to St Honoré, he remained for a while gently chatting.

'A very nice man,' thought Miss Marple to herself, 'and I really feel rather ashamed of having to tell him lies. But I don't quite see what else I can do.'

Miss Marple had been brought up to have a proper regard for truth and was indeed by nature a very truthful person. But on certain occasions, when she considered it her duty so to do, she could tell lies with a really astonishing verisimilitude.

She cleared her throat, uttered an apologetic little cough, and said, in an old ladyish and slightly twittering manner:

'There is something, Dr Graham, I would like to ask you. I don't really like mentioning it – but I don't quite see what else I am to do – although of course it's *quite* unimportant really. But you see, it's important to *me*. And I hope you will understand and not think what I am asking is tiresome or – or unpardonable in any way.'

To this opening Dr Graham replied kindly: 'Something is worrying you? Do let me help.'

'It's connected with Major Palgrave. *So* sad about his dying. It was quite a shock when I heard it this morning.'

'Yes,' said Dr Graham, 'it was very sudden, I'm afraid. He seemed in such good spirits yesterday.' He spoke kindly, but conventionally. To him, clearly, Major Palgrave's death was nothing out of the way. Miss Marple wondered whether she was really making something out of nothing. Was this suspicious habit of mind growing on her? Perhaps she could no longer trust her own judgment. Not that it was judgment really, only suspicion. Anyway she was in for it now! She must go ahead.

'We were sitting talking together yesterday afternoon,' she said. 'He was telling me about his very varied and interesting life. So many strange parts of the globe.'

'Yes indeed,' said Dr Graham, who had been bored many times by the Major's reminiscences.

'And then he spoke of his family, boyhood rather, and I told him a little about my own nephews and nieces and he listened very sympathetically. And I showed him a snapshot I had with me of one of my nephews. Such a dear boy – at least not exactly a boy now, but always a boy to *me* if you understand.'

'Quite so,' said Dr Graham, wondering how long it would be before the old lady was going to come to the point.

'I had handed it to him and he was examining it when quite suddenly those people – those very nice people – who collect wild flowers and butterflies, Colonel and Mrs Hillingdon I think the name is –'

'Oh yes? The Hillingdons and the Dysons.'

'Yes, that's right. They came suddenly along laughing and

talking. They sat down and ordered drinks and we all talked together. Very pleasant it was. But without thinking, Major Palgrave must have put back my snapshot into his wallet and returned it to his pocket. I wasn't paying very much attention at the time but I remembered afterward and I said to myself – "I mustn't forget to ask the Major to give me back my picture of Denzil." I *did* think of it last night while the dancing and the band was going on, but I didn't like to interrupt him just then, because they were having such a merry party together and I thought "I will remember to ask him for it in the morning." Only this morning –' Miss Marple paused – out of breath.

'Yes, yes,' said Dr Graham, 'I quite understand. And you – well, naturally you want the snapshot back. Is that it?'

Miss Marple nodded her head in eager agreement.

'Yes. That's it. You see, it is the only one I have got and I haven't got the negative. And I would hate to lose that snapshot, because poor Denzil died some five or six years ago and he was my favourite nephew. This is the only picture I have to remind me of him. I wondered – I hoped – it is rather tiresome of me to ask – whether you could possibly manage to get hold of it for me? I don't really know who else to ask, you see. I don't know who'll attend to all his belongings and things like that. It is all so difficult. They would think it such a nuisance of me. You see, they don't understand. Nobody could quite understand what this snapshot means to me.'

'Of course, of course,' said Dr Graham. 'I quite understand. A most natural feeling on your part. Actually, I am meeting the local authorities shortly – the funeral is tomorrow – and someone will be coming from the Administrator's office to look over his papers and effects before communicating with the next of kin – all that sort of thing – If you could describe this snapshot.'

'It was just the front of a house,' said Miss Marple. 'And someone – Denzil, I mean – was just coming out of the front door. As I say it was taken by one of my other nephews who is very keen on flower shows – and he was photographing a hibiscus, I think, or one of those beautiful – something like antipasto – lilies.

Denzil just happened to come out of the front door at that time. It wasn't a very good photograph of him – just a trifle blurred – But I liked it and have always kept it.'

'Well,' said Dr Graham, 'that seems clear enough. I think we'll have no difficulty in getting back your picture for you, Miss Marple.'

He rose from his chair. Miss Marple smiled up at him.

'You are very kind, Dr Graham, very kind *indeed*. You do understand, don't you?'

'Of course I do, of course I do,' said Dr Graham, shaking her warmly by the hand. 'Now don't you worry. Exercise that knee every day gently but not too much, and I'll send you round these tablets. Take one three times a day.'

Chapter Five

Miss Marple makes a Decision

The funeral service was said over the body of the late Major Palgrave on the following day. Miss Marple attended in company with Miss Prescott. The Canon read the service – after that life went on as usual.

Major Palgrave's death was already only an incident, a slightly unpleasant incident, but one that was soon forgotten. Life here was sunshine, sea, and social pleasures. A grim visitor had interrupted these activities, casting a momentary shadow, but the shadow was now gone. After all, nobody had known the deceased very well. He had been rather a garrulous elderly man of the club-bore type, always telling you personal reminiscences that you had no particular desire to hear. He had had little to anchor himself to any particular part of the world. His wife had died many years ago. He had had a lonely life and a lonely death. But it had been the kind of loneliness that spends itself in living amongst people, and in passing the time that way not unpleasantly. Major Palgrave might have been a lonely man, he had also been quite a cheerful one. He had enjoyed himself in his own particular way. And now he was dead, buried, and nobody cared very much, and in another week's time nobody would even remember him or spare him a passing thought.

The only person who could possibly be said to miss him was Miss Marple. Not indeed out of any personal affection, but he represented a kind of life that she knew. As one grew older, so she reflected to herself, one got more and more into the habit of listening; listening possibly without any great interest, but there had been between her and the Major the gentle give and take of two old people. It had had a cheerful, human quality. She did not actually mourn Major Palgrave but she missed him.

On the afternoon of the funeral, as she was sitting knitting in her favourite spot, Dr Graham came and joined her. She put her needles down and greeted him. He said at once, rather apologetically:

'I am afraid I have rather disappointing news, Miss Marple.'

'Indeed? About my –'

'Yes. We haven't found that precious snapshot of yours. I'm afraid that will be a disappointment to you.'

'Yes. Yes it is. But of course it does not *really* matter. It was a sentimentality. I do realise that now. It wasn't in Major Palgrave's wallet?'

'No. Nor anywhere else among his things. There were a few letters and newspaper clippings and odds and ends, and a few old photographs, but no sign of a snapshot such as you mentioned.'

'Oh dear,' said Miss Marple. 'Well, it can't be helped... Thank you very much, Dr Graham, for the trouble you've taken.'

'Oh it was no trouble, indeed. But I know quite well from my own experience how much family trifles mean to one, especially as one is getting older.'

The old lady was really taking it very well, he thought. Major Palgrave, he presumed, had probably come across the snapshot when taking something out of his wallet, and not even realising how it had come there, had torn it up as something of no importance. But of course it was of great importance to this old lady. Still, she seemed quite cheerful and philosophical about it.

Internally, however, Miss Marple was far from being either cheerful or philosophical. She wanted a little time in which to think things out, but she was also determined to use her present opportunities to the fullest effect.

She engaged Dr Graham in conversation with an eagerness which she did not attempt to conceal. That kindly man, putting down her flow of talk to the natural loneliness of an old lady, exerted himself to divert her mind from the loss of the snapshot, by conversing easily and pleasantly about life in St Honoré, and the various interesting places perhaps Miss Marple might like to visit. He hardly knew himself how the conversation drifted back to Major Palgrave's decease.

'It seems so sad,' said Miss Marple. 'To think of anyone dying like this away from home. Though I gather, from what he himself told me, that he had no immediate family. It seems he lived by himself in London.'

'He travelled a fair amount, I believe,' said Dr Graham. 'At any rate in the winters. He didn't care for our English winters. Can't say I blame him.'

'No, indeed,' said Miss Marple. 'And perhaps he had some special reason like a weakness of the lungs or something which made it necessary for him to winter abroad?'

'Oh no, I don't think so.'

'He had high blood pressure, I believe. So sad nowadays. One hears so much of it.'

'He spoke about it to you, did he?'

'Oh no. No, *he* never mentioned it. It was somebody else who told me.'

'Ah, really.'

'I suppose,' went on Miss Marple, 'that death was to be expected under those circumstances.'

'Not necessarily,' said Dr Graham. 'There are methods of controlling blood pressure nowadays.'

'His death *seemed* very sudden – but I suppose *you* weren't surprised.'

'Well I wasn't particularly surprised in a man of that age. But I certainly didn't expect it. Frankly, he always seemed to me in very good form, but I hadn't ever attended him professionally. I'd never taken his blood pressure or anything like that.'

'Does one know – I mean, does a doctor know – when a man has high blood pressure just by looking at him?' Miss Marple inquired with a kind of dewy innocence.

'Not just by looking,' said the doctor, smiling. 'One has to do a bit of testing.'

'Oh I see. That dreadful thing when you put a rubber band round somebody's arm and blow it up – I dislike it *so* much. But my doctor said that my blood pressure was really very good for my age.'

'Well that's good hearing,' said Dr Graham.

'Of course, the Major *was* rather fond of Planters Punch,' said Miss Marple thoughtfully.

'Yes. Not the best thing with blood pressure – alcohol.'

'One takes tablets, doesn't one, or so I have heard?'

'Yes. There are several on the market. There was a bottle of one of them in his room – Serenite.'

'How wonderful science is nowadays,' said Miss Marple. 'Doctors can do so much, can't they?'

'We all have one great competitor,' said Dr Graham. 'Nature, you know. And some of the good old-fashioned home remedies come back from time to time.'

'Like putting cobwebs on a cut?' said Miss Marple. 'We always used to do that when I was a child.'

'Very sensible,' said Dr Graham.

'And a linseed poultice on the chest and rubbing in camphorated oil for a bad cough.'

'I see you know it all!' said Dr Graham laughing. He got up. 'How's the knee? Not been too troublesome?'

'No, it seems much, much better.'

'Well, we won't say whether that's Nature or my pills,' said Dr Graham. 'Sorry I couldn't have been of more help to you.'

'But you have been most kind – I am really ashamed of taking up your time – Did you say that there were no photographs in the Major's wallet?'

'Oh yes – a very old one of the Major himself as quite a young man on a polo pony – and one of a dead tiger – He was standing with his foot on it. Snaps of that sort – memories of his younger days – But I looked very carefully, I assure you, and the one you describe of your nephew was definitely not there –'

'Oh I'm sure you looked carefully – I didn't mean that – I was just interested – We all tend to keep such very odd things –'

'Treasures from the past,' said the doctor smiling.

He said goodbye and departed.

Miss Marple remained looking thoughtfully at the palm trees and the sea. She did not pick up her knitting again for some minutes. She had a fact now. She had to think about that fact and what it meant. The snapshot that the Major had brought out of his wallet and replaced so hurriedly was *not there after he died*. It was not the sort of thing the Major would throw away. He had replaced it in his wallet and it ought to have been in his wallet after his death. Money might have been stolen, but no one would want to steal a snapshot. Unless, that is, they had a special reason for so doing...

Miss Marple's face was grave. She had to take a decision. Was she, or was she not, going to allow Major Palgrave to remain quietly in his grave? Might it not be better to do just that? She quoted under her breath. 'Duncan is dead. After Life's fitful fever he sleeps well!' Nothing could hurt Major Palgrave now. He had gone where danger could not touch him. Was it just a coincidence that he should have died on that particular night? Or was it just possibly *not* a coincidence? Doctors accepted the deaths of elderly men so easily. Especially since in his room there had been a bottle of the tablets that people with high blood pressure had to take every day of their lives. But if someone had taken the snapshot from the Major's wallet, that same person could have put that bottle of tablets in the Major's room. She herself never remembered *seeing* the Major take tablets; he had never spoken about his blood pressure to her. The only thing he had ever said about his health was the admission – 'Not as young as I was.' He had been occasionally a little short of breath, a trifle asthmatic, nothing else. But someone had mentioned that Major Palgrave had high blood pressure – Molly? Miss Prescott? She couldn't remember.

Miss Marple sighed, then admonished herself in words, though she did not speak those words aloud.

'Now, Jane, what are you suggesting or thinking? Are you,

perhaps, just making the whole thing up? Have you *really* got anything to build on?'

She went over, step by step, as nearly as she could, the conversation between herself and the Major on the subject of murder and murderers.

'Oh dear,' said Miss Marple. 'Even if – really, I *don't* see how I *can* do anything about it –'

But she knew that she meant to try.

Chapter Six

In the Small Hours

I

Miss Marple woke early. Like many old people she slept lightly and had periods of wakefulness which she used for the planning of some action or actions to be carried out on the next or following days. Usually, of course, these were of a wholly private or domestic nature, of little interest to anybody but herself. But this morning Miss Marple lay thinking soberly and constructively of murder, and what, if her suspicions were correct, she could do about it. It wasn't going to be easy. She had one weapon and one weapon only, and that was conversation.

Old ladies were given to a good deal of rambling conversation. People were bored by this, but certainly did not suspect them of ulterior motives. It would not be a case of asking direct questions. (Indeed, she would have found it difficult to know what questions to ask!) It would be a question of finding out a little more about certain people. She reviewed these certain people in her mind.

She could find out, possibly, a little more about Major Palgrave, but would that really help her? She doubted if it would. If Major Palgrave had been killed it was not because of secrets in his life or to inherit his money or for revenge upon him. In fact, although he was the victim, it was one of those rare cases where a greater knowledge of the victim does not help you or lead you in any way to his murderer. The point, it seemed to her, and the sole point, was that Major Palgrave talked too much!

She had learnt one rather interesting fact from Dr Graham. He had had in his wallet various photographs: one of himself in company with a polo pony, one of a dead tiger, also one or two other shots of the same nature. Now why did Major Palgrave carry these about with him? Obviously, thought Miss Marple, with long experience of old admirals, brigadier-generals and mere majors behind her, because he had certain stories which he enjoyed telling to people. Starting off with 'Curious thing happened once when I was out tiger shooting in India...' Or a reminiscence of himself and a polo pony. Therefore this story about a suspected murderer would in due course be illustrated by the production of the snapshot from his wallet.

He had been following that pattern in his conversation with her. The subject of murder having come up, and to focus interest on his story, he had done what he no doubt usually did, produced his snapshot and said something in the nature of 'Wouldn't think this chap was a murderer, would you?'

The point was that it had been a *habit* of his. This murderer story was one of his regular repertoire. If any reference to murder came up, then away went the Major, full steam ahead.

In that case, reflected Miss Marple, he might *already* have told his story to someone else here. Or to more than one person – If that were so, then she herself might learn from that person what the further details of the story had been, possibly what the person in the snapshot had looked like.

She nodded her head in satisfaction – That would be a beginning.

And, of course, there were the people she called in her mind the 'Four Suspects'. Though really, since Major Palgrave had been talking about a *man* – there were only two. Colonel Hillingdon or Mr Dyson, very unlikely-looking murderers, but then murderers so often *were* unlikely. Could there have been anyone else? She had seen no one when she turned her head to look. There was the bungalow of course. Mr Rafiel's bungalow. Could somebody have come out of the bungalow and gone in again before she had had time to turn her head? If so, it could only have been the valet-attendant. What was his name? Oh yes, Jackson. Could it have been *Jackson* who had come out of the door? That would have been the same pose as the photograph. *A man coming out of a door.* Recognition might have struck suddenly. Up till then, Major Palgrave would not have looked at Arthur Jackson, valet-attendant, with any interest. His roving and curious eye was essentially a snobbish eye – Arthur Jackson was not a *pukka sahib* – Major Palgrave would not have glanced at him twice.

Until, perhaps, he had had the snapshot in his hand, and had looked over Miss Marple's right shoulder and had seen a man coming out of a door...?

Miss Marple turned over on her pillow – Programme for tomorrow – or rather for today – Further investigation of the Hillingdons, the Dysons and Arthur Jackson, valet-attendant.

II

Dr Graham also woke early. Usually he turned over and went to sleep again. But today he was uneasy and sleep failed to come. This anxiety that made it so difficult to go to sleep again was a thing he had not suffered from for a long time. What was causing this anxiety? Really, he couldn't make it out. He lay there thinking it over. Something to do with – something to do with – yes, Major Palgrave. Major Palgrave's death? He didn't see, though, what there could be to make him uneasy there. Was it something that that twittery old lady had said? Bad luck for her about her snapshot. She'd taken it very well. But now what was it she had said, what chance word of hers had it been, that had given him this funny feeling of uneasiness? After all, there was nothing *odd* about the Major's death. Nothing at all. At least he supposed there was nothing at all.

It was quite clear that in the Major's state of health – a faint check came in his thought process. Did he really know much *about* Major Palgrave's state of health? Everybody *said* that he'd suffered from high blood pressure. But he himself had never had any conversation with the Major about it. But then he'd never had much conversation with Major Palgrave anyway. Palgrave was an old bore and he avoided old bores. Why on earth should he have this idea that perhaps everything *mightn't* be all right? Was it that old woman? But after all she hadn't *said* anything. Anyway, it was none of his business. The local authorities were quite satisfied. There had been that bottle of Serenite tablets, and the old boy had apparently talked to people about his blood pressure quite freely.

Dr Graham turned over in bed and soon went to sleep again.

III

Outside the hotel grounds, in one of a row of shanty cabins beside a creek, the girl Victoria Johnson rolled over and sat up in bed. The St Honoré girl was a magnificent creature with a torso of black marble such as a sculptor would have enjoyed. She ran her fingers through her dark, tightly curling hair. With her foot she nudged her sleeping companion in the ribs.

'Wake up, man.'

The man grunted and turned.

'What you want? It's not morning.'

'Wake up, man. I want to talk to you.'

The man sat up, stretched, showed a wide mouth and beautiful teeth.

'What's worrying you, woman?'

'That Major man who died. Something I don't like. Something wrong about it.'

'Ah, what d'you want to worry about that? He was old. He died.'

'Listen, man. It's them pills. Them pills the doctor asked me about.'

44

'Well, what about them? He took too many maybe.'

'No. It's not that. Listen.' She leant towards him, talking vehemently. He yawned and lay down again.

'There's nothing in that. What're you talking about?'

'All the same, I'll speak to Mrs Kendal about it in the morning. I think there's something wrong there somewhere.'

'Shouldn't bother,' said the man who, without benefit of ceremony, she considered as her present husband. 'Don't let's look for trouble,' he said and rolled over on his side yawning.

Chapter Seven

Morning on the Beach

I

It was mid-morning on the beach below the hotel.

Evelyn Hillingdon came out of the water and dropped on the warm golden sand. She took off her bathing cap and shook her dark head vigorously. The beach was not a very big one. People tended to congregate there in the mornings and about 11.30 there was always something of a social reunion. To Evelyn's left in one of the exotic-looking modern basket chairs lay Señora de Caspearo, a handsome woman from Venezuela. Next to her was old Mr Rafiel who was by now the doyen of the Golden Palm Hotel and held the sway that only an elderly invalid of great wealth could attain. Esther Walters was in attendance on him. She usually had her shorthand notebook and pencil with her in case Mr Rafiel should suddenly think of urgent business cables which must be got off at once. Mr Rafiel in beach attire was incredibly desiccated, his bones draped with festoons of dry skin. Though looking like a man on the point of death, he had looked exactly the same for at least the last eight years – or so it was said in the islands. Sharp blue eyes peered out of his wrinkled cheeks, and his prinicipal pleasure in life was denying robustly anything that anyone else said.

Miss Marple was also present. As usual she sat and knitted and listened to what went on, and very occasionally joined in the conversation. When she did so, everyone was surprised because they had usually forgotten that she was there! Evelyn Hillingdon looked at her indulgently, and thought that she was a nice old pussy.

Señora de Caspearo rubbed some more oil on her long beautiful legs and hummed to herself. She was not a woman who spoke much. She looked discontentedly at the flask of sun oil.

'This is not so good as Frangipanio,' she said, sadly. 'One cannot get it here. A pity.' Her eyelids drooped again.

'Are you going in for your dip now, Mr Rafiel?' asked Esther Walters.

'I'll go in when I'm ready,' said Mr Rafiel, snappishly.

'It's half past eleven,' said Mrs Walters.

'What of it?' said Mr Rafiel. 'Think I'm the kind of man to be tied by the clock? Do this at the hour, do this at twenty minutes past, do that at twenty to – bah!'

Mrs Walters had been in attendance on Mr Rafiel long enough to have adopted her own formula for dealing with him. She knew that he liked a good space of time in which to recover from the exertion of bathing and she had therefore reminded him of the time, allowing a good ten minutes for him to rebut her suggestion and then be able to adopt it without seeming to do so.

'I don't like these espadrilles,' said Mr Rafiel raising a foot and looking at it. 'I told that fool Jackson so. The man never pays attention to a word I say.'

'I'll fetch you some others, shall I, Mr Rafiel?'

'No, you won't, you'll sit here and keep quiet. I hate people rushing about like clucking hens.'

Evelyn shifted slightly in the warm sand, stretching out her arms.

Miss Marple, intent on her knitting – or so it seemed – stretched out a foot, then hastily she apologised.

'I'm so sorry, so very sorry, Mrs Hillingdon. I'm afraid I kicked you.'

'Oh, it's quite all right,' said Evelyn. 'This beach gets rather crowded.'

'Oh, please don't move. Please. I'll move my chair a little back so that I won't do it again.'

As Miss Marple resettled herself, she went on talking in a childish and garrulous manner.

'It still seems so wonderful to be *here!* I've never been to the West Indies before, you know. I thought it was the kind of place I never should come to and here I am. All by the kindness of my dear nephew. I suppose you know this part of the world very well, don't you, Mrs Hillingdon?'

'I have been in this island once or twice before and of course in most of the others.'

'Oh yes. Butterflies isn't it, and wild flowers? You and your – your friends – or are they relations?'

'Friends. Nothing more.'

'And I suppose you go about together a great deal because of your interests being the same?'

'Yes. We've travelled together for some years now.'

'I suppose you must have had some rather exciting adventures sometimes?'

'I don't think so,' said Evelyn. Her voice was unaccentuated, slightly bored. 'Adventures always seem to happen to other people.' She yawned.

'No dangerous encounters with snakes or with wild animals or with natives gone berserk?'

('What a fool I sound,' thought Miss Marple.)

'Nothing worse than insect bites,' Evelyn assured her.

'Poor Major Palgrave, you know, was bitten by a snake once,' said Miss Marple, making a purely fictitious statement.

'Was he?'

'Did he never tell you about it?'

'Perhaps. I don't remember.'

'I suppose you knew him quite well, didn't you?'

'Major Palgrave? No, hardly at all.'

'He always had so many interesting stories to tell.'

'Ghastly old bore,' said Mr Rafiel. 'Silly fool, too. He needn't have died if he'd looked after himself properly.'

'Oh come now, Mr Rafiel,' said Mrs Walters.

'I know what I'm talking about. If you look after your health properly you're all right anywhere. Look at me. The doctors gave *me* up years ago. All right, I said, I've got my own rules of health and I shall keep to them. And here I am.'

He looked round proudly.

It did indeed seem rather a mistake that he should be there.

'Poor Major Palgrave had high blood pressure,' said Mrs Walters.

'Nonsense,' said Mr Rafiel.

'Oh, but he did,' said Evelyn Hillingdon. She spoke with sudden, unexpected authority.

'Who says so?' said Mr Rafiel. 'Did he tell you so?'

'Somebody said so.'

'He looked very red in the face,' Miss Marple contributed.

'Can't go by that,' said Mr Rafiel. 'And anyway he *didn't* have high blood pressure because he told me so.'

'What do you mean, he told you so?' said Mrs Walters. 'I mean, you can't exactly tell people you *haven't* got a thing.'

'Yes you can. I said to him once when he was downing all those Planters Punches, and eating too much, I said, "You ought to watch your diet and your drink. You've got to think of your blood pressure at your age." And he said he'd nothing to look out for in that line, that his blood pressure was very good for his age.'

'But he took some stuff for it, I believe,' said Miss Marple, entering the conversation once more. 'Some stuff called – oh, something like – was it Serenite?'

'If you ask me,' said Evelyn Hillingdon, 'I don't think he ever liked to admit that there could be anything the matter with him or that he could be ill. I think he was one of those people who are afraid of illness and therefore deny there's ever anything wrong with them.'

It was a long speech for her. Miss Marple looked thoughtfully down at the top of her dark head.

'The trouble is,' said Mr Rafiel dictatorially, 'everybody's too fond of knowing other people's ailments. They think everybody over fifty is going to die of hypertension or coronary thrombosis or one of those things – poppycock! If a man says there's nothing much wrong with him I don't suppose there is. A man ought to know about his own health. What's the time? Quarter to twelve? I ought to have had my dip long ago. Why can't you remind me about these things, Esther?'

Mrs Walters made no protest. She rose to her feet and with some deftness assisted Mr Rafiel to his. Together they went down the beach, she supporting him carefully. Together they stepped into the sea.

Señora de Caspearo opened her eyes and murmured: 'How ugly are old men! Oh how they are ugly! They should all be put to death at forty, or perhaps thirty-five would be better. Yes?'

Edward Hillingdon and Gregory Dyson came crunching down the beach.

'What's the water like, Evelyn?'

'Just the same as always.'

'Never much variation, is there? Where's Lucky?'

'I don't know,' said Evelyn.

Again Miss Marple looked down thoughtfully at the dark head.

'Well, now I give my imitation of a whale,' said Gregory. He threw off his gaily patterned Bermuda shirt and tore down the beach, flinging himself, puffing and panting, into the sea, doing a fast crawl. Edward Hillingdon sat down on the beach by his wife. Presently he asked, 'Coming in again?'

She smiled – put on her cap – and they went down the beach together in a much less spectacular manner.

Señora de Caspearo opened her eyes again.

'I think at first those two they are on their honeymoon, he is so charming to her, but I hear they have been married eight – nine years. It is incredible, is it not?'

'I wonder where Mrs Dyson is?' said Miss Marple.

'That Lucky? She is with some man.'

'You – you think so?'

'It is certain,' said Señora de Caspearo. 'She is that type. But she is not so young any longer – Her husband – already his eyes go elsewhere – He makes passes – here, there, all the time. I know.'

'Yes,' said Miss Marple. 'I expect you would know.'

Señora de Caspearo shot a surprised glance at her. It was clearly not what she had expected from that quarter.

Miss Marple, however, was looking at the waves with an air of gentle innocence.

II

'May I speak to you, ma'am, Mrs Kendal?'

'Yes, of course,' said Molly. She was sitting at her desk in the office.

Victoria Johnson, tall and buoyant in her crisp white uniform, came in farther and shut the door behind her with a somewhat mysterious air.

'I like to tell you something, please, Mrs Kendal.'

'Yes, what is it? Is anything wrong?'

'I don't know that. Not for sure. It's the old gentleman who died. The Major gentleman. He die in his sleep.'

'Yes, yes. What about it?'

'There was a bottle of pills in his room. Doctor, he asked me about them.'

'Yes?'

'The doctor said – "Let me see what he has here on the bathroom shelf," and he looked, you see. He see there was tooth powder and indigestion pills and aspirin and cascara pills, and then these pills in a bottle called Serenite.'

'Yes,' repeated Molly yet again.

'And the doctor looked at them. He seemed quite satisfied, and nodded his head. But I get to thinking afterwards. Those pills weren't there before. I've not seen them in his bathroom before. The others, yes. The tooth powder and the aspirin and the aftershave lotion and all the rest. But those pills, those Serenite pills, I never noticed them before.'

'So you think –' Molly looked puzzled.

'I don't know what to think,' said Victoria. 'I just think it's not right, so I think I better tell you about it. Perhaps you tell doctor? Perhaps it means something. Perhaps *someone* put those pills there so he take them and he died.'

'Oh, I don't think that's likely at all,' said Molly.

Victoria shook her dark head. 'You never know. People do bad things.'

Molly glanced out of the window. The place looked like an earthly paradise. With its sunshine, its sea, its coral reef, its music, its dancing, it seemed a Garden of Eden. But even in the Garden of Eden, there had been a shadow – the shadow of the Serpent – *Bad things* – how hateful to hear those words.

'I'll make inquiries, Victoria,' she said sharply. 'Don't worry. And above all don't go starting a lot of silly rumours.'

Tim Kendal came in, just as Victoria was, somewhat unwillingly, leaving.

'Anything wrong, Molly?'

She hesitated – but Victoria might go to him – She told him what the girl had said.

'I don't see what all this rigmarole – what *were* these pills anyway?'

'Well, I don't really know, Tim. Dr Robertson when he came said they – were something to do with blood pressure, I think.'

'Well, that would be all right, wouldn't it? I mean, he *had* high blood pressure, and he *would* be taking things for it, wouldn't he? People do. I've seen them, lots of times.'

'Yes,' Molly hesitated, 'but Victoria seemed to think that he might have taken one of these pills and it would have killed him.'

'Oh darling, that is a bit *too* melodramatic! You mean that somebody might have changed his blood pressure pills for something else, and that they poisoned him?'

'It does sound absurd,' said Molly apologetically, 'when you say it like that. But that seemed to be what Victoria thought!'

'Silly girl! We *could* go and ask Dr Graham about it, I suppose he'd know. But really it's such nonsense that it's not worth bothering him.'

'That's what I think.'

'What on earth made the girl think anybody would have changed the pills? You mean, put different pills into the same bottle?'

'I didn't quite gather,' said Molly, looking rather helpless. 'Victoria seemed to think that was the first time that Serenite bottle had been there.'

'Oh but that's nonsense,' said Tim Kendal. 'He had to take those pills all the time to keep his blood pressure down.' And he went off cheerfully to consult with Fernando the *maître d'hôtel*.

But Molly could not dismiss the matter so lightly. After the stress of lunch was over she said to her husband:

'Tim – I've been thinking – If Victoria is going around talking about this perhaps we ought just to ask someone about it?'

'My dear girl! Robertson and all the rest of them came and looked at everything and asked all the questions they wanted at the time.'

'Yes, but you know how they work themselves up, these girls –'

'Oh, all right! I'll tell you what – we'll go and ask Graham – he'll know.'

Dr Graham was sitting on his loggia with a book. The young couple came in and Molly plunged into her recital. It was a little incoherent and Tim took over.

'Sounds rather idiotic,' he said apologetically, 'but as far as I can make out, this girl has got it into her head that someone put some poison tablets in the – what's the name of the stuff – Sera – something bottle.'

'But why should she get this idea into her head?' asked Dr Graham. 'Did she see anything or hear anything or – I mean, why should she think so?'

'I don't know,' said Tim rather helplessly. 'Was it a different bottle? Was that it, Molly?'

'No,' said Molly. 'I think what she said was that there was a bottle there labelled – Seven – Seren –'

'Serenite,' said the doctor. 'That's quite right. A well-known preparation. He'd been taking it regularly.'

'Victoria said she'd never seen it in his room before.'

'Never seen it in his room before?' said Graham sharply. 'What does she mean by that?'

'Well, that's what she *said*. She said there were all sorts of things on the bathroom shelf. You know, tooth powder, aspirin and aftershave and – oh – she rattled them off gaily. I suppose she's always cleaning them and so she knows them all off by heart. But this one – the Serenite – she hadn't seen it there until the day after he died.'

'That's very odd,' said Dr Graham, rather sharply. 'Is she sure?'

The unusual sharpness of his tone made both of the Kendals look up at him. They had not expected Dr Graham to take up quite this attitude.

'She sounded sure,' said Molly slowly.

'Perhaps she just wanted to be sensational,' suggested Tim.

'I think perhaps,' said Dr Graham, 'I'd better have a few words with the girl myself.'

Victoria displayed a distinct pleasure at being allowed to tell her story.

'I don't want to get in no trouble,' she said. '*I* didn't put that bottle there and I don't know who did.'

'But you think it *was* put there?' asked Graham.

'Well, you see, Doctor, it *must* have been put there if it wasn't there before.'

'Major Palgrave could have kept it in a drawer – or a dispatch-case, something like that.'

Victoria shook her head shrewdly.

'Wouldn't do that if he was taking it all the time, would he?'

'No,' said Graham reluctantly. 'No, it was stuff he would have to take several times a day. You never saw him taking it or anything of that kind?'

'He didn't have it there before. I just thought – word got round as that stuff had something to do with his death, poisoned his blood or something, and I thought maybe he had an enemy put it there so as to kill him.'

'Nonsense, my girl,' said the doctor robustly. 'Sheer nonsense.'

Victoria looked shaken.

'You say as this stuff was medicine, good medicine?' she asked doubtfully.

'Good medicine, and what is more, *necessary* medicine,' said Dr Graham. 'So you needn't worry, Victoria. I can assure you there was nothing wrong with that medicine. It was the proper thing for a man to take who had his complaint.'

'Surely you've taken a load off my mind,' said Victoria. She showed white teeth at him in a cheerful smile.

But the load was not taken off Dr Graham's mind. That uneasiness of his that had been so nebulous was now becoming tangible.

Chapter Eight

A Talk with Esther Walters

'THIS PLACE ISN'T what it used to be,' said Mr Rafiel, irritably, as he observed Miss Marple approaching the spot where he and his secretary were sitting. 'Can't move a step without some old hen getting under your feet. What do old ladies want to come to the West Indies for?'

'Where do you suggest they should go?' asked Esther Walters.

'To Cheltenham,' said Mr Rafiel promptly. 'Or Bournemouth,' he offered, 'or Torquay or Llandrindod Wells. Plenty of choice. They like it there – they're quite happy.'

'They can't often afford to come to the West Indies, I suppose,' said Esther. 'It isn't everyone who is as lucky as you are.'

'That's right,' said Mr Rafiel. 'Rub it in. Here am I, a mass of aches and pains and disjoints. You grudge me any alleviation! And you don't do any work – Why haven't you typed out those letters yet?'

'I haven't had time.'

'Well, get on with it, can't you? I bring you out here to do a bit of work, not to sit about sunning yourself and showing off your figure.'

Some people would have considered Mr Rafiel's remarks quite insupportable but Esther Walters had worked for him for some years and she knew well enough that Mr Rafiel's bark was a great deal worse than his bite. He was a man who suffered almost continual pain, and making disagreeable remarks was one of his ways of letting off steam. No matter what he said she remained quite imperturbable.

'Such a lovely evening, isn't it?' said Miss Marple, pausing beside them.

'Why not?' said Mr Rafiel. 'That's what we're here for, isn't it?'

Miss Marple gave a tinkly little laugh.

'You're so severe – of course the weather *is* a very English subject of conversation – one forgets – Oh dear – this is the wrong coloured wool.' She deposited her knitting bag on the garden table and trotted towards her own bungalow.

'Jackson!' yelled Mr Rafiel.

Jackson appeared.

'Take me back inside,' said Mr Rafiel. 'I'll have my massage now before that chattering hen comes back. Not that massage does me a bit of good,' he added. Having said which, he allowed himself to be deftly helped to his feet and went off with the masseur beside him into his bungalow.

Esther Walters looked after them and then turned her head as Miss Marple came back with a ball of wool to sit down near her.

'I hope I'm not disturbing you?' said Miss Marple.

'Of course not,' said Esther Walters, 'I've got to go off and do some typing in a minute, but I'm going to enjoy another ten minutes of the sunset first.'

Miss Marple sat down and in a gentle voice began to talk. As she talked, she summed up Esther Walters. Not at all glamorous, but could be attractive-looking if she tried. Miss Marple wondered why she didn't try. It could be, of course, because Mr Rafiel would not have liked it, but Miss Marple didn't think Mr Rafiel would really mind in the least. He was so completely taken up with himself that so long as he was not personally neglected, his secretary might have got herself up like a houri in Paradise without his objecting. Besides, he usually went to bed early and in the evening hours of steel bands and dancing, Esther Walters might easily have – Miss Marple paused to select a word in her mind, at the same time conversing cheerfully about her visit to Jamestown – Ah yes, *blossomed*. Esther Walters might have blossomed in the evening hours.

She led the conversation gently in the direction of Jackson.

On the subject of Jackson Esther Walters was rather vague.

'He's very competent,' she said. 'A fully trained masseur.'

'I suppose he's been with Mr Rafiel a long time?'

'Oh no – about nine months, I think –'

'Is he married?' Miss Marple hazarded.

'Married? I don't think so,' said Esther slightly surprised. 'He's never mentioned it if so –

' No,' she added. 'Definitely *not* married, I should say.' And she showed amusement.

Miss Marple interpreted that by adding to it in her own mind the following sentence – 'At any rate he doesn't behave as though he were married.'

But then, how many married men there were who behaved as though they weren't married! Miss Marple could think of a dozen examples!

'He's quite good-looking,' she said thoughtfully.

'Yes – I suppose he is,' said Esther without interest.

Miss Marple considered her thoughtfully. Uninterested in men? The kind of woman, perhaps, who was only interested in one man – A widow, they had said.

She asked – 'Have you worked for Mr Rafiel long?'

'Four or five years. After my husband died, I had to take a job again. I've got a daughter at school and my husband left me very badly off.'

'Mr Rafiel must be a difficult man to work for?' Miss Marple hazarded.

'Not really, when you get to know him. He flies into rages and is very contradictory. I think the real trouble is he gets tired of people. He's had five different valet-attendants in two years. He likes having someone new to bully. But he and I have always got on very well.'

'Mr Jackson seems a very obliging young man?'

'He's very tactful and resourceful,' said Esther. 'Of course, he's sometimes a little –' She broke off.

Miss Marple considered. 'Rather a difficult position sometimes?' she suggested.

'Well, yes. Neither one thing nor the other. However –' she smiled – 'I think he manages to have quite a good time.'

Miss Marple considered this also. It didn't help her much. She continued her twittering conversation and soon she was hearing a good deal about that nature-loving quartet, the Dysons and the Hillingdons.

'The Hillingdons have been here for the last three or four years at least,' said Esther, 'but Gregory Dyson has been here much longer than that. He knows the West Indies very well. He came here, originally, I believe, with his first wife. She was delicate and had to go abroad in the winters, or go somewhere warm, at any rate.'

'And she died? Or was it divorce?'

'No. She died. Out here, I believe. I don't mean this particular island but one of the West Indies islands. There was some sort of trouble, I believe, some kind of scandal or other. He never talks about her. Somebody else told me about it. They didn't, I gather, get on very well together.'

'And then he married this wife. "Lucky".' Miss Marple said the word with faint dissatisfaction as if to say 'Really, a most incredible name!'

'I believe she was a relation of his first wife.'

'Have they known the Hillingdons a great many years?'

'Oh, I think only since the Hillingdons came out here. Three or four years, not more.'

'The Hillingdons seem very pleasant,' said Miss Marple. 'Quiet, of course.'

'Yes. They're both quiet.'

'Everyone says they're very devoted to each other,' said Miss Marple. The tone of her voice was quite non-committal but Esther Walters looked at her sharply.

'But you don't think they are?' she said.

'You don't really think so yourself, do you, my dear?'

'Well, I've wondered sometimes…'

'Quiet men, like Colonel Hillingdon,' said Miss Marple, 'are often attracted to flamboyant types.' And she added, after a significant pause, 'Lucky – such a curious name. Do you think Mr Dyson has any idea of – of what might be going on?'

'Old scandal-monger,' thought Esther Walters. 'Really, these old women!'

She said rather coldly, 'I've no idea.'

Miss Marple shifted to another subject. 'It's very sad about poor Major Palgrave isn't it?' she said.

Esther Walters agreed, though in a somewhat perfunctory fashion.

'The people I'm really sorry for are the Kendals,' she said.

'Yes, I suppose it is really rather unfortunate when something of that kind happens in a hotel.'

'People come here, you see, to enjoy themselves, don't they?' said Esther. 'To forget about illnesses and deaths and income tax and frozen pipes and all the rest of it. They don't like –' she went on, with a sudden flash of an entirely different manner – 'any reminders of mortality.'

Miss Marple laid down her knitting. 'Now that is very well put, my dear,' she said, 'very well put indeed. Yes, it is as you say.'

'And you see they're quite a young couple,' went on Esther Walters. 'They only just took over from the Sandersons six months ago and they're terribly worried about whether they're going to succeed or not, because they haven't had much experience.'

'And you think this might be really disadvantageous to them?'

'Well, no, I don't, frankly,' said Esther Walters. 'I don't think people remember anything for more than a day or two, not in this atmosphere of "we've-all-come-out-here-to-enjoy-ourselves-let's-get-on-with-it." I think a death just gives them a jolt for about twenty-four hours or so and then they don't think of it again once the funeral is over. Not unless they're reminded of it, that is. I've told Molly so, but of course she is a worrier.'

'Mrs Kendal is a worrier? She always seems so carefree.'

'I think a lot of that is put on,' said Esther slowly. 'Actually, I think she's one of those anxious sort of people who can't help worrying all the time that things *may* go wrong.'

'I should have thought *he* worried more than she did.'

'No, I don't think so. I think she's the worrier and he worries because she worries if you know what I mean.'

'That is interesting,' said Miss Marple.

'I think Molly wants desperately to try and appear very gay and to be enjoying herself. She works at it very hard but the effort exhausts her. Then she has these odd fits of depression. She's not – well, not really well-balanced.'

'Poor child,' said Miss Marple. 'There certainly are people like that, and very often outsiders don't suspect it.'

'No, they put on such a good show, don't they? However,' Esther added, 'I don't think Molly has really anything to worry about in this case. I mean, people are dying of coronary thrombosis or cerebral hæmorrhage or things of that kind all the time nowadays. Far more than they used to, as far as I can see. It's only food poisoning or typhoid or something like that, that makes people get het up.'

'Major Palgrave never mentioned to *me* that he had high blood pressure,' said Miss Marple. 'Did he to you?'

'He said so to somebody – I don't know who – it may have been to Mr Rafiel. I know Mr Rafiel says just the opposite – but then he's like that! Certainly Jackson mentioned it to me once. He said the Major ought to be more careful over the alcohol he took.'

'I see,' said Miss Marple, thoughtfully. She went on: 'I expect you found him rather a boring old man? He told a lot of stories and I expect repeated himself a good deal.'

'That's the worst of it,' said Esther. 'You do hear the same story again and again unless you can manage to be quick enough to fend it off.'

'Of course *I* didn't mind so much,' said Miss Marple, 'because I'm used to that sort of thing. If I get stories told to me rather often, I don't really mind hearing them again because I've usually forgotten them.'

'There is that,' said Esther and laughed cheerfully.

'There was one story he was very fond of telling,' said Miss Marple, 'about a murder. I expect he told you that, didn't he?'

Esther Walters opened her handbag and started searching through it. She drew out her lipstick saying, 'I thought I'd lost it.' Then she asked, 'I beg your pardon, what did you say?'

'I asked if Major Palgrave told you his favourite murder story?'

'I believe he did, now I come to think of it. Something about someone who gassed themselves, wasn't it? Only really it was the *wife* who gassed him. I mean she'd given him a sedative of some kind and then stuck his head in the gas oven. Was that it?'

'I don't think that was exactly it,' said Miss Marple. She looked at Esther Walters thoughtfully.

'He told such a lot of stories,' said Esther Walters, apologetically, 'and as I said, one didn't always listen.'

'He had a snapshot,' said Miss Marple, 'that he used to show people.'

'I believe he did... I can't remember what it was now. Did he show it to you?'

'No,' said Miss Marple. 'He didn't show it to me. We were interrupted –'

Chapter Nine

Miss Prescott and Others

'THE STORY *I* heard,' began Miss Prescott, lowering her voice, and looking carefully around.

Miss Marple drew her chair a little closer. It had been some time before she had been able to get together with Miss Prescott for a heart-to-heart chat. This was owing to the fact that clergymen are very strong family men so that Miss Prescott was nearly always accompanied by her brother, and there was no doubt that Miss Marple and Miss Prescott found it less easy to take their back hair down in a good gossip when the jovial Canon was of their company.

'It seems,' said Miss Prescott, 'though of course I don't want to talk any scandal and I really know *nothing* about it –'

'Oh, I *quite* understand,' said Miss Marple.

'It seems there was some scandal when his first wife was still alive! Apparently this woman, Lucky – such a name! – who I think was a cousin of his first wife, came out here and joined them and I think did some work with him on flowers or butterflies or whatever it was. And people talked a lot because they got on so well together – if you know what I mean.'

'People do *notice* things so much, don't they?' said Miss Marple.

'And then of course, when his wife died rather suddenly –'

'She died here, on this island?'

'No. No, I think they were in Martinique or Tobago at the time.'

'I see.'

'But I gathered from some other people who were there at the time, and who came on here and talked about things, that the doctor wasn't very satisfied.'

'Indeed,' said Miss Marple, with interest.

'It was only *gossip*, of course, but – well, Mr Dyson certainly married again *very quickly.*' She lowered her voice again. 'Only a *month* I believe.'

'Only a month,' said Miss Marple.

The two women looked at each other. 'It seemed – unfeeling,' said Miss Prescott.

'Yes,' said Miss Marple. 'It certainly did.' She added delicately, 'Was there – any money?'

'I don't really know. He makes his little joke – perhaps you've heard him – about his wife being his "lucky piece" –'

'Yes, I've heard him,' said Miss Marple.

'And some people think that means that he was lucky to marry a rich wife. Though, of course,' said Miss Prescott with the air of one being entirely fair, 'she's very good-looking too, if you care for that type. And I think myself that it was the *first* wife who had the money.'

'Are the Hillingdons well off?'

'Well, I think they're *well off.* I don't mean fabulously rich, I just mean well off. They have two boys at public school and a very nice place in England, I believe, and they travel most of the winter.'

The Canon appearing at this moment to suggest a brisk walk, Miss Prescott rose to join her brother. Miss Marple remained sitting there.

A few minutes later Gregory Dyson passed her striding along towards the hotel. He waved a cheerful hand as he passed.

'Penny for your thoughts,' he called out.

Miss Marple smiled gently, wondering how he would have reacted if she had replied:

'I was wondering if you were a murderer.'

It really seemed most probable that he was. It all fitted in so nicely – This story about the death of the first Mrs Dyson – Major Palgrave had certainly been talking about a wife killer – with special reference to the 'Brides in the Bath Case'.

Yes – it fitted – the only objection was that it fitted almost too well. But Miss Marple reproved herself for this thought – who was she to demand Murders Made to Measure?

A voice made her jump – a somewhat raucous one.

'Seen Greg any place, Miss – er –'

Lucky, Miss Marple thought, was not in a good temper.

'He passed by just now – going towards the hotel.'

'I'll bet!' Lucky uttered an irritated ejaculation and hurried on.

'Forty, if she's a day, and looks it this morning,' thought Miss Marple.

Pity invaded her – pity for the Luckys of the world – who were so vulnerable to Time –

At the sound of a noise behind her, she turned her chair round –

Mr Rafiel, supported by Jackson, was making his morning appearance and coming out of his bungalow –

Jackson settled his employer in his wheelchair and fussed round him. Mr Rafiel waved his attendant away impatiently and Jackson went off in the direction of the hotel.

Miss Marple lost no time – Mr Rafiel was never left alone for long – Probably Esther Walters would come and join him. Miss Marple wanted a word alone with Mr Rafiel and now, she thought, was her chance. She would have to be quick about what she wanted to say. There could be no leading up to things. Mr Rafiel was not a man who cared for the idle twittering conversation of old ladies. He would probably retreat again into his bungalow, definitely regarding himself the victim of persecution. Miss Marple decided to plump for downrightness.

She made her way to where he was sitting, drew up a chair, sat down, and said:

'I want to ask you something, Mr Rafiel.'

'All right, all right,' said Mr Rafiel, 'let's have it. What do you want – a subscription, I suppose? Missions in Africa or repairing a church, something of that kind?'

'Yes,' said Miss Marple. 'I am interested in several objects of that nature, and I shall be delighted if you will give me a subscription for them. But that wasn't actually what I was going to ask you. What I was going to ask you was if Major Palgrave ever told you a story about a murder.'

'Oho,' said Mr Rafiel. 'So he told it to you too, did he? And I suppose you fell for it, hook, line and sinker.'

'I didn't really know what to think,' said Miss Marple. 'What exactly did he tell you?'

'He prattled on,' said Mr Rafiel, 'about a lovely creature, Lucrezia Borgia reincarnated. Beautiful, young, golden-haired, everything.'

'Oh,' said Miss Marple slightly taken aback, 'and who did she murder?'

'Her husband, of course,' said Mr Rafiel, 'who do you think?'

'Poison?'

'No, I think she gave him a sleeping draught and then stuck him in a gas oven. Resourceful female. Then she said it was suicide. She got off quite lightly. Diminished responsibility or something. That's what it's called nowadays if you're a good-looking woman, or some miserable young hooligan whose mother's been too fond of him. Bah!'

'Did the Major show you a snapshot?'

'What – a snapshot of the woman? No. Why should he?'

'Oh –' said Miss Marple.

She sat there, rather taken aback. Apparently Major Palgrave spent his life telling people not only about tigers he had shot and elephants he had hunted but also about murderers he had met. Perhaps he had a whole repertoire of murder stories. One had to face it – She was startled by Mr Rafiel suddenly giving a roar of 'Jackson!' There was no response.

'Shall I find him for you?' said Miss Marple rising.

'You won't find him. Tom-catting somewhere, that's what he does. No good, that fellow. Bad character. But he suits me all right.'

'I'll go and look for him,' said Miss Marple.

Miss Marple found Jackson sitting on the far side of the hotel terrace having a drink with Tim Kendal.

'Mr Rafiel is asking for you,' she said.

Jackson made an expressive grimace, drained his glass, and rose to his feet.

'Here we go again,' he said. 'No peace for the wicked – Two telephone calls and a special diet order – I thought that might give me a quarter of an hour's alibi – Apparently not! Thank you, Miss Marple. Thanks for the drink, Mr Kendal.'

He strode away.

'I feel sorry for that chap,' said Tim. 'I have to stand him a drink now and then, just to cheer him up – Can I offer you something, Miss Marple – How about fresh lime? I know you're fond of that.'

'Not just now, thank you – I suppose looking after someone like Mr Rafiel must always be rather exacting. Invalids are frequently difficult –'

'I didn't mean only that – It's very well paid and you expect to put up with a good deal of crotchetiness – old Rafiel's not really a bad sort. I mean more that –' he hesitated.

Miss Marple looked inquiring.

'Well – how shall I put it – it's difficult for him socially. People are so damned snobbish – there's no one here of his class. He's better than a servant – and below the average visitor – or they think he is. Rather like the Victorian governess. Even the secretary woman, Mrs Walters – feels she's a cut above him. Makes things difficult.' Tim paused, then said with feeling: 'It's really awful the amount of social problems there are in a place like this.'

Dr Graham passed them – he had a book in his hand. He went and sat at a table overlooking the sea.

'Dr Graham looks rather worried,' remarked Miss Marple.

'Oh! We're all worried.'

'You too? Because of Major Palgrave's death?'

'I've left off worrying about that. People seem to have forgotten it – taken it in their stride. No – it's my wife – Molly – Do you know anything about dreams?'

'Dreams?' Miss Marple was surprised.

'Yes – bad dreams – nightmares, I suppose. Oh, we all get that sort of thing sometimes. But Molly – she seems to have them nearly all the time. They frighten her. Is there anything one can do about them? Take for them? She's got some sleeping pills, but she says they make it worse – she struggles to wake up and can't.'

'What are the dreams about?'

'Oh, something or someone chasing her – Or watching her and spying on her – she can't shake off the feeling even when she's awake.'

'Surely a doctor –'

'She's got a thing against doctors. Won't hear of it – Oh well – I dare say it will all pass off – But we were so happy. It was all such fun – And now, just lately – Perhaps old Palgrave's death upset her. She seems like a different person since...'

He got up.

'Must get on with the daily chores – are you sure you won't have that fresh lime?'

Miss Marple shook her head.

She sat there, thinking. Her face was grave and anxious.

She glanced over at Dr Graham.

Presently she came to a decision.

She rose and went across to his table.

'I have got to apologise to you, Dr Graham,' she said.

'Indeed?' The doctor looked at her in kindly surprise. He pulled forward a chair and she sat down.

'I am afraid I have done the most disgraceful thing,' said Miss Marple. 'I told you, Dr Graham, a deliberate lie.'

She looked at him apprehensively.

Dr Graham did not look at all shattered, but he did look a little surprised.

'Really?' he said. 'Ah well, you mustn't let that worry you too much.'

What had the dear old thing been telling lies about, he wondered; her age? Though as far as he could remember she hadn't mentioned her age. 'Well, let's hear about it,' he said, since she clearly wished to confess.

'You remember my speaking to you about a snapshot of my nephew, one that I showed to Major Palgrave, and that he didn't give back to me?'

'Yes, yes, of course I remember. Sorry we couldn't find it for you.'

'There wasn't any such thing,' said Miss Marple, in a small frightened voice.

'I beg your pardon?'

'There wasn't any such thing. I made up that story, I'm afraid.'

'You made it up?' Dr Graham looked slightly annoyed. 'Why?'

Miss Marple told him. She told him quite clearly, without twittering. She told him about Major Palgrave's murder story and how he'd been about to show her this particular snapshot and his sudden confusion and then she went on to her own anxiety and to her final decision to try somehow to obtain a view of it.

'And really, I couldn't see any way of doing so without telling you something that was quite untrue,' she said, 'I do hope you will forgive me.'

'You thought that what he had been about to show you was a picture of a murderer?'

'That's what he said it was,' said Miss Marple. 'At least he said it was given him by this acquaintance who had told him the story about a man who was a murderer.'

'Yes, yes. And – excuse me – you believed him?'

'I don't know if I really believed him or not at the time,' said Miss Marple. 'But then, you see, the next day he died.'

'Yes,' said Dr Graham, struck suddenly by the clarity of that one sentence. *The next day he died...*

'And the snapshot had disappeared.'

Dr Graham looked at her. He didn't know quite what to say.

'Excuse me, Miss Marple,' he said at last, 'but is what you're telling me now – is it really true this time?'

'I don't wonder your doubting me,' said Miss Marple. 'I should, in your place. Yes, it is true what I am telling you now, but I quite realise that you have only my word for it. Still, even if you don't believe me, I thought I ought to tell you.'

'Why?'

'I realised that you ought to have the fullest information possible – in case –'

'In case what?'

'In case you decided to take any steps about it.'

Chapter Ten

A Decision In Jamestown

Dr Graham was in Jamestown, in the Administrator's office, sitting at a table opposite his friend Daventry, a grave young man of thirty-five.

'You sounded rather mysterious on the phone, Graham,' said Daventry. 'Anything special the matter?'

'I don't know,' said Dr Graham, 'but I'm worried.'

Daventry looked at the other's face, then he nodded as drinks were brought in. He spoke lightly of a fishing expedition he had made lately. Then when the servant had gone away, he sat back in his chair and looked at the other man.

'Now then,' he said, 'let's have it.'

Dr Graham recounted the facts that had worried him. Daventry gave a slow long whistle.

'I see. You think maybe there's something funny about old Palgrave's death? You're no longer sure that it was just natural causes? Who certified the death? Robertson, I suppose. He didn't have any doubts, did he?'

'No, but I think he may have been influenced in giving the certificate by the fact of the Serenite tablets in the bathroom. He asked me if Palgrave had mentioned that he suffered from hypertension, and I said No, I'd never had any medical conversation with him myself, but apparently he had talked about it to other people in the hotel. The whole thing – the bottle of tablets, and what Palgrave had said to people – it all fitted in – no earthly reason to suspect anything else. It was a perfectly natural inference to make – but I think now it may not have been

71

correct. If it had been my business to give the certificate, I'd have given it without a second thought. The appearances are quite consistent with his having died from that cause. I'd never have thought about it since if it hadn't been for the odd disappearance of that snapshot…'

'But look here, Graham,' said Daventry, 'if you will allow me to say so, aren't you relying a little too much on a rather fanciful story told you by an elderly lady? You know what these elderly ladies are like. They magnify some small detail and work the whole thing up.'

'Yes, I know,' said Dr Graham, unhappily. 'I know that. I've said to myself that it may be so, that it probably *is* so. But I can't quite convince myself. She was so very clear and detailed in her statement.'

'The whole thing seems wildly improbable to me,' said Daventry. 'Some old lady tells a story about a snapshot that ought not to be there – no, I'm getting mixed myself – I mean the other way about, don't I? – but the only thing you've really got to go on is that a chambermaid says that a bottle of pills which the authorities had relied on for evidence, wasn't in the Major's room the day before his death. But there are a hundred explanations for that. He might always have carried those pills about in his pocket.'

'It's possible, I suppose, yes.'

'Or the chambermaid may have made a mistake and she simply hadn't noticed them before –'

'That's possible, too.'

'Well, then.'

Graham said slowly:

'The girl was very positive.'

'Well, the St Honoré people are very excitable. You know. Emotional. Work themselves up easily. Are you thinking that she knows – a little more than she has said?'

'I think it might be so,' said Dr Graham slowly.

'You'd better try and get it out of her, if so. We don't want to make an unnecessary fuss – unless we've something definite to go on. If he didn't die of blood pressure, what do you think it was?'

'There are too many things it might be nowadays,' said Dr Graham.

'You mean things that don't leave recognisable traces?'

'Not everyone,' said Dr Graham dryly, 'is so considerate as to use arsenic.'

'Now let's get things quite clear – what's the suggestion? That a bottle of pills was substituted for the real ones? And that Major Palgrave was poisoned in that way?'

'No – it's not like that. That's what the girl – Victoria Something thinks – But she's got it all wrong – If it was decided to get rid of the Major – quickly – he would have been given something – most likely in a drink of some kind. Then to make it appear a natural death, a bottle of the tablets prescribed to relieve blood pressure was put in his room. And the rumour was put about that he suffered from high blood pressure.'

'Who put the rumour about?'

'I've tried to find out – with no success – It's been too cleverly done. A says "I *think* B told me" – B, asked, says "No, I didn't say so but I do remember C mentioning it one day." C says "Several people talked about it – one of them, I think, was A." And there we are, back again.'

'Someone was clever?'

'Yes. As soon as the death was discovered, everybody seemed to be talking about the Major's high blood pressure and repeating round what other people had said.'

'Wouldn't it have been simpler just to poison him and let it go at that?'

'No. That might have meant an inquiry – possibly an autopsy – This way, a doctor would accept the death and give a certificate – as he did.'

'What do you want me to do? Go to the CID? Suggest they dig the chap up? It'd make a lot of stink –'

'It could be kept quite quiet.'

'Could it? In St Honoré? Think again! The grapevine would be on to it before it had happened. All the same,' Daventry sighed – 'I suppose we'll have to do something. But if you ask me, it's all a mare's nest!'

'I devoutly hope it is,' said Dr Graham.

Chapter Eleven

Evening at the Golden Palm

I

Molly rearranged a few of the table decorations in the dining-room, removed an extra knife, straightened a fork, reset a glass or two, stood back to look at the effect and then walked out on to the terrace outside. There was no one about just at present and she strolled to the far corner and stood by the balustrade. Soon another evening would begin. Chattering, talking, drinking, all so gay and carefree, the sort of life she had longed for and, up to a few days ago, had enjoyed so much. Now even Tim seemed anxious and worried. Natural, perhaps, that he should worry a little. It was important that this venture of theirs should turn out all right. After all, he had sunk all he had in it.

But that, thought Molly, is not *really* what's worrying him. It's *me*. But I don't see, said Molly to herself, why he should worry about *me*. Because he did worry about her. That she was quite sure of. The questions he put, the quick nervous glance he shot at her from time to time. 'But why?' thought Molly. 'I've been very careful.' She summed up things in her mind. She didn't understand it really herself. She couldn't remember when it had begun. She wasn't even very sure what it was. She'd begun to be frightened of people. She didn't know why. What could they do to her? What should they want to do to her?

She nodded her head, then started violently as a hand touched her arm. She spun round to find Gregory Dyson, slightly taken aback, looking apologetic.

'Ever so sorry. Did I startle you, little girl?'

Molly hated being called 'little girl'. She said quickly and brightly: 'I didn't hear you coming, Mr Dyson, so it made me jump.'

'Mr Dyson? We're very formal tonight. Aren't we all one great happy family here? Ed and me and Lucky and Evelyn and you and Tim and Esther Walters and old Rafiel. All the lot of us one happy family.'

'He's had plenty to drink already,' thought Molly. She smiled at him pleasantly.

'Oh! I come over the heavy hostess sometimes,' she said, lightly. 'Tim and I think it's more polite not to be too handy with Christian names.'

'Aw! we don't want any of that stuffed-shirt business. Now then, Molly my lovely, have a drink with me.'

'Ask me later,' said Molly. 'I have a few things to get on with.'

'Now don't run away.' His arm fastened round her arm. 'You're a lovely girl, Molly. I hope Tim appreciates his good luck.'

'Oh, I see to it that he does,' said Molly cheerfully.

'I could go for you, you know, in a big way.' He leered at her – 'though I wouldn't let my wife hear me say so.'

'Did you have a good trip this afternoon?'

'I suppose so. Between you and me I get a bit fed up sometimes. You can get tired of the birds and butterflies. What say you and I go for a little picnic on our own one day?'

'We'll have to see about that,' said Molly gaily. 'I'll be looking forward to it.'

With a light laugh she escaped, and went back into the bar.

'Hallo, Molly,' said Tim, 'you seem in a hurry. Who's that you've been with out there?'

He peered out.

'Gregory Dyson.'

'What does he want?'

'Wanted to make a pass at me,' said Molly.

'Blast him,' said Tim.

'Don't worry,' said Molly, 'I can do all the blasting necessary.'

Tim started to answer her, caught sight of Fernando and went over to him shouting out some directions. Molly slipped away through the kitchen door and down the steps to the beach.

Gregory Dyson swore under his breath. Then he walked slowly back in the direction of his bungalow. He had nearly got there when a voice spoke to him from the shadow of one of the bushes. He turned his head, startled. In the gathering dusk he thought for a moment that it was a ghostly figure that stood there. Then he laughed. It had looked like a faceless apparition but that was because, though the dress was white, the face was black.

Victoria stepped out of the bushes on to the path.

'Mr Dyson, please?'

'Yes. What is it?'

Ashamed of being startled, he spoke with a touch of impatience.

'I brought you this, sir.' She held out her hand. In it was a bottle of tablets. 'This belongs to you, doesn't it? Yes?'

'Oh, my bottle of Serenite tablets. Yes, of course. Where did you find it?'

'I found it where it had been put. In the gentleman's room.'

'What do you mean – in the gentleman's room?'

'The gentleman who is dead,' she added gravely. 'I do not think he sleeps very well in his grave.'

'Why the devil not?' asked Dyson.

Victoria stood looking at him.

'I still don't know what you're talking about. You mean you found this bottle of tablets in Major Palgrave's bungalow?'

'That's right, yes. After the doctor and the Jamestown people go away, they give me all the things in his bathroom to throw away. The toothpaste and the lotions, and all the other things – including this.'

'Well, why didn't you throw it away?'

'Because these are yours. You missed them. You remember, you asked about them?'

'Yes – well – yes, I did. I – I thought I'd just mislaid them.'

'No, you did not mislay them. They were taken from your

bungalow and put in Major Palgrave's bungalow.'

'How do you know?' He spoke roughly.

'I know. I saw.' She smiled at him in a sudden flash of white teeth. 'Someone put them in the dead gentleman's room. Now I give them back to you.'

'Here – wait. What do you mean? What – who did you see?'

She hurried away, back into the darkness of the bushes. Greg made as to move after her and then stopped. He stood stroking his chin.

'What's the matter, Greg? Seen a ghost?' asked Mrs Dyson, as she came along the path from their bungalow.

'Thought I had for a minute or two.'

'Who was that you were talking to?'

'The coloured girl who does our place. Victoria, her name is, isn't it?'

'What did she want? Making a pass at you?'

'Don't be stupid, Lucky. That girl's got some idiotic idea into her head.'

'Idea about what?'

'You remember I couldn't find my Serenite the other day?'

'You said you couldn't.'

'What do you mean "I said I couldn't"?'

'Oh, for heck's sake, have you got to take me up on everything?'

'I'm sorry,' said Greg. 'Everybody goes about being so damn' mysterious.' He held out his hand with the bottle in it. 'That girl brought them back to me.'

'Had she pinched them?'

'No. She – found them somewhere I think.'

'Well, what of it? What's the mystery about?'

'Oh, nothing,' said Greg. 'She just riled me, that's all.'

'Look here, Greg, what is this stuff all about? Come along and have a drink before dinner.'

II

Molly had gone down to the beach. She pulled out one of the old basket chairs, one of the more rickety ones that were seldom used. She sat in it for a while looking at the sea, then suddenly she dropped her head in her hands and burst into tears. She sat there sobbing unrestrainedly for some time. Then she heard a rustle close by her and glanced up sharply to see Mrs Hillingdon looking down at her.

'Hallo, Evelyn, I didn't hear you. I – I'm sorry.'

'What's the matter, child?' said Evelyn. 'Something gone wrong?' She pulled another chair forward and sat down. 'Tell me.'

'There's nothing wrong,' said Molly. 'Nothing at all.'

'Of course there is. You wouldn't sit and cry here for nothing. Can't you tell me? Is it – some trouble between you and Tim?'

'Oh *no.*'

'I'm glad of that. You always look so happy together.'

'Not more than you do,' said Molly. 'Tim and I always think how wonderful it is that you and Edward should seem so happy together after being married so many years.'

'Oh, that,' said Evelyn. Her voice was sharp as she spoke but Molly hardly noticed.

'People bicker so,' she said, 'and have such rows. Even if they're quite fond of each other they still seem to have rows and not to mind a bit whether they have them in public or not.'

'Some people like living that way,' said Evelyn. 'It doesn't really mean anything.'

'Well, I think it's horrid,' said Molly.

'So do I, really,' said Evelyn.

'But to see you and Edward –'

'Oh it's no good, Molly. I can't let you go on thinking things of that kind. Edward and I –' she paused. 'If you want to know the truth, we've hardly said a word to each other in private for the last three years.'

'What!' Molly stared at her, appalled. 'I – I can't believe it.'

'Oh, we both put up quite a good show,' said Evelyn. 'We're neither of us the kind that like having rows in public. And anyway there's nothing really to have a row about.'

'But what went wrong?' asked Molly.

'Just the usual.'

'What do you mean by the usual? Another –'

'Yes, another woman in the case, and I don't suppose it will be difficult for you to guess who the woman is.'

'Do you mean Mrs Dyson – Lucky?'

Evelyn nodded.

'I know they always flirt together a lot,' said Molly, 'but I thought that was just…'

'Just high spirits?' said Evelyn. 'Nothing behind it?'

'But why –' Molly paused and tried again. 'But didn't you – oh I mean, well I suppose I oughtn't to ask.'

'Ask anything you like,' said Evelyn. 'I'm tired of never saying a word, tired of being a well-bred happy wife. Edward just lost his head completely about Lucky. He was stupid enough to come and tell me about it. It made him feel better I suppose. Truthful. Honourable. All that sort of stuff. It didn't occur to him to think that it wouldn't make *me* feel better.'

'Did he want to leave you?'

Evelyn shook her head. 'We've got two children, you know,' she said. 'Children whom we're both very fond of. They're at school in England. We didn't want to break up the home. And then of course, Lucky didn't want a divorce either. Greg's a very rich man. His first wife left a lot of money. So we agreed to live and let live – Edward and Lucky in happy immorality, Greg in blissful ignorance, and Edward and I just good friends.' She spoke with scalding bitterness.

'How – how can you bear it?'

'One gets used to anything. But sometimes –'

'Yes?' said Molly.

'Sometimes I'd like to kill that woman.'

The passion behind her voice startled Molly.

'Don't let's talk any more about me,' said Evelyn. 'Let's talk about you. I want to know what's the matter.'

Molly was silent for some moments and then she said, 'It's only – it's only that I think there's something wrong about me.'

'Wrong? What do you mean?'

Molly shook her head unhappily. 'I'm frightened,' she said. 'I'm terribly frightened.'

'Frightened of what?'

'Everything,' said Molly. 'It's – growing on me. Voices in the bushes, footsteps – or things that people say. As though someone were watching me all the time, spying on me. Somebody hates me. That's what I keep feeling. Somebody hates me.'

'My dear child.' Evelyn was shocked and startled. 'How long has this been going on?'

'I don't know. It came – it started by degrees. And there have been other things too.'

'What sort of things?'

'There are times,' said Molly slowly, 'that I can't account for, that I can't remember.'

'Do you mean you have blackouts – that sort of thing?'

'I suppose so. I mean sometimes it's – oh, say it's five o'clock – and I can't remember anything since about half past one or two.'

'Oh my dear, but that's just that you've been asleep. Had a doze.'

'No,' said Molly, 'it's not like that at all. Because you see, at the end of the time it's not as though I'd just dozed off. I'm in a different *place*. Sometimes I'm wearing different clothes and sometimes I seem to have been doing things – even saying things to people, talked to someone, and not remembering that I've done so.'

Evelyn looked shocked. 'But Molly, my dear, if this is so, then you ought to see a doctor.'

'I won't see a doctor! I don't want to. I wouldn't go *near* a doctor.'

Evelyn looked sharply down into her face, then she took the girl's hand in hers.

'You may be frightening yourself for nothing, Molly. You know there are all kinds of nervous disorders that aren't really serious at all. A doctor would soon reassure you.'

'He mightn't. He might say that there was something really wrong with me.'

'Why should there be anything wrong with you?'

'Because –' Molly spoke and then was silent '– no reason, I suppose,' she said.

'Couldn't your family – haven't you any family, any mother or sisters or someone who could come out here?'

'I don't get on with my mother. I never have. I've got sisters. They're married but I suppose – I suppose they could come if I wanted them. But I don't want them. I don't want anyone – anyone except Tim.'

'Does Tim know about this? Have you told him?'

'Not really,' said Molly. 'But he's anxious about me and he watches me. It's as though he were trying to – to help me or to shield me. But if he does that it means I want shielding, doesn't it?'

'I think a lot of it may be imagination but I still think you ought to see a doctor.'

'Old Dr Graham? He wouldn't be any good.'

'There are other doctors on the island.'

'It's all right, really,' said Molly. 'I just – mustn't think of it. I expect, as you say, it's all imagination. Good gracious, it's getting frightfully late. I ought to be on duty now in the dining-room. I – I must go back.'

She looked sharply and almost offensively at Evelyn Hillingdon, and then hurried off. Evelyn stared after her.

CHAPTER TWELVE

OLD SINS CAST LONG SHADOWS

I

'I THINK AS I am on to something, man.'

'What's that you say, Victoria?'

'I think I'm on to something. It may mean money. Big money.'

'Now look, girl, you be careful, you'll not tangle yourself up in something. Maybe I'd better tackle what it is.'

Victoria laughed, a deep rich chuckle.

'You wait and see,' she said. 'I know how to play this hand. It's money, man, it's big money. Something I see, and something I guess. I think I guess right.'

And again the soft rich chuckle rolled out on the night.

II

'Evelyn...'

'Yes?'

Evelyn Hillingdon spoke mechanically, without interest. She did not look at her husband.

'Evelyn, would you mind if we chucked all this and went home to England?'

She had been combing her short dark hair. Now her hands came down from her head sharply. She turned towards him.

'You mean – but we've only just come. We've not been out

here in the islands for more than three weeks.'

'I know. But – would you mind?'

Her eyes searched him incredulously.

'You really want to go back to England? Back home?'

'Yes.'

'Leaving – Lucky?'

He winced.

'You've known all the time, I suppose, that – that it was going on?'

'Pretty well. Yes.'

'You've never said anything.'

'Why should I? We had the whole thing out years ago. Neither of us wanted to make a break. So we agreed to go our separate ways – but keep up the show in public.' Then she added before he could speak, 'But why are you so set on going back to England *now?*'

'Because I'm at breaking point. I can't stick it any longer, Evelyn. I can't.' The quiet Edward Hillingdon was transformed. His hands shook, he swallowed, his calm unemotional face seemed distorted by pain.

'For God's sake, Edward, what's the *matter?*'

'Nothing's the matter except that I want to get out of here –'

'You fell wildly in love with Lucky. And now you've got over it. Is that what you're telling me?'

'Yes. I don't suppose you'll ever feel the same.'

'Oh let's not go into that now! I want to understand what's upsetting you so much, Edward.'

'I'm not particularly upset.'

'But you are. Why?'

'Isn't it obvious?'

'No, it isn't,' said Evelyn. 'Let's put it in plain concrete terms. You've had an affair with a woman. That happens often enough. And now it's over. Or isn't it over? Perhaps it isn't over on *her* side. Is that it? Does Greg know about it? I've often wondered.'

'I don't know,' said Edward. 'He's never said anything. He always seems friendly enough.'

'Men can be extraordinarily obtuse,' said Evelyn thoughtfully. 'Or else – Perhaps Greg has got an outside interest of his own!'

'He's made passes at you, hasn't he?' said Edward. 'Answer me – I know he has –'

'Oh yes,' said Evelyn, carelessly, 'but he makes passes at everyone. That's just Greg. It doesn't ever really mean much, I imagine. It's just part of the Greg he-man act.'

'Do you care for him, Evelyn? I'd rather know the truth.'

'Greg? I'm quite fond of him – he amuses me. He's a good friend.'

'And that's all? I wish I could believe you.'

'I can't really see how it can possibly matter to you,' said Evelyn dryly.

'I suppose I deserve that.'

Evelyn walked to the window, looked out across the veranda and came back again.

'I wish you would tell me what's *really* upsetting you, Edward.'

'I've told you.'

'I wonder.'

'You can't understand, I suppose, how extraordinary a temporary madness of this kind can seem to you after you've got over it.'

'I can try, I suppose. But what's worrying me now is that Lucky seems to have got some kind of stranglehold upon you. She's not just a discarded mistress. She's a tigress with claws. You *must* tell me the truth, Edward. It's the only way if you want me to stand by you.'

Edward said in a low voice: 'If I don't get away from her soon – I shall kill her.'

'Kill Lucky? Why?'

'Because of what she made me do…'

'What did she make you do?'

'I helped her to commit a murder –'

The words were out – There was silence – Evelyn stared at him.

'Do you know what you are saying?'

'Yes. I didn't know I was doing it. There were things she asked me to get for her – at the chemist's. I didn't know – I hadn't the least idea what she wanted them for – She got me to copy out a prescription she had…'

'When was this?'

'Four years ago. When we were in Martinique. When – when Greg's wife –'

'You mean Greg's first wife – Gail? You mean Lucky poisoned her?'

'Yes – and I helped her. When I realised –'

Evelyn interrupted him.

'When you realised what had happened, Lucky pointed out to you that *you* had written out the prescription, that *you* had got the drugs, that you and she were in it together? Is that right?'

'Yes. She said she had done it out of pity – that Gail was suffering – that she had begged Lucky to get something that would end it all.'

'A mercy killing! I see. And you believed *that?*'

Edward Hillingdon was silent a moment – then he said:

'No – I didn't really – not deep down – I accepted it because I *wanted* to believe it – because I was infatuated with Lucky.'

'And afterwards – when she married Greg – did you still believe it?'

'I'd made myself believe it by then.'

'And Greg – how much did he know about it all?'

'Nothing at all.'

'That I find hard to believe!'

Edward Hillingdon broke out –

'Evelyn, I've *got* to get free of it all! That woman taunts me still with what I did. She knows I don't care for her any longer. Care for her? – I've come to hate her – But she makes me feel I'm tied to her – by the thing we did together –'

Evelyn walked up and down the room – then she stopped and faced him.

'The entire trouble with you, Edward, is that you are ridiculously sensitive – and also incredibly suggestible. That devil of a woman has got you just where she wants you by playing on your sense of guilt – And I'll tell you this in plain Bible terms, the guilt that weighs on you is the guilt of adultery – not murder – you were guilt-stricken about your affair with Lucky – and then she made a cat's-paw of you for her murder scheme, and managed to make you feel you shared her guilt. You *don't.*'

'Evelyn...' He stepped towards her –

She stepped back a minute – and looked at him searchingly.

'Is this all true, Edward – *Is* it? Or are you making it up?'

'Evelyn! Why on earth should I do such a thing?'

'I don't know,' said Evelyn Hillingdon slowly – 'It's just perhaps – because I find it hard to trust – anybody. And because – Oh! I don't know – I've got, I suppose, so that I don't know the truth when I hear it.'

'Let's chuck all this – Go back home to England.'

'Yes – We will – But not now.'

'Why not?'

'We must carry on as usual – just for the present. It's important. Do you understand, Edward? Don't let Lucky have an inkling of what we're up to –'

Chapter Thirteen

Exit Victoria Johnson

THE EVENING WAS drawing to a close. The steel band was at last relaxing its efforts. Tim stood by the dining-room looking over the terrace. He extinguished a few lights on tables that had been vacated.

A voice spoke behind him. 'Tim, can I speak to you a moment?'

Tim Kendal started.

'Hallo, Evelyn, is there anything I can do for you?'

Evelyn looked round.

'Come to this table here, and let's sit down a minute.'

She led the way to a table at the extreme end of the terrace. There were no other people near them.

'Tim, you must forgive me talking to you, but I'm worried about Molly.'

His face changed at once.

'What about Molly?' he said stiffly.

'I don't think she's awfully well. She seems upset.'

'Things do seem to upset her rather easily just lately.'

'She ought to see a doctor, I think.'

'Yes, I know, but she doesn't want to. She'd hate it.'

'Why?'

'Eh? What d'you mean?'

'I said why? Why should she hate seeing a doctor?'

'Well,' said Tim rather vaguely, 'people do sometimes, you know. It's – well, it sort of makes them feel frightened about themselves.'

'You're worried about her yourself, aren't you, Tim?'

'Yes. Yes, I am rather.'

'Isn't there anyone of her family who could come out here to be with her?'

'No. That'd make things worse, far worse.'

'What *is* the trouble – with her family, I mean?'

'Oh, just one of those things. I suppose she's just highly strung and – she didn't get on with them – particularly her mother. She never has. They're – they're rather an odd family in some ways and she cut loose from them. Good thing she did, I think.'

Evelyn said hesitantly – 'She seems to have had blackouts, from what she told me, and to be frightened of people. Almost like persecution mania.'

'Don't say that,' said Tim angrily. 'Persecution mania! People always say that about people. Just because she – well – maybe she's a bit nervy. Coming out here to the West Indies. All the dark faces. You know, people are rather queer, sometimes, about the West Indies and coloured people.'

'Surely not girls like Molly?'

'Oh, how does one know the things people are frightened of? There are people who can't be in the room with cats. And other people who faint if a caterpillar drops on them.'

'I hate suggesting it – but don't you think perhaps she ought to see a – well, a psychiatrist?'

'*No!*' said Tim explosively. 'I won't have people like that monkeying about with her. I don't believe in them. They make people worse. If her mother had left psychiatrists alone…'

'So there *was* trouble of that kind in her family – was there? I mean a history of –' she chose the word carefully – 'instability.'

'I don't want to talk about it – I took her away from it all and she was all right, quite all right. She has just got into a nervous state… But these things aren't hereditary. Everybody knows that nowadays. It's an exploded idea. Molly's perfectly sane. It's just that – oh! I believe it was that wretched old Palgrave dying that started it all off.'

'I see,' said Evelyn thoughtfully. 'But there was nothing really to worry anyone in Major Palgrave's death, was there?'

'No, of course there wasn't. But it's a kind of shock when somebody dies suddenly.'

He looked so desperate and defeated that Evelyn's heart smote her. She put her hand on his arm.

'Well, I hope you know what you're doing, Tim, but if I could help in any way – I mean if I could go with Molly to New York – I could fly with her there or Miami or somewhere where she could get really first-class medical advice.'

'It's very good of you, Evelyn, but Molly's all right. She's getting over it, anyway.'

Evelyn shook her head in doubt. She turned away slowly and looked along the line of the terrace. Most people had gone by now to their bungalows. Evelyn was walking towards her table to see if she'd left anything behind there, when she heard Tim give an exclamation. She looked up sharply. He was staring towards the steps at the end of the terrace and she followed his gaze. Then she too caught her breath.

Molly was coming up the steps from the beach. She was breathless with deep, sobbing breaths, her body swayed to and fro as she came, in a curious directionless run. Tim cried:

'*Molly!* What's the matter?'

He ran towards her and Evelyn followed him, Molly was at the top of the steps now and she stood there, both hands behind her back. She said in sobbing breaths:

'I found her... She's there in the bushes... There in the bushes... And look at my hands – look at my *hands*.' She held them out and Evelyn caught her breath as she saw the queer dark stains. They looked dark in the subdued lighting but she knew well enough that their real colour was red.

'What's happened, Molly?' cried Tim.

'Down there,' said Molly. She swayed on her feet. 'In the bushes...'

Tim hesitated, looked at Evelyn, then shoved Molly a little towards Evelyn and ran down the steps. Evelyn put her arm round the girl.

'Come. Sit down, Molly. Here. You'd better have something to drink.'

Molly collapsed in a chair and leaned forward on the table, her forehead on her crossed arm. Evelyn did not question her any more. She thought it better to leave her time to recover.

'It'll be all right, you know,' said Evelyn gently. 'It'll be all right.'

'I don't know,' said Molly. 'I don't know what happened. I don't know anything. I can't remember. I –' she raised her head suddenly. 'What's the matter with me? What's the *matter* with me?'

'It's all right, child. It's all right.'

Tim was coming slowly up the steps. His face was ghastly. Evelyn looked up at him, raising her eyebrows in a query.

'It's one of our girls,' he said. 'What's-her-name – Victoria. Somebody's put a knife in her.'

CHAPTER FOURTEEN

INQUIRY

I

MOLLY LAY ON her bed. Dr Graham and Dr Robertson, the West Indian police doctor, stood on one side – Tim on the other. Robertson had his hand on Molly's pulse – He nodded to the man at the foot of the bed, a slender dark man in police uniform, Inspector Weston of the St Honoré Police Force.

'A bare statement – no more,' the doctor said.

The other nodded.

'Now, Mrs Kendal – just tell us how you came to find this girl.'

For a moment or two it was as though the figure on the bed had not heard. Then she spoke in a faint, faraway voice.

'In the bushes – white…'

'You saw something white – and you looked to see what it was? Is that it?'

'Yes – white – lying there – I tried – tried to lift – she it – blood – blood all over my hands.'

She began to tremble.

Dr Graham shook his head at them. Robertson whispered – 'She can't stand much more.'

'What were you doing on the beach path, Mrs Kendal?'

'Warm – nice – by the sea –'

'You knew who the girl was?'

'Victoria – nice – nice girl – laughs – she used to laugh – oh! and now she won't – She won't ever laugh again. I'll never forget it – I'll never forget it –' Her voice rose hysterically.

'Molly – don't.' It was Tim.

'Quiet – Quiet –' Dr Robertson spoke with a soothing authority – 'Just relax – relax – Now just a small prick –' He withdrew the hypodermic.

'She'll be in no fit condition to be questioned for at least twenty-four hours,' he said – 'I'll let you know when.'

II

The big handsome negro looked from one to the other of the men sitting at the table.

'Ah declare to God,' he said. 'That's all Ah know. Ah don't know nothing but what Ah've told you.'

The perspiration stood out on his forehead. Daventry sighed. The man presiding at the table, Inspector Weston of the St Honoré CID, made a gesture of dismissal. Big Jim Ellis shuffled out of the room.

'It's not all he knows, of course,' Weston said. He had the soft Island voice. 'But it's all we shall learn from him.'

'You think he's in the clear himself?' asked Daventry.

'Yes. They seem to have been on good terms together.'

'They weren't married?'

A faint smile appeared on Lieutenant Weston's lips. 'No,' he said, 'they weren't married. We don't have so many marriages on the Island. They christen the children, though. He's had two children by Victoria.'

'Do you think he was in it, whatever it was, with her?'

'Probably not. I think he'd have been nervous of anything of that kind. And I'd say, too, that what she did know wasn't very much.'

'But enough for blackmail?'

'I don't know that I'd even call it that. I doubt if the girl would even understand that word. Payment for being discreet isn't thought of as blackmail. You see, some of the people who stay here are the rich playboy lot and their morals won't bear much investigation.' His voice was slightly scathing.

'We get all kinds, I agree,' said Daventry. 'A woman, maybe, doesn't want it known that she's sleeping around, so she gives a present to the girl who waits on her. It's tacitly understood that the payment's for discretion.'

'Exactly.'

'But this,' objected Daventry, 'wasn't anything of *that* kind. It was murder.'

'I should doubt, though, if the girl knew it was serious. She saw something, some puzzling incident, something to do presumably with this bottle of pills. It belonged to Mr Dyson, I understand. We'd better see him next.'

Gregory came in with his usual hearty air.

'Here I am,' he said, 'what can I do to help? Too bad about this girl. She was a nice girl. We both liked her, I suppose it was some sort of quarrel or other with a man, but she seemed quite happy and no signs of being in trouble about anything. I was kidding her only last night.'

'I believe you take a preparation, Mr Dyson, called Serenite?'

'Quite right. Little pink tablets.'

'You have them on prescription from a physician?'

'Yes. I can show it to you if you like. Suffer a bit from high blood pressure, like so many people do nowadays.'

'Very few people seem to be aware of that fact.'

'Well, I don't go talking about it. I – well, I've always been well and hearty and I never like people who talk about their ailments all the time.'

'How many of the pills do you take?'

'Two, three times a day.'

'Do you have a fairly large stock with you?'

'Yes. I've got about half a dozen bottles. But they're locked up, you know, in a suitcase. I only keep out one, the one that's in current use.'

'And you missed this bottle a short time ago, so I hear?'

'Quite right.'

'And you asked this girl, Victoria Johnson, whether she'd seen it?'

'Yes, I did.'

'And what did she say?'

'She said the last time she'd seen it was on the shelf in our bathroom. She said she'd looked around.'

'And after that?'

'She came and returned the bottle to me some time later. She said was this the bottle that was missing?'

'And you said?'

'I said "That's it, all right, where did you find it?" and she said it was in old Major Palgrave's room. I said "How on earth did it get there?"'

'And what did she answer to that?'

'She said she didn't know, but –' he hesitated.

'Yes, Mr Dyson?'

'Well, she gave me the feeling that she did know a little more than she was saying, but I didn't pay much attention. After all, it wasn't very important. As I say, I've got other bottles of the pills with me. I thought perhaps I'd left it around in the restaurant or somewhere and old Palgrave picked it up for some reason. Perhaps he put it in his pocket meaning to return it to me, then forgot.'

'And that's all you know about it, Mr Dyson?'

'That's all I know. Sorry to be so unhelpful. Is it important? Why?'

Weston shrugged his shoulders. 'As things are, anything may be important.'

'I don't see where pills come in. I thought you'd want to know about what my movements were when this wretched girl was stabbed. I've written them all down as carefully as I can.'

Weston looked at him thoughtfully.

'Indeed? That was very helpful of you, Mr Dyson.'

'Save everybody trouble, I thought,' said Greg. He shoved a piece of paper across the table.

Weston studied it and Daventry drew his chair a little closer and looked over his shoulder.

'That seems very clear,' said Weston, after a moment or two.

'You and your wife were together changing for dinner in your bungalow until ten minutes to nine. You then went along to the terrace where you had drinks with Señora de Caspearo. At quarter past nine Colonel and Mrs Hillingdon joined you and you went in to dine. As far as you can remember, you went off to bed at about half past eleven.'

'Of course,' said Greg, 'I don't know what time the girl was actually killed –?'

There was a faint semblance of a question in the words. Lieutenant Weston, however, did not appear to notice it.

'Mrs Kendal found her, I understand? Must have been a very nasty shock for her.'

'Yes. Dr Robertson had to give her a sedative.'

'This was quite late, wasn't it, when most people had trundled off to bed?'

'Yes.'

'Had she been dead long? When Mrs Kendal found her, I mean?'

'We're not quite certain of the exact time yet,' said Weston smoothly.

'Poor little Molly. It must have been a nasty shock for her. Matter of fact, I didn't notice *her* about last night. Thought she might have had a headache or something and was lying down.'

'When was the last time you *did* see Mrs Kendal?'

'Oh, quite early, before I went to change. She was playing about with some of the table decorations and things. Rearranging the knives.'

'I see.'

'She was quite cheerful then,' said Greg. 'Kidding and all that. She's a great girl. We're all very fond of her. Tim's a lucky fellow.'

'Well, thank you, Mr Dyson. You can't remember anything more than you've told us about what the girl Victoria said when she returned the tablets?'

'No… It was just as I say. Asked me were these the tablets I'd been asking for. Said she'd found them in old Palgrave's room.'

'She'd no idea who put them there?'

'Don't think so – can't remember, really.'

'Thank you, Mr Dyson.'

Gregory went out.

'Very thoughtful of him,' said Weston, gently tapping the paper with his fingernail, 'to be so anxious to want us to know for sure exactly where he was last night.'

'A little over-anxious do you think?' asked Daventry.

'That's very difficult to tell. There are people, you know, who are naturally nervous about their own safety, about being mixed up with anything. It isn't necessarily because they have any guilty knowledge. On the other hand it might be just that.'

'What about opportunity? Nobody's really got much of an alibi, what with the band and the dancing and the coming and going. People are getting up, leaving their tables, coming back. Women go to powder their noses. Men take a stroll. Dyson could have slipped away. Anybody could have slipped away. But he does seem rather anxious to prove that *he* didn't.' He looked thoughtfully down at the paper. 'So Mrs Kendal was rearranging knives on the table,' he said. 'I rather wonder if he dragged that in on purpose.'

'Did it sound like it to you?'

The other considered. 'I think it's possible.'

Outside the room where the two men were sitting, a noise had arisen. A high voice was demanding admittance shrilly.

'I've got something to tell. I've got something to tell. You take me in to where the gentlemen are. You take me in to where the policeman is.'

A uniformed policeman pushed open the door.

'It's one of the cooks here,' he said, 'very anxious to see you. Says he's got something you ought to know.'

A frightened dark man in a cook's cap pushed past him and came into the room. It was one of the minor cooks. A Cuban, not a native of St Honoré.

'I tell you something. I tell you,' he said. 'She come through my kitchen, she did, and she had a knife with her. A knife, I tell

97

you. She had a knife in her hand. She come through my kitchen and out the door. Out into the garden. I saw her.'

'Now calm down,' said Daventry, 'calm down. Who are you talking about?'

'I tell you who I'm talking about. I'm talking about the boss's wife. Mrs Kendal. I'm talking about her. She have a knife in her hand and she go out into the dark. Before dinner that was – and *she didn't come back.*'

CHAPTER FIFTEEN

INQUIRY CONTINUED

I

'CAN WE HAVE a word with you, Mr Kendal?'

'Of course.' Tim looked up from his desk. He pushed some papers aside and indicated chairs. His face was drawn and miserable. 'How are you getting on? Got any forwarder? There seems to be a doom in this place. People are wanting to leave, you know, asking about air passages. Just when it seemed everything was being a success. Oh Lord, you don't know what it means, this place, to me and to Molly. We staked everything on it.'

'It's very hard on you, I know,' said Inspector Weston. 'Don't think that we don't sympathise.'

'If it all could be cleared up quickly,' said Tim. 'This wretched girl Victoria – Oh! I oughtn't to talk about her like that. She was quite a good sort, Victoria was. But – but there must be some quite simple reason, some – kind of intrigue, or love affair she had. Perhaps her husband –'

'Jim Ellis wasn't her husband, and they seemed a settled sort of couple.'

'If it could only be cleared up *quickly*,' said Tim again. 'I'm sorry. You wanted to talk to me about something, ask me something.'

'Yes. It was about last night. According to medical evidence Victoria was killed some time between 10.30 pm and midnight. Alibis under the circumstances that prevail here are not very easy to prove. People are moving about, dancing, walking away from the terrace, coming back. It's all very difficult.'

'I suppose so. But does that mean that you definitely consider Victoria was killed by one of the guests here?'

'Well, we have to examine that possibility, Mr Kendal. What I want to ask you particularly about, is a statement made by one of your cooks.'

'Oh? Which one? What does he say?'

'He's a Cuban, I understand.'

'We've got two Cubans and a Puerto Rican.'

'This man Enrico states that your wife passed through the kitchen on her way from the dining-room, and went out into the garden and that she was carrying a knife.'

Tim stared at him.

'Molly, carrying a knife? Well, why shouldn't she? I mean – why – you don't think – what are you trying to suggest?'

'I am talking of the time before people had come into the dining-room. It would be, I suppose, some time about 8.30. You yourself were in the dining-room talking to the head waiter, Fernando, I believe.'

'Yes.' Tim cast his mind back. 'Yes, I remember.'

'And your wife came in from the terrace?'

'Yes, she did,' Tim agreed. 'She always went out to look over the tables. Sometimes the boys set things wrong, forgot some of the cutlery, things like that. Very likely that's what it was. She may have been rearranging cutlery or something. She might have had a spare knife or a spoon, something like that in her hand.'

'And she came from the terrace into the dining-room. Did she speak to you?'

'Yes, we had a word or two together.'

'What did she say? Can you remember?'

'I think I asked her who she'd been talking to. I heard her voice out there.'

'And who did she say she'd been talking to?'

'Gregory Dyson.'

'Ah, Yes. That is what *he* said.'

Tim went on, 'He'd been making a pass at her, I understand. He was a bit given to that kind of thing. It annoyed me and I said "Blast him" and Molly laughed and said she could do all the blasting that needed to be done. Molly's a very clever girl that way. It's not always an easy position, you know. You can't offend guests, and so an attractive girl like Molly has to pass things off with a laugh and a shrug. Gregory Dyson finds it difficult to keep his hands off any good-looking woman.'

'Had there been an altercation between them?'

'No, I don't think so. I think, as I say, she just laughed it off as usual.'

'You can't say definitely whether she had a knife in her hand or not?'

'I can't remember – I'm almost sure she didn't – in fact quite sure she didn't.'

'But you said just now…'

'Look here, what I meant was that if she was in the dining-room or in the kitchen it's quite likely she might have picked up a knife or had one in her hand. Matter of fact I can remember quite well, she came in from the dining-room and she had *nothing* in her hand. Nothing at all. That's definite.'

'I see,' said Weston.

Tim looked at him uneasily.

'What on earth is this you're getting at? What did that damn' fool Enrico – Manuel – whoever it was – say?'

'He said your wife came out into the kitchen, that she looked upset, that she had a knife in her hand.'

'He's just dramatising.'

'Did you have any further conversation with your wife during dinner or after?'

'No, I don't think I did really. Matter of fact I was rather busy.'

'Was your wife there in the dining-room during the meal?'

'I – oh – yes, we always move about among the guests and things like that. See how things are going on.'

'Did you speak to her at all?'

'No, I don't think I did… We're usually fairly busy. We don't always notice what the other one's doing and we certainly haven't got time to talk to each other.'

'Actually you don't remember speaking to her until she came up the steps three hours later, after finding the body?'

'It was an awful shock for her. It upset her terribly.'

'I know. A very unpleasant experience. How did she come to be walking along the beach path?'

'After the stress of dinner being served, she often does go for a turn. You know, get away from the guests for a minute or two, get a breather.'

'When she came back, I understand you were talking to Mrs Hillingdon.'

'Yes. Practically everyone else had gone to bed.'

'What was the subject of your conversation with Mrs Hillingdon?'

'Nothing particular. Why? What's she been saying?'

'So far she hasn't said anything. We haven't asked her.'

'We were just talking of this and that. Molly, and hotel running, and one thing and another.'

'And then – your wife came up the steps of the terrace and told you what had happened?'

'Yes.'

'There was blood on her hands?'

'Of course there was! She'd been over the girl, tried to lift her, couldn't understand what had happened, what was the matter with her. Of course there was blood on her hands! Look here, what the hell are you suggesting? You *are* suggesting something?'

'Please calm down,' said Daventry. 'It's all a great strain on you I know, Tim, but we have to get the facts clear. I understand your wife hasn't been feeling very well lately?'

'Nonsense – she's all right. Major Palgrave's death upset her a bit. Naturally. She's a sensitive girl.'

'We shall have to ask her a few questions as soon as she's fit enough,' said Weston.

'Well, you can't now. The doctor gave her a sedative and said she wasn't to be disturbed. I won't have her upset and brow-beaten, d'you hear?'

'We're not going to do any brow-beating,' said Weston. 'We've just got to get the facts clear. We won't disturb her at present, but as soon as the doctor allows us, we'll have to see her.' His voice was gentle – inflexible.

Tim looked at him, opened his mouth, but said nothing.

II

Evelyn Hillingdon, calm and composed as usual, sat down in the chair indicated. She considered the few questions asked her, taking her time over it. Her dark, intelligent eyes looked at Weston thoughtfully.

'Yes,' she said, 'I was talking to Mr Kendal on the terrace when his wife came up the steps and told us about the murder.'

'Your husband wasn't there?'

'No, he had gone to bed.'

'Had you any special reason for your conversation with Mr Kendal?'

Evelyn raised her finely pencilled eyebrows – It was a definite rebuke.

She said coldly:

'What a very odd question. No – there was nothing special about our conversation.'

'Did you discuss the matter of his wife's health?'

Again Evelyn took her time.

'I really can't remember,' she said at last.

'Are you sure of that?'

'Sure that I can't remember? What a curious way of putting it – one talks about so many things at different times.'

'Mrs Kendal has not been in good health lately, I understand.'

'She looked quite all right – a little tired perhaps. Of course running a place like this means a lot of worries, and she is quite inexperienced. Naturally, she gets flustered now and then.'

'Flustered.' Weston repeated the word. 'That was the way you would describe it?'

'It's an old-fashioned word, perhaps, but just as good as the modern jargon we use for everything – A "virus infection" for a bilious attack – an "anxiety neurosis" for the minor bothers of daily life –'

Her smile made Weston feel slightly ridiculous. He thought to himself that Evelyn Hillingdon was a clever woman. He looked at Daventry, whose face remained unmoved, and wondered what he thought.

'Thank you, Mrs Hillingdon,' said Weston.

III

'We don't want to worry you, Mrs Kendal, but we have to have your account of just how you came to find this girl. Dr Graham says you are sufficiently recovered to talk about it now.'

'Oh yes,' said Molly, 'I'm really quite all right again.' She gave them a small nervous smile. 'It was just the shock – It *was* rather awful, you know.'

'Yes, indeed it must have been – I understand you went for a walk after dinner.'

'Yes – I often do.'

Her eyes shifted, Daventry noticed, and the fingers of her hands twined and untwined about each other.

'What time would that have been, Mrs Kendal?' asked Weston.

'Well, I don't really know – we don't go much by the time.'

'The steel band was still playing?'

'Yes – at least – I think so – I can't really remember.'

'And you walked – which way?'

'Oh, along the beach path.'

'To the left or the right?'

'Oh! First one way – and then the other – I – I – really didn't notice.'

'Why didn't you notice, Mrs Kendal?'

She frowned.

'I suppose I was – well – thinking of things.'

'Thinking of anything particular?'

'No – No – Nothing particular – Just things that had to be done – seen to – in the hotel.' Again that nervous twining and untwining of fingers. 'And then – I noticed something white – in a clump of hibiscus bushes – and I wondered what it was. I stopped and – and pulled –' She swallowed convulsively – 'And it was her – Victoria – all huddled up – and I tried to raise her head up and I got – blood – on my hands.'

She looked at them and repeated wonderingly as though recalling something impossible:

'Blood – on my hands.'

'Yes – Yes – A very dreadful experience. There is no need for you to tell us more about that part of it – How long had you been walking, do you think, when you found her –'

'I don't know – I have no idea.'

'An hour? Half an hour? Or more than an hour –'

'I don't know,' Molly repeated.

Daventry asked in a quiet everyday voice:

'Did you take a knife with you on your – walk?'

'A knife?' Molly sounded surprised. 'Why should I take a knife?'

'I only ask because one of the kitchen staff mentioned that you had a knife in your hand when you went out of the kitchen into the garden.'

Molly frowned.

'But I didn't go out of the kitchen – oh you mean earlier – before dinner – I – I don't *think* so –'

'You had been rearranging the cutlery on the tables, perhaps.'

'I have to, sometimes. They lay things wrong – not enough knives – or too many. The wrong number of forks and spoons – that sort of thing.'

'So you may have gone out of the kitchen that evening carrying a knife in your hand?'

'I don't think I did – I'm sure I didn't –' She added – 'Tim was there – he would know. Ask him.'

'Did you like this girl – Victoria – was she good at her work?' asked Weston.

'Yes – she was a very nice girl.'

'You had no dispute with her?'

'Dispute? No.'

'She had never threatened you – in any way?'

'Threatened me? What do you mean?'

'It doesn't matter – You have no idea of who could have killed her? No idea at all?'

'None.' She spoke positively.

'Well, thank you, Mrs Kendal.' He smiled. 'It wasn't so terrible, was it?'

'That's all?'

'That's all for now.'

Daventry got up, opened the door for her, and watched her go out.

'Tim would know,' he quoted as he returned to his chair. 'And Tim says definitely that she *didn't* have a knife.'

Weston said gravely:

'I think that that is what any husband would feel called upon to say.'

'A table knife seems a very poor type of knife to use for murder.'

'But it was a *steak* knife, Mr Daventry. Steaks were on the menu that evening. Steak knives are kept sharp.'

'I really can't bring myself to believe that that girl we've just been talking to is a red-handed murderess, Weston.'

'It is not necessary to believe it yet. It could be that Mrs Kendal went out into the garden before dinner, clasping a knife she had taken off one of the tables because it was superfluous – she might not even have noticed she was holding it, and she could have put it down somewhere – or dropped it – It could have been found and used by someone else – I, too, think her an unlikely murderess.'

'All the same,' said Daventry thoughtfully, 'I'm pretty sure she is not telling all she knows. Her vagueness over time is odd – where was she – what was she doing out there? Nobody, so far, seems to have noticed her in the dining-room that evening.'

'The husband was about as usual – but not the wife –'

'You think she went to meet someone – Victoria Johnson?'

'Perhaps – or perhaps she saw whoever it was who did go to meet Victoria.'

'You're thinking of Gregory Dyson?'

'We know he was talking to Victoria earlier – He may have arranged to meet her again later – everyone moved around freely on the terrace, remember – dancing, drinking – in and out of the bar.'

'No alibi like a steel band,' said Daventry wryly.

Chapter Sixteen

Miss Marple seeks Assistance

IF ANYBODY HAD been there to observe the gentle-looking elderly lady who stood meditatively on the loggia outside her bungalow, they would have thought she had nothing more on her mind than deliberation on how to arrange her time that day – An expedition, perhaps, to Castle Cliff – a visit to Jamestown – a nice drive and lunch at Pelican Point – or just a quiet morning on the beach –

But the gentle old lady was deliberating quite other matters – she was in militant mood.

'*Something has got to be done*,' said Miss Marple to herself.

Moreover, she was convinced that there was no time to be lost – There was urgency.

But who was there that she could convince of that fact? Given time, she thought she could find out the truth by herself.

She had found out a good deal. But not enough – not nearly enough. And time was short.

She realised, bitterly, that here on this Paradise of an island, she had none of her usual allies.

She thought regretfully of her friends in England – Sir Henry Clithering – always willing to listen indulgently – his godson Dermot, who in spite of his increased status at Scotland Yard was still ready to believe that when Miss Marple voiced an opinion there was usually something behind it.

But would that soft-voiced native police officer pay any attention to an old lady's urgency? Dr Graham? But Dr Graham was not what she needed – too gentle and hesitant, certainly not a man of quick decisions and rapid actions.

Miss Marple, feeling rather like a humble deputy of the Almighty, almost cried aloud her need in Biblical phrasing.

Who will go for me?

Whom shall I send?

The sound that reached her ears a moment later was not instantly recognised by her as an answer to prayer – far from it – At the back of her mind it registered only as a man possibly calling his dog.

'Hi!'

Miss Marple, lost in perplexity, paid no attention.

'Hi!' The volume thus increased, Miss Marple looked vaguely round.

'HI!' called Mr Rafiel impatiently. He added – 'You there –'

Miss Marple had not at first realised that Mr Rafiel's 'Hi You' was addressed to her. It was not a method that anyone had ever used before to summon her. It was certainly not a gentlemanly mode of address. Miss Marple did not resent it, because people seldom did resent Mr Rafiel's somewhat arbitrary method of doing things. He was a law unto himself and people accepted him as such. Miss Marple looked across the intervening space between her bungalow and his. Mr Rafiel was sitting outside on his loggia and he beckoned her.

'You were calling me?' she asked.

'Of course I was calling you,' said Mr Rafiel. 'Who did you think I was calling – a cat? Come over here.'

Miss Marple looked round for her handbag, picked it up, and crossed the intervening space.

'I can't come to you unless someone helps me,' explained Mr Rafiel, 'so you've got to come to me.'

'Oh yes,' said Miss Marple, 'I quite understand *that*.'

Mr Rafiel pointed to an adjacent chair. 'Sit down,' he said, 'I want to talk to you. Something damned odd is going on in this island.'

'Yes, indeed,' agreed Miss Marple, taking the chair as indicated. By sheer habit she drew her knitting out of her bag.

'Don't start knitting again,' said Mr Rafiel, 'I can't stand it. I hate women knitting. It irritates me.'

Miss Marple returned her knitting to her bag. She did this with no undue air of meekness, rather with the air of one who makes allowances for a fractious patient.

'There's a lot of chit-chat going on,' said Mr Rafiel, 'and I bet you're in the forefront of it. You and the parson and his sister.'

'It is, perhaps, only natural that there should be chit-chat,' said Miss Marple with spirit, 'given the circumstances.'

'This Island girl gets herself knifed. Found in the bushes. *Might* be ordinary enough. That chap she was living with might have got jealous of another man – or he'd got himself another girl and she got jealous and they had a row. Sex in the tropics. That sort of stuff. What do you say?'

'No,' said Miss Marple, shaking her head.

'The authorities don't think so, either.'

'They would say more to you,' pointed out Miss Marple, 'than they would say to me.'

'All the same, I bet you know more about it than I do. You've listened to the tittle-tattle.'

'Certainly I have,' said Miss Marple.

'Nothing much else to do, have you, except listen to tittle-tattle?'

'It is often informative and useful.'

'D'you know,' said Mr Rafiel, studying her attentively. 'I made a mistake about you. I don't often make mistakes about people. There's a lot more to you than I thought there was. All these rumours about Major Palgrave and the stories he told. You think he was bumped off, don't you?'

'I very much fear so,' said Miss Marple.

'Well, he was,' said Mr Rafiel.

Miss Marple drew a deep breath. 'That is definite, is it?' she asked.

'Yes, it's definite enough. I had it from Daventry. I'm not breaking a confidence because the facts of the autopsy will have to come out. You told Graham something, he went to Daventry, Daventry went to the Administrator, the CID were informed, and between them they agreed that things looked fishy, so they dug up old Palgrave and had a look.'

'And they found?' Miss Marple paused interrogatively.

'They found he'd had a lethal dose of something that only a doctor could pronounce properly. As far as I remember it sounds vaguely like di-flor, hexagonalethylcarbenzol. That's not the right name. But that's roughly what it *sounds* like. The police doctor put it that way so that nobody should know, I suppose, what it really *was*. The stuff's probably got some quite simple nice easy name like Evipan or Veronal or Easton's Syrup or something of that kind. This is its official name to baffle laymen with. Anyway, a sizeable dose of it, I gather, would produce death, and the signs would be much the same as those of high blood pressure aggravated by over-indulgence in alcohol on a gay evening. In fact, it all looked perfectly natural and nobody questioned it for a moment. Just said "poor old chap" and buried him quick. Now they wonder if he ever had high blood pressure at all. Did he ever say he had to you?'

'No.'

'Exactly! And yet everyone seems to have taken it as a fact.'

'Apparently he told people he had.'

'It's like seeing ghosts,' said Mr Rafiel. 'You never meet the chap who's seen the ghost himself. It's always the second cousin of his aunt, or a friend, or a friend of a friend. But leave that for a moment. They thought he had blood pressure, because there was a bottle of tablets controlling blood pressure found in his room but – and now we're coming to the point – I gather that this girl who was killed went about saying that that bottle was put there by somebody else, and that *actually* it belonged to that fellow Greg.'

'Mr Dyson *has* got blood pressure. His wife mentioned it,' said Miss Marple.

'So it was put in Palgrave's room to suggest that he suffered from blood pressure and to make his death seem natural.'

'Exactly,' said Miss Marple. 'And the story was put about, very cleverly, that he had frequently mentioned to people that he had high blood pressure. But you know, it's very easy to put about a story. Very easy. I've seen a lot of it in my time.'

'I bet you have,' said Mr Rafiel.

'It only needs a murmur here and there,' said Miss Marple. 'You don't say it of your own knowledge, you just say that Mrs B. told you that Colonel C. told her. It's always at second hand or third hand or fourth hand and it's very difficult to find out who was the original whisperer. Oh yes, it can be done. And the people you say it to go on and repeat it to others as if they know it of their own knowledge.'

'Somebody's been clever,' said Mr Rafiel thoughtfully.

'Yes,' said Miss Marple, 'I think somebody's been quite clever.'

'This girl saw something, or knew something and tried blackmail, I suppose,' said Mr Rafiel.

'She mayn't have thought of it as blackmail,' said Miss Marple. 'In these large hotels, there are often things the maids know that some people would rather not have repeated. And so they hand out a larger tip or a little present of money. The girl possibly didn't realise at first the importance of what she knew.'

'Still, she got a knife in her back all right,' said Mr Rafiel brutally.

'Yes. Evidently, someone couldn't afford to let her talk.'

'Well? Let's hear what you think about it all.'

Miss Marple looked at him thoughtfully.

'Why should you think I know any more than you do, Mr Rafiel?'

'Probably you don't,' said Mr Rafiel, 'but I'm interested to hear your ideas about what you do know.'

'But why?'

'There's not very much to do out here,' said Mr Rafiel, 'except make money.'

Miss Marple looked slightly surprised.

'Make money? Out here?'

'You can send out half a dozen cables in code every day if you like,' said Mr Rafiel. 'That's how I amuse myself.'

'Take-over bids?' Miss Marple asked doubtfully, in the tone of one who speaks a foreign language.

'That kind of thing,' agreed Mr Rafiel. 'Pitting your wits against other people's wits. The trouble is it doesn't occupy enough time, so I've got interested in this business. It's aroused my curiosity. Palgrave spent a good deal of his time talking to you. Nobody else would be bothered with him, I expect. What did be say?'

'He told me a good many stories,' said Miss Marple.

'I know he did. Damn' boring, most of them. And you hadn't only got to hear them once. If you got anywhere within range you heard them three or four times over.'

'I know,' said Miss Marple. 'I'm afraid that does happen when gentlemen get older.'

Mr Rafiel looked at her very sharply.

'I don't tell stories,' he said. 'Go on. It started with one of Palgrave's stories, did it?'

'He said he knew a murderer,' said Miss Marple. 'There's nothing really special about that,' she added in her gentle voice, 'because I suppose it happens to nearly everybody.'

'I don't follow you,' said Mr Rafiel.

'I don't mean specifically,' said Miss Marple, 'but surely, Mr Rafiel, if you cast over in your mind your recollections of various events in your life, hasn't there nearly always been an occasion when somebody has made some careless reference such as "Oh yes I knew the So-and-So's quite well – he died very suddenly and they always say his wife did him in, but I dare say that's just gossip." You've heard people say something like that, haven't you?'

'Well, I suppose so – yes, something of the kind. But not – well, not seriously.'

'Exactly,' said Miss Marple, 'but Major Palgrave was a very serious man. I think he enjoyed telling this story. He said he had a snapshot of the murderer. He was going to show it to me but – actually – he didn't.'

'Why?'

'Because he saw something,' said Miss Marple. 'Saw someone, I suspect. His face got very red and he shoved back the snapshot into his wallet and began talking on another subject.'

'Who did he see?'

'I've thought about that a good deal,' said Miss Marple. 'I was sitting outside my bungalow, and he was sitting nearly opposite me and – whatever he saw, he saw over my right shoulder.'

'Someone coming along the path then from behind you on the right, the path from the creek and the car park –'

'Yes.'

'*Was* anyone coming along the path?'

'Mr and Mrs Dyson and Colonel and Mrs Hillingdon.'

'Anybody else?'

'Not that I can find out. Of course, your bungalow would also be in his line of vision…'

'Ah, Then we include – shall we say – Esther Walters and my chap, Jackson. Is that right? Either of them, I suppose, *might* have come out of the bungalow and gone back inside again without your seeing them.'

'They might have,' said Miss Marple, 'I didn't turn my head at once.'

'The Dysons, the Hillingdons, Esther, Jackson. One of them's a murderer. Or, of course, myself,' he added; obviously as an afterthought.

Miss Marple smiled faintly.

'And he spoke of the murderer as a *man?*'

'Yes.'

'Right. That cuts out Evelyn Hillingdon, Lucky and Esther Walters. So your murderer, allowing that all this far-fetched nonsense is true, your murderer is Dyson, Hillingdon or my smooth-tongued Jackson.'

'Or yourself,' said Miss Marple.

Mr Rafiel ignored this last point.

'Don't say things to irritate me,' he said. 'I'll tell you the first thing that strikes me, and which you don't seem to have thought of. *If* it's one of those three, why the devil didn't old Palgrave recognise him before? Dash it all, they've all been sitting round looking at each other for the last two weeks. That doesn't seem to make sense.'

'I think it could,' said Miss Marple.

'Well, tell me how.'

'You see, in Major Palgrave's story he hadn't seen this man *himself* at any time. It was a story told to him by a doctor. The doctor gave him the snapshot as a curiosity. Major Palgrave may have looked at the snapshot fairly closely at the time but after that he'd just stack it away in his wallet and keep it as a souvenir. Occasionally, perhaps, he'd take it out and show it to someone he was telling the story to. And another thing, Mr Rafiel, we don't know how long ago this happened. He didn't give me any indication of that when he was telling the story. I mean this may have been a story he's been telling to people for *years*. Five years – ten years – longer still perhaps. Some of his tiger stories go back about twenty years.'

'They would!' said Mr Rafiel.

'So I don't suppose for a moment that Major Palgrave would recognise the face in the snapshot if he came across the man casually. What I think happened, what I'm almost sure *must* have happened, is that as he told his story he fumbled for the snapshot, took it out, looked down at it studying the face and then looked up to see *the same face*, or one with a strong resemblance, coming towards him from a distance of about ten or twelve feet away.'

'Yes,' said Mr Rafiel consideringly, 'yes, that's possible.'

'He was taken aback,' said Miss Marple, 'and he shoved it back in his wallet and began to talk loudly about something else.'

'He couldn't have been sure,' said Mr Rafiel, shrewdly.

'No,' said Miss Marple, 'he couldn't have been sure. But of course afterwards he would have studied the snapshot very carefully and would have looked at the man and tried to make up his mind whether it was just a likeness or whether it could actually be the same person.

Mr Rafiel reflected a moment or two, then he shook his head.

'There's something wrong here. The motive's inadequate. Absolutely inadequate. He was speaking to you loudly, was he?'

'Yes,' said Miss Marple, 'quite loudly. He always did.'

'True enough. Yes, he did shout. So whoever was approaching would hear what he said?'

'I should imagine you could hear it for quite a good radius round.'

Mr Rafiel shook his head again. He said, 'It's fantastic, too fantastic. Anybody would laugh at such a story. Here's an old booby telling a story about another story somebody told him, and showing a snapshot, and all of it centring round a murder which had taken place years ago! Or at any rate, a year or two. How on earth can *that* worry the man in question? No evidence, just a bit of hearsay, a story at third hand. He could even admit a likeness, he could say: "Yes, I *do* look rather like that fellow, don't I! Ha, ha!" Nobody's going to take old Palgrave's identification seriously. Don't tell me so, because I won't believe it. No, the chap, if it *was* the chap, had nothing to fear – nothing whatever. It's the kind of accusation he can just laugh off. Why on earth should he proceed to murder old Palgrave? It's absolutely unnecessary. You must see that.'

'Oh I do see that,' said Miss Marple. 'I couldn't agree with you more. That's what makes me uneasy. So very uneasy that I really couldn't sleep last night.'

Mr Rafiel stared at her. 'Let's hear what's on your mind,' he said quietly.

'I may be entirely wrong,' said Miss Marple hesitantly.

'Probably you are,' said Mr Rafiel with his usual lack of courtesy, 'but at any rate let's hear what you've thought up in the small hours.'

'There could be a very powerful motive if –'

'If what?'

'If there was going to be – quite soon – *another murder.*'

Mr Rafiel stared at her. He tried to pull himself up a little in his chair.

'Let's get this clear,' he said.

'I am so bad at explaining.' Miss Marple spoke rapidly and rather incoherently. A pink flush rose to her cheeks. 'Supposing there was a murder planned. If you remember, the story Major Palgrave told me concerned a man whose wife died under suspicious circumstances. Then, after a certain lapse of time, there was another murder under exactly the same circumstances. A man of a different name had a wife who died in much the same way and the doctor who was telling it recognised him as the same man, although he'd changed his name. Well, it does look, doesn't it, as though this murderer might be the kind of murderer who made a habit of the thing?'

'You mean like Smith, Brides in the Bath, that kind of thing. Yes.'

'As far as I can make out,' said Miss Marple, 'and from what I have heard and read, a man who does a wicked thing like this and gets away with it the first time, is, alas, *encouraged*. He thinks it's easy, he thinks he's clever. And so he repeats it. And in the end, as you say, like Smith and the Brides in the Bath, it becomes a *habit*. Each time in a different place and each time the man changes his name. But the crimes themselves are all very much alike. So it seems to me, although I may be quite wrong –'

'But you don't think you are wrong, do you?' Mr Rafiel put in shrewdly.

Miss Marple went on without answering. '– that if that *were* so and if this – this person had got things all lined up for a murder out here, for getting rid of *another* wife, say, and if this is crime three or four, well then, the Major's story *would* matter because the murderer couldn't afford to have any similarity pointed out. If you remember, that was exactly the way Smith got caught. The circumstances of a crime attracted the attention of somebody who compared it with a newspaper clipping of some other case. So you do see, don't you, that if this wicked person has got a crime planned, arranged, and shortly about to take place, he couldn't afford to let Major Palgrave go about telling this story and showing that snapshot.'

She stopped and looked appealingly at Mr Rafiel.

'So you see he had to do something very quickly, as quickly as possible.'

Mr Rafiel spoke. 'In fact, that very same night, eh?'

'Yes,' said Miss Marple.

'Quick work,' said Mr Rafiel, 'but it could be done. Put the tablets in old Palgrave's room, spread the blood pressure rumour about and add a little of our fourteen-syllable drug to a Planters Punch. Is that it?'

'Yes – But that's all over – we needn't worry about it. It's the *future*. It's now. With Major Palgrave out of the way and the snapshot destroyed, *this man will go on with his murder as planned.*'

Mr Rafiel whistled.

'You've got it all worked out, haven't you?'

Miss Marple nodded. She said in a most unaccustomed voice, firm and almost dictatorial, 'And we've got to stop it. *You've* got to stop it, Mr Rafiel.'

'Me?' said Mr Rafiel, astonished, 'Why me?'

'Because you're rich and important,' said Miss Marple, simply. 'People will take notice of what you say or suggest. They wouldn't listen to me for a moment. They would say that I was an old lady imagining things.'

'They might at that,' said Mr Rafiel. 'More fools if they did. I must say, though, that nobody would think you had any brains in your head to hear your usual line of talk. Actually, you've got a logical mind. Very few women have.' He shifted himself uncomfortably in his chair. 'Where the hell's Esther or Jackson?' he said. 'I need resettling. No, it's no good your doing it. You're not strong enough. I don't know what they mean, leaving me alone like this.'

'I'll go and find them.'

'No, you won't. You'll stay here – and thrash this out. Which of them is it? The egregious Greg? The quiet Edward Hillingdon or my fellow Jackson? It's got to be one of the three, hasn't it?'

Chapter Seventeen

Mr Rafiel takes Charge

'I DON'T KNOW,' said Miss Marple.

'What do you mean? What have we been talking about for the last twenty minutes?'

'It has occurred to me that I may have been wrong.'

Mr Rafiel stared at her.

'Scatty after all!' he said disgustedly. 'And you sounded so sure of yourself.'

'Oh, I am sure – about the *murder*. It's the *murderer* I'm not sure about. You see I've found out that Major Palgrave had more than one murder story – you told me yourself he'd told you one about a kind of Lucrezia Borgia –'

'So he did – at that. But that was quite a different kind of story.'

'I know. And Mrs Walters said he had one about someone being gassed in a gas oven –'

'But the story he told you –'

Miss Marple allowed herself to interrupt – a thing that did not often happen to Mr Rafiel.

She spoke with desperate earnestness and only moderate incoherence.

'Don't you see – it's so difficult to be *sure*. The whole point is that – so often – one doesn't *listen*. Ask Mrs Walters – she said the same thing – you listen to begin with – and then your attention flags – your mind wanders – and suddenly you find you've missed a bit. I just wonder if possibly there may have been a gap – a very small one – between the story he was telling me – about a *man* – and the moment when he was getting out his

119

wallet and saying – "Like to see a picture of a murderer."'

'But you thought it was a picture of the man he had been talking about?'

'I thought so – yes. It never occurred to me that it mightn't have been. But now – how can I be *sure?*'

Mr Rafiel looked at her very thoughtfully…

'The trouble with you is,' he said, 'that you're too conscientious. Great mistake – Make up your mind and don't shilly shally. You didn't shilly shally to begin with. If you ask me, in all this chit-chat you've been having with the parson's sister and the rest of them, you've got hold of something that's unsettled you.'

'Perhaps you're right.'

'Well, cut it out for the moment. Let's go ahead with what you had to begin with. Because, nine times out of ten, one's original judgments are right – or so I've found. We've got three suspects. Let's take 'em out and have a good look at them. Any preference?'

'I really haven't,' said Miss Marple, 'all three of them seem so very unlikely.'

'We'll take Greg first,' said Mr Rafiel. 'Can't stand the fellow. Doesn't make him a murderer, though. Still, there *are* one or two points against him. Those blood pressure tablets belonged to him. Nice and handy to make use of.'

'That would be a little obvious, wouldn't it?' Miss Marple objected.

'I don't know that it would,' said Mr Rafiel. 'After all, the main thing was to do something *quickly,* and he'd got the tablets. Hadn't much time to go looking round for tablets that somebody else might have. Let's say it's Greg. All right. *If* he wanted to put his dear wife Lucky out of the way – (Good job, too, I'd say. In fact I'm in sympathy with him.) I can't actually see his motive. From all accounts he's rich. Inherited money from his first wife who had pots of it. He qualifies on that as a possible wife murderer all right. But that's over and done with. He got away with it. But Lucky was his first wife's poor relation. No money there, so if he wants to put *her* out of the way it must be in order to marry somebody else. Any gossip going around about that?'

Miss Marple shook her head.

'Not that I have heard. He – er – has a very gallant manner with *all* the ladies.'

'Well, that's a nice, old-fashioned way of putting it,' said Mr Rafiel. 'All right, he's a stoat. He makes passes. Not enough! We want more than that. Let's go on to Edward Hillingdon. Now there's a dark horse, if ever there was one.'

'He is not, I think, a happy man,' offered Miss Marple.

Mr Rafiel looked at her thoughtfully.

'Do you think a murderer ought to be a happy man?'

Miss Marple coughed.

'Well, they usually have been in my experience.'

'I don't suppose your experience has gone very far,' said Mr Rafiel.

In this assumption, as Miss Marple could have told him, he was wrong. But she forbore to contest his statement. Gentlemen, she knew, did not like to be put right in their facts.

'I rather fancy Hillingdon myself,' said Mr Rafiel. 'I've an idea that there is something a bit odd going on between him and his wife. You noticed it at all?'

'Oh yes,' said Miss Marple, 'I have noticed it. Their behaviour is perfect in public, of course, but that one would expect.'

'You probably know more about those sort of people than I would,' said Mr Rafiel. 'Very well, then, everything is in perfectly good taste but it's a probability that, in a gentlemanly way, Edward Hillingdon is contemplating doing away with Evelyn Hillingdon. Do you agree?'

'If so,' said Miss Marple, 'there must be another woman.'

Miss Marple shook her head in a dissatisfied manner.

'I can't help feeling – I really can't – that it's not all quite as simple as that.'

'Well, who shall we consider next – Jackson? We leave me out of it.'

Miss Marple smiled for the first time.

'And why do we leave you out of it, Mr Rafiel?'

'Because if you want to discuss the possibilities of my being a murderer you'd have to do it with somebody else. Waste of time talking about it to me. And anyway, I ask you, am I cut out for the part? Helpless, hauled out of bed like a dummy, dressed, wheeled about in a chair, shuffled along for a walk. What earthly chance have *I* of going and murdering anyone?'

'Probably as good a chance as anyone else,' said Miss Marple vigorously.

'And how do you make that out?'

'Well, you would agree yourself, I think, that you have brains?'

'Of course I've got brains,' declared Mr Rafiel. 'A good deal more than anybody else in this community, I'd say.'

'And having brains,' went on Miss Marple, 'would enable you to overcome the physical difficulties of being a murderer.'

'It would take some doing!'

'Yes,' said Miss Marple, 'it would take some doing. But then, I think, Mr Rafiel, you would enjoy that.'

Mr Rafiel stared at her for a long time and then he suddenly laughed.

'You've got a nerve!' he said. 'Not quite the gentle fluffy old lady you look, are you? So you really think I'm a murderer?'

'No,' said Miss Marple, 'I do not.'

'And why?'

'Well, really, I think just *because* you have got brains. Having brains, you can get most things you want without having recourse to murder. Murder is stupid.'

'And anyway who the devil should I want to murder?'

'That would be a very interesting question,' said Miss Marple. 'I have not yet had the pleasure of sufficient conversation with you to evolve a theory as to that.'

Mr Rafiel's smile broadened.

'Conversations with you might be dangerous,' he said.

'Conversations are always dangerous, if you have something to hide,' said Miss Marple.

'You may be right. Let's get on to Jackson. What do you think of Jackson?'

'It is difficult for me to say. I have not had the opportunity really of *any* conversation with him.'

'So you've no views on the subject?'

'He reminds me a little,' said Miss Marple reflectively, 'of a young man in the Town Clerk's office near where I live, Jonas Parry.'

'And?' Mr Rafiel asked and paused.

'He was not,' said Miss Marple, 'very satisfactory.'

'Jackson's not wholly satisfactory either. He suits me all right. He's first class at his job, and he doesn't mind being sworn at. He knows he's damn' well paid and so he puts up with things. I wouldn't employ him in a position of trust, but I don't have to trust him. Maybe his past is blameless, maybe it isn't. His references were all right but I discern – shall I say – a note of reserve. Fortunately, I'm not a man who has any guilty secrets, so I'm not a subject for blackmail.'

'No secrets?' said Miss Marple, thoughtfully. 'Surely, Mr Rafiel, you have business secrets?'

'Not where Jackson can get at them. No. Jackson is a smooth article, one might say, but I really don't see him as a murderer. I'd say that wasn't his line at all.'

He paused a minute and then said suddenly, 'Do you know, if one stands back and takes a good look at all this fantastic business, Major Palgrave and his ridiculous stories and all the rest of it, the *emphasis* is entirely wrong. *I'm* the person who ought to be murdered.'

Miss Marple looked at him in some surprise.

'Proper type casting,' explained Mr Rafiel. 'Who's the victim in murder stories? Elderly men with lots of money.'

'And lots of people with a good reason for wishing him out of the way, so as to get that money,' said Miss Marple. 'Is that true also?'

'Well –' Mr Rafiel considered. 'I can count up to five or six men in London who wouldn't burst into tears if they read my obituary in *The Times*. But they wouldn't go so far as to do anything to bring about my demise. After all, why should they?

I'm expected to die any day. In fact the bug – blighters are astonished that I've lasted so long. The doctors are surprised too.'

'You have, of course, a great will to live,' said Miss Marple.

'You think that's odd, I suppose,' said Mr Rafiel.

Miss Marple shook her head.

'Oh no,' she said, 'I think it's quite natural. Life is more worth living, more full of interest when you are likely to lose it. It shouldn't be, perhaps, but it is. When you're young and strong and healthy, and life stretches ahead of you, living isn't really important at all. It's young people who commit suicide easily, out of despair from love, sometimes from sheer anxiety and worry. But old people know how valuable life is and how interesting.'

'Hah!' said Mr Rafiel, snorting. 'Listen to a couple of old crocks.'

'Well, what I said is true, isn't it?' demanded Miss Marple.

'Oh, yes,' said Mr Rafiel, 'it's true enough. But don't you think I'm right when I say that I ought to be cast as the victim?'

'It depends on who has reason to gain by your death,' said Miss Marple.

'Nobody, really,' said Mr Rafiel. 'Apart, as I've said, from my competitors in the business world who, as I have also said, can count comfortably on my being out of it before very long. I'm not such a fool as to leave a lot of money divided up among my relations. Precious little they'd get of it after the Government had taken practically the lot. Oh, no, I've attended to all that years ago. Settlements, trusts and all the rest of it.'

'Jackson, for instance, wouldn't profit by your death?'

'He wouldn't get a penny,' said Mr Rafiel cheerfully. 'I pay him double the salary that he'd get from anyone else. That's because he has to put up with my bad temper; and he knows quite well that he will be the loser when I die.'

'And Mrs Walters?'

'The same goes for Esther. She's a good girl. First-class secretary, intelligent, good-tempered, understands my ways, doesn't turn a hair if I fly off the handle, couldn't care less if I insult her. Behaves like a nice nursery governess in charge of an outrageous and obstreperous child. She irritates me a bit sometimes, but who doesn't? There's nothing outstanding about her. She's rather a commonplace young woman in many ways, but I couldn't have anyone who suited me better. She's had a lot of trouble in her life. Married a man who wasn't much good. I'd say she never had much judgment when it came to men. Some women haven't. They fall for anyone who tells them a hard-luck story. Always convinced that all the man needs is proper female understanding. That, once married to her, he'll pull up his socks and make a go of life! But of course that type of man never does. Anyway, fortunately her unsatisfactory husband died; drank too much at a party one night and stepped in front of a bus. Esther had a daughter to support and she went back to her secretarial job. She's been with me five years. I made it quite clear to her from the start that she need have no expectations from me in the event of my death. I paid her from the start a very large salary, and that salary I've augmented by as much as a quarter as much again each year. However decent and honest people are, one should never trust *anybody* – that's why I told Esther quite clearly that she'd nothing to hope for from my death. Every year I live she'll get a bigger salary. If she puts most of that aside every year – and that's what I think she has done – she'll be quite a well-to-do woman by the time I kick the bucket. I've made myself responsible for her daughter's schooling and I've put a sum in trust for the daughter which she'll get when she comes of age. So Mrs Esther Walters is very comfortably placed. My death, let me tell you, would mean a serious financial loss to her.' He looked very hard at Miss Marple. 'She fully realises all that. She's very sensible, Esther is.'

'Do she and Jackson get on?' asked Miss Marple.

Mr Rafiel shot a quick glance at her.

'Noticed something, have you?' he said. 'Yes, I think Jackson's done a bit of tom-catting around, with an eye in her direction, especially lately. He's a good-looking chap, of course, but he hasn't cut any ice in that direction. For one thing, there's class distinction. She's just a cut above him. Not very much. If she was *really* a cut above him it wouldn't matter, but the lower middle class – they're very particular. Her mother was a school teacher and her father a bank clerk. No, she won't make a fool of herself about Jackson. Dare say he's after her little nest egg, but he won't get it.'

'Hush – she's coming now!' said Miss Marple.

They both looked at Esther Walters as she came along the hotel path towards them.

'She's quite a good-looking girl, you know,' said Mr Rafiel, 'but not an atom of glamour. I don't know why, she's quite nicely turned out.'

Miss Marple sighed, a sigh that any woman will give however old at what might be considered wasted opportunities. What was lacking in Esther had been called by so many names during Miss Marple's span of existence. 'Not really attractive to me.' 'No SA.' 'Lacks Come-hither in her eye.' Fair hair, good complexion, hazel eyes, quite a good figure, pleasant smile, but lacking that something that makes a man's head turn when he passes a woman in the street.

'She ought to get married again,' said Miss Marple, lowering her voice.

'Of course she ought. She'd make a man a good wife.'

Esther Walters joined them and Mr Rafiel said, in a slightly artificial voice:

'So there you are at last! What's been keeping you?'

'Everyone seemed to be sending cables this morning,' said Esther. 'What with that, and people trying to check out –'

'Trying to check out, are they? A result of this murder business?'

'I suppose so. Poor Tim Kendal is worried to death.'

'And well he might be. Bad luck for that young couple, I must say.'

'I know. I gather it was rather a big undertaking for them to take on this place. They've been worried about making a success of it. They were doing very well, too.'

'They were doing a good job,' agreed Mr Rafiel. 'He's very capable and a damned hard worker. She's a very nice girl – attractive too. They've both worked like blacks, though that's an odd term to use out here, for blacks don't work themselves to death at all, so far as I can see. Was looking at a fellow shinning up a coconut tree to get his breakfast, then he goes to sleep for the rest of the day. Nice life.'

He added, 'We've been discussing the murder here.'

Esther Walters looked slightly startled. She turned her head towards Miss Marple.

'I've been wrong about her,' said Mr Rafiel, with characteristic frankness. 'Never been much of a one for the old pussies. All knitting wool and tittle-tattle. But this one's got something. Eyes and ears, and she uses them.'

Esther Walters looked apologetically at Miss Marple, but Miss Marple did not appear to take offence.

'That's really meant to be a compliment, you know,' Esther explained.

'I quite realise that,' said Miss Marple. 'I realise, too, that Mr Rafiel is privileged, or thinks he is.'

'What do you mean – privileged?' asked Mr Rafiel.

'To be rude if you want to be rude,' said Miss Marple.

'Have I been rude?' said Mr Rafiel, surprised. 'I'm sorry if I've offended you.'

'You haven't offended me,' said Miss Marple, 'I make allowances.'

'Now, don't be nasty. Esther, get a chair and bring it here. Maybe you can help.'

Esther walked a few steps to the balcony of the bungalow and brought over a light basket chair.

'We'll go on with our consultation,' said Mr Rafiel. 'We started with old Palgrave, deceased, and his eternal stories.'

'Oh, dear,' sighed Esther. 'I'm afraid I used to escape from him whenever I could.'

'Miss Marple was more patient,' said Mr Rafiel. 'Tell me, Esther, did he ever tell you a story about a murderer?'

'Oh yes,' said Esther. 'Several times.'

'What was it exactly? Let's have *your* recollection.'

'Well –' Esther paused to think. 'The trouble is,' she said apologetically, 'I didn't really listen very closely. You see, it was rather like that terrible story about the lion in Rhodesia which used to go on and on. One did get rather in the habit of not listening.'

'Well, tell us what you *do* remember.'

'I think it arose out of some murder case that had been in the papers. Major Palgrave said that he'd had an experience not every person had had. He'd actually met a murderer face to face.'

'Met?' Mr Rafiel exclaimed. 'Did he actually use the word "met"?'

Esther looked confused.

'I think so.' She was doubtful. 'Or he may have said, "I can point you out a murderer."'

'Well, which was it? There's a difference.'

'I can't really be sure… I *think* he said he'd show me a picture of someone.'

'That's better.'

'And then he talked a lot about Lucrezia Borgia.'

'Never mind Lucrezia Borgia. We know all about her.'

'He talked about poisoners and that Lucrezia was very beautiful and had red hair. He said there were probably far more women poisoners going about the world than anyone knew.'

'That I fear is *quite* likely,' said Miss Marple.

'And he talked about poison being a woman's weapon.'

'Seems to have been wandering from the point a bit,' said Mr Rafiel.

'Well, of course, he always did wander from the point in his stories. And then one used to stop listening and just say "Yes" and "Really?" And "You don't say so".'

'What about this picture he was going to show you?'

'I don't remember. It may have been something he'd seen in the paper –'

'He didn't actually show you a snapshot?'

'A snapshot? No.' She shook her head. 'I'm quite sure of that.

He did say that she was a good-looking woman, and you'd never think she was a murderer to look at her.'

'She?'

'There you are,' exclaimed Miss Marple. 'It makes it all so confusing.'

'He was talking about a woman?' Mr Rafiel asked.

'Oh, yes.'

'The snapshot was a snapshot of a woman?'

'Yes.'

'It can't have been!'

'But it was,' Esther persisted. 'He said "She's here in this island. I'll point her out to you, and then I'll tell you the whole story."'

Mr Rafiel swore. In saying what he thought of the late Major Palgrave he did not mince his words.

'The probabilities are,' he finished, 'that not a word of anything he said was true!'

'One does begin to wonder,' Miss Marple murmured.

'So there we are,' said Mr Rafiel. 'The old booby started telling you hunting tales. Pig sticking, tiger shooting, elephant hunting, narrow escapes from lions. One or two of them might have been fact. Several of them were fiction, and others had happened to somebody else! Then he gets on to the subject of murder and he tells one murder story to cap another murder story. And what's more he tells them all as if they'd happened to *him*. Ten to one most of them were a hash-up of what he'd read in the paper, or seen on TV.'

He turned accusingly on Esther. 'You admit that you weren't listening closely. Perhaps you misunderstood what he was saying.'

'I'm certain he was talking about a woman,' said Esther obstinately, 'because of course I wondered who it was.'

'Who do you think it was?' asked Miss Marple.

Esther flushed and looked slightly embarrassed.

'Oh, I didn't really – I mean, I wouldn't like to –'

Miss Marple did not insist. The presence of Mr Rafiel, she thought, was inimical to her finding out exactly what suppositions Esther Walters had made. That could only be cosily brought out in a *tête-à-tête* between two women. And there was, of course, the possibility that Esther Walters was lying. Naturally, Miss Marple did not suggest this aloud. She registered it as a possibility but she was not inclined to believe in it. For one thing she did not think that Esther Walters was a liar (though one never knew) and for another, she could see no point in such a lie.

'But *you* say,' Mr Rafiel was now turning upon Miss Marple, '*you* say that he told you this yarn about a murderer and that he then said he had a picture of him which he was going to show you.'

'I thought so, yes.'

'You thought so? You were sure enough to begin with!'

Miss Marple retorted with spirit.

'It is never easy to repeat a conversation and be entirely accurate in what the other party to it has said. One is always inclined to jump at what you think they *meant*. Then, afterwards, you put actual words into their mouths. Major Palgrave told me this story, yes. He told me that the man who told it to him, this doctor, had shown him a snapshot of the murderer; but if I am to be quite honest I must admit that what he actually said to me was "Would you like to see a snapshot of a murderer?" and naturally I assumed that it was the same snapshot he had been talking about. That it was the snapshot of that particular murderer. But I have to admit that it is possible – only remotely possible, but still possible – that by an association of ideas in his mind he leaped from the snapshot he had been shown in the past, to a snapshot he had taken recently of someone here who he was convinced was a murderer.'

'Women!' snorted Mr Rafiel in exasperation. 'You're all the same, the whole blinking lot of you! Can't be accurate. You're never exactly *sure* of what a thing was. And now,' he added irritably, 'where does *that* leave us?' He snorted. 'Evelyn Hillingdon, or Greg's wife, Lucky? The whole thing is a mess.'

There was a slight apologetic cough. Arthur Jackson was standing at Mr Rafiel's elbow. He had come so noiselessly that nobody had noticed him.

'Time for your massage, sir,' he said.

Mr Rafiel displayed immediate temper.

'What do you mean by sneaking up on me in that way and making me jump? I never heard you.'

'Very sorry, sir.'

'I don't think I'll have any massage today. It never does me a damn' bit of good.'

'Oh, come sir, you mustn't say that.' Jackson was full of professional cheerfulness. 'You'd soon notice if you left it off.'

He wheeled the chair deftly round.

Miss Marple rose to her feet, smiled at Esther and went down to the beach.

Chapter Eighteen

Without Benefit of Clergy

I

THE BEACH WAS rather empty this morning. Greg was splashing in the water in his usual noisy style, Lucky was lying on her face on the beach with a sun-tanned back well oiled and her blonde hair splayed over her shoulders. The Hillingdons were not there. Señora de Caspearo, with an assorted bag of gentlemen in attendance, was lying face upwards and talking deep-throated, happy Spanish. Some French and Italian children were playing at the water's edge and laughing. Canon and Miss Prescott were sitting in beach chairs observing the scene. The Canon had his hat tilted forward over his eyes and seemed half asleep. There was a convenient chair next to Miss Prescott and Miss Marple made for it and sat down.

'Oh dear,' she said with a deep sigh.

'I know,' said Miss Prescott.

It was their joint tribute to violent death.

'That poor girl,' said Miss Marple.

'Very sad,' said the Canon. 'Most deplorable.'

'For a moment or two,' said Miss Prescott, 'we really thought of leaving, Jeremy and I. But then we decided against it. It would not really be fair, I felt, on the Kendals. After all, it's not *their* fault – It might have happened anywhere.'

'In the midst of life we are in death,' said the Canon solemnly.

'It's very important, you know,' said Miss Prescott, 'that they should make a go of this place. They have sunk all their capital in it.'

'A very sweet girl,' said Miss Marple, 'but not looking at all well lately.'

'Very nervy,' agreed Miss Prescott. 'Of course her family –' she shook her head.

'I really think, Joan,' said the Canon in mild reproof, 'that there are some things –'

'Everybody knows about it,' said Miss Prescott. 'Her family live in our part of the world. A great-aunt – most peculiar – and one of her uncles took off all his clothes in one of the tube stations. Green Park, I believe it was.'

'Joan, that is a thing that should *not* be repeated.'

'Very sad,' said Miss Marple, shaking her head, 'though I believe not an uncommon form of madness. I know when we were working for the Armenian relief, a most respectable elderly clergyman was afflicted the same way. They telephoned his wife and she came along at once and took him home in a cab, wrapped in a blanket.'

'Of course, Molly's immediate family's all right,' said Miss Prescott. 'She never got on very well with her mother, but then so few girls seem to get on with their mothers nowadays.'

'Such a pity,' said Miss Marple, shaking her head, 'because really a young girl needs her mother's knowledge of the world and experience.'

'Exactly,' said Miss Prescott with emphasis. 'Molly, you know, took up with some man – *quite* unsuitable, I understand.'

'It so often happens,' said Miss Marple.

'Her family disapproved, naturally. *She* didn't tell them about it. They heard about it from a complete outsider. Of course her mother said she must bring him along so that they met him properly. This, I understand, the girl refused to do. She said it was humiliating to him. Most insulting to be made to come and meet her family and be looked over. Just as though you were a horse, she said.'

Miss Marple sighed. 'One does need so much *tact* when dealing with the young,' she murmured.

'Anyway, there it was! They forbade her to see him.'

'But you can't *do* that nowadays,' said Miss Marple. 'Girls have jobs and they meet people whether anyone forbids them or not.'

'But then, very fortunately,' went on Miss Prescott, 'she met Tim Kendal, and the other man sort of faded out of the picture. I can't *tell* you how relieved the family was.'

'I hope they didn't show it too plainly,' said Miss Marple. 'That so often puts girls off from forming suitable attachments.'

'Yes, indeed.'

'One remembers oneself –' murmured Miss Marple, her mind going back to the past. A young man she had met at a croquet party. He had seemed so nice – rather gay, almost *Bohemian* in his views. And then he had been unexpectedly warmly welcomed by her father. He had been suitable, eligible; he had been asked freely to the house more than once, and Miss Marple had found that, after all, he was *dull*. Very dull.

The Canon seemed safely comatose and Miss Marple advanced tentatively to the subject she was anxious to pursue.

'Of course you know so much about this place,' she murmured. 'You have been here several years running, have you not?'

'Well, last year and two years before that. We like St Honoré very much. Always such nice people here. Not the flashy, ultra-rich set.'

'So I suppose you know the Hillingdons and the Dysons well?'

'Yes, fairly well.'

Miss Marple coughed and lowered her voice slightly.

'Major Palgrave told me such an interesting story,' she said.

'He had a great repertoire of stories, hadn't he? Of course he had travelled very widely. Africa, India, even China I believe.'

'Yes indeed,' said Miss Marple. 'But I didn't mean one of *those* stories. This was a story concerned with – well, with one of the people I have just mentioned.'

'Oh!' said Miss Prescott. Her voice held meaning.

'Yes. Now I wonder –' Miss Marple allowed her eyes to travel gently round the beach to where Lucky lay sunning her back. 'Very beautifully tanned, isn't she,' remarked Miss Marple. 'And her hair. Most attractive. Practically the same colour as Molly Kendal's, isn't it?'

'The only difference,' said Miss Prescott, 'is that Molly's is natural and Lucky's comes out of a bottle!'

'Really, Joan,' the Canon protested, unexpectedly awake again. 'Don't you think that is *rather* an uncharitable thing to say?'

'It's not uncharitable,' said Miss Prescott, acidly. 'Merely a *fact*.'

'It looks very nice to *me*,' said the Canon.

'Of course. That's why she does it. But I assure you, my dear Jeremy, it wouldn't deceive any *woman* for a moment. Would it?' She appealed to Miss Marple.

'Well, I'm afraid –' said Miss Marple, 'of course I haven't the experience that you have – but I'm afraid – yes I should say definitely *not natural*. The appearance at the roots every fifth or sixth day –' She looked at Miss Prescott and they both nodded with quiet female assurance.

The Canon appeared to be dropping off again.

'Major Palgrave told me a really extraordinary story,' murmured Miss Marple, 'about – well I couldn't quite make out. I am a little deaf sometimes. He appeared to be saying or hinting –' she paused.

'I know what you mean. There was a great deal of talk at the time –'

'You mean at the time that –'

'When the first Mrs Dyson died. Her death was quite unexpected. In fact, everybody thought she was a *malade imaginaire* – a hypochondriac. So when she had the attack and died so unexpectedly, well, of course, people did talk.'

'There wasn't – any – trouble at the time?'

'The doctor was puzzled. He was quite a young man and he hadn't had much experience. He was what I call one of those antibiotics-for-all men. You know, the kind that doesn't bother to look at the patient much, or worry what's the matter with him. They just give them some kind of pill out of a bottle and if they don't get better, then they try a different pill. Yes, I believe he *was* puzzled, but it seemed she had had gastric trouble before.

At least her husband said so, and there seemed no reason for believing anything was *wrong.*'

'But you yourself think –'

'Well, I always try to keep an open mind, but one does wonder, you know. And what with various things people said –'

'Joan!' The Canon sat up. He looked belligerent. 'I don't like – I really don't like to hear this kind of ill-natured gossip being repeated. We've always set our faces against that kind of thing. See no evil, hear no evil, speak no evil – and what is more, *think* no evil! That should be the motto of every Christian man and woman.'

The two women sat in silence. They were rebuked, and in deference to their training they deferred to the criticism of a man. But inwardly they were frustrated, irritated and quite unrepentant. Miss Prescott threw a frank glance of irritation towards her brother. Miss Marple took out her knitting and looked at it. Fortunately for them Chance was on their side.

'*Mon père,*' said a small shrill voice. It was one of the French children who had been playing at the water's edge. She had come up unnoticed, and was standing by Canon Prescott's chair.

'*Mon père,*' she fluted.

'Eh? Yes, my dear? *Oui, qu'est-ce qu'il y a, ma petite?*'

The child explained. There had been a dispute about who should have the water-wings next and also other matters of seaside etiquette. Canon Prescott was extremely fond of children, especially small girls. He was always delighted to be summoned to act as arbiter in their disputes. He rose willingly now and accompanied the child to the water's edge. Miss Marple and Miss Prescott breathed deep sighs and turned avidly towards each other.

II

'Jeremy, of course rightly, is very against ill-natured gossip,' said Miss Prescott, 'but one cannot really ignore what people are saying. And there was, as I say, a great deal of talk at the time.'

'Yes?' Miss Marple's tone urged her forward.

'This young woman, you see, Miss Greatorex I think her name was then, I can't remember now, was a kind of cousin and she looked after Mrs Dyson. Gave her all her medicines and things like that.' There was a short, meaningless pause. 'And of course there had, I understand' – Miss Prescott's voice was lowered – 'been goings-on between Mr Dyson and Miss Greatorex. A lot of people had noticed them. I mean things like that are quickly observed in a place like this. Then there was some curious story about some stuff that Edward Hillingdon got for her at a chemist.'

'Oh, Edward Hillingdon came into it?'

'Oh yes, he was very much attracted. People noticed it. And Lucky – Miss Greatorex – played them off against each other. Gregory Dyson and Edward Hillingdon. One has to face it, she has always been an attractive woman.'

'Though not as young as she was,' Miss Marple replied.

'Exactly. But she was always very well turned out and made up. Of course not so flamboyant when she was just the poor relation. She always *seemed* very devoted to the invalid. But, well, you see how it was.'

'What was this story about the chemist – how did that get known?'

'Well, it wasn't in Jamestown, I think it was when they were in Martinique. The French, I believe, are more lax than we are in the matter of drugs – This chemist talked to someone, and the story got around – Well, you know how these things happen.'

Miss Marple did. None better.

'He said something about Colonel Hillingdon asking for something and not seeming to know what it was he was asking for. Consulting a piece of paper, you know, on which it was written down. Anyway, as I say, there was *talk*.'

'But I don't see quite why Colonel Hillingdon –' Miss Marple frowned in perplexity.

'I suppose he was just being used as a *cat's-paw*. Anyway, Gregory Dyson married again in an almost indecently short time. Barely a month later, I understand.'

They looked at each other.

'But there was no *real* suspicion?' Miss Marple asked.

'Oh no, it was just – well, *talk*. Of course there may have been absolutely nothing in it.'

'Major Palgrave thought there was.'

'Did he say so to you?'

'I wasn't really listening very closely,' confessed Miss Marple. 'I just wondered if – er – well, if he'd said the same thing to you?'

'He did point her out to me one day,' said Miss Prescott.

'Really? He actually pointed her out?'

'Yes. As a matter of fact, I thought at first it was Mrs Hillingdon he was pointing out. He wheezed and chuckled a bit and said, "Look at that woman over there. In my opinion that's a woman who's done murder and got away with it." I was very shocked, of course. I said, "Surely you're joking, Major Palgrave," and he said, "Yes, yes, dear lady, let's call it joking." The Dysons and the Hillingdons were sitting at a table quite near to us, and I was afraid they'd overhear. He chuckled and said "Wouldn't care to go to a drinks party and have a certain person mix me a cocktail. Too much like supper with the Borgias."'

'How *very* interesting,' said Miss Marple. 'Did he mention – a – a photograph?'

'I don't remember… Was it some newspaper cutting?'

Miss Marple, about to speak, shut her lips. The sun was momentarily obscured by a shadow. Evelyn Hillingdon paused beside them.

'Good morning,' she said.

'I was wondering where you were,' said Miss Prescott, looking up brightly.

'I've been to Jamestown, shopping.'

'Oh, I see.'

Miss Prescott looked round vaguely and Evelyn Hillingdon said:

'Oh, I didn't take Edward with me. Men hate shopping.'

'Did you find anything of interest?'

'It wasn't that sort of shopping. I just had to go to the chemist.'

With a smile and a slight nod she went on down the beach.

'Such nice people, the Hillingdons,' said Miss Prescott, 'though she's not really very easy to know, is she? I mean, she's always very pleasant and all that, but one never seems to get to know her any better.'

Miss Marple agreed thoughtfully.

'One never knows what she is thinking,' said Miss Prescott.

'Perhaps that is just as well,' said Miss Marple.

'I beg your pardon?'

'Oh nothing really, only that I've always had the feeling that perhaps her thoughts might be rather disconcerting.'

'Oh,' said Miss Prescott, looking puzzled. 'I see what you mean.' She went on with a slight change of subject. 'I believe they have a very charming place in Hampshire, and a boy – or is it two boys – who have just gone – or one of them – to Winchester.'

'Do you know Hampshire well?'

'No. Hardly at all. I believe their house is somewhere near Alton.'

'I see.' Miss Marple paused and then said, 'And where do the Dysons live?'

'California,' said Miss Prescott. 'When they are at home, that is. They are great travellers.'

'One really knows so little about the people one meets when one is travelling,' said Miss Marple. 'I mean – how shall I put it – one only knows, doesn't one, what they choose to tell you about themselves. For instance, you don't *really* know that the Dysons live in California.'

Miss Prescott looked startled.

'I'm sure Mr Dyson mentioned it.'

'Yes. Yes, exactly. That's what I mean. And the same thing perhaps with the Hillingdons. I mean when you say that they live in Hampshire, you're really repeating what *they* told *you*, aren't you?'

Miss Prescott looked slightly alarmed. 'Do you mean that they don't live in Hampshire?' she asked.

'No, no, not for one moment,' said Miss Marple, quickly apologetic. 'I was only using them as an instance as to what one knows or doesn't know about people.' She added, '*I* have told you that I live at St Mary Mead, which is a place, no doubt, of which you have never heard. But you don't, if I may say so, know it of your *own* knowledge, do you?'

Miss Prescott forbore from saying that she really couldn't care less *where* Miss Marple lived. It was somewhere in the country and in the South of England and that is all she knew. 'Oh, I do see what you mean,' she agreed hastily, 'and I know that one can't possibly be too careful when one is abroad.'

'I didn't exactly mean *that*,' said Miss Marple.

There were some odd thoughts going through Miss Marple's mind. Did she really know, she was asking herself, that Canon Prescott and Miss Prescott were really Canon Prescott and Miss Prescott? They said so. There was no evidence to contradict them. It would really be easy, would it not, to put on a dog-collar, to wear the appropriate clothes, to make the appropriate conversation. If there was a motive...

Miss Marple was fairly knowledgeable about the clergy in her part of the world, but the Prescotts came from the north. Durham, wasn't it? She had no doubt they were the Prescotts, but still, it came back to the same thing – one believed what people said to one.

Perhaps one ought to be on one's guard against that. Perhaps... She shook her head thoughtfully.

Chapter Nineteen

Uses of a Shoe

Canon Prescott came back from the water's edge slightly short of breath (playing with children is always exhausting).

Presently he and his sister went back to the hotel, finding the beach a little too hot.

'But,' said Señora de Caspearo scornfully as they walked away – 'how can a beach be too hot? It is nonsense that – And look what she wears – her arms and her neck are all covered up. Perhaps it is as well, that. Her skin it is hideous, like a plucked chicken!'

Miss Marple drew a deep breath. Now or never was the time for conversation with Señora de Caspearo. Unfortunately she did not know what to say. There seemed to be no common ground on which they could meet.

'You have children, Señora?' she inquired.

'I have three angels,' said Señora de Caspearo, kissing her fingertips.

Miss Marple was rather uncertain as to whether this meant that Señora de Caspearo's offspring were in Heaven or whether it merely referred to their characters.

One of the gentlemen in attendance made a remark in Spanish and Señora de Caspearo flung back her head appreciatively and laughed loudly and melodiously.

'You understand what he said?' she inquired of Miss Marple.

'I'm afraid not,' said Miss Marple apologetically.

'It is just as well. He is a wicked man.'

A rapid and spirited interchange of Spanish badinage followed.

'It is infamous – infamous,' said Señora de Caspearo, reverting to English with sudden gravity, 'that the police do not let us go from this island. I storm, I scream, I stamp my foot – but all they say is No – No. You know how it will end – we shall all be killed.'

Her bodyguard attempted to reassure her.

'But yes – I tell you it is unlucky here. I knew it from the first – That old Major, the ugly one – he had the Evil Eye – you remember? His eyes they crossed – It is bad, that! I make the Sign of the Horns every time when he looks my way.' She made it in illustration. 'Though since he is cross-eyed I am not always sure when he does look my way –'

'He had a glass eye,' said Miss Marple in an explanatory voice. 'An accident, I understand, when he was quite young. It was not his fault.'

'I tell you he brought bad luck – I say it is the Evil Eye he had.'

Her hand shot out again in the well-known Latin gesture – the first finger and the little finger sticking out, the two middle ones doubled in. 'Anyway,' she said cheerfully, 'he is dead – I do not have to look at him any more. I do not like to look at things that are ugly.'

It was, Miss Marple thought, a somewhat cruel epitaph on Major Palgrave.

Farther down the beach Gregory Dyson had come out of the sea. Lucky had turned herself over on the sand. Evelyn Hillingdon was looking at Lucky, and her expression, for some reason, made Miss Marple shiver.

'Surely I can't be cold – in this hot sun,' she thought.

What was the old phrase – '*A goose walking over your grave –*'

She got up and went slowly back to her bungalow.

On the way she passed Mr Rafiel and Esther Walters coming down the beach. Mr Rafiel winked at her. Miss Marple did not wink back. She looked disapproving.

She went into her bungalow and lay down on her bed. She felt old and tired and worried.

She was quite certain that there was no time to be lost – no time – to – be lost… It was getting late. The sun was going to set – the sun – one must always look at the sun through smoked glass – Where was that piece of smoked glass that someone had given her?…

No, she wouldn't need it after all. A shadow had come over the sun blotting it out. A shadow. Evelyn Hillingdon's shadow – No, not Evelyn Hillingdon – The Shadow (what were the words?) the *Shadow of the Valley of Death*. That was it. She must – what was it? Make the Sign of the Horns – to avert the Evil Eye – Major Palgrave's Evil Eye.

Her eyelids flickered open – she had been asleep. But there *was* a shadow – someone peering in at her window.

The shadow moved away – and Miss Marple saw who it was – It was Jackson.

'Impertinence – peering in like that,' she thought – and added parenthetically, 'Just like Jonas Parry.'

The comparison reflected no credit on Jackson.

Then she wondered *why* Jackson had been peering into her bedroom. To see if she was there? Or to note that she was there, but was asleep.

She got up, went into the bathroom and peered cautiously through the window.

Arthur Jackson was standing by the door of the bungalow next door. Mr Rafiel's bungalow. She saw him give a rapid glance round and then slip quickly inside. Interesting, thought Miss Marple. Why did he have to look round in that furtive manner? Nothing in the world could have been more natural than his going into Mr Rafiel's bungalow since he himself had a room at the back of it. He was always going in and out of it on some errand or other. So why that quick, guilty glance round? 'Only one reason,' said Miss Marple answering her own question, 'he wanted to be sure that nobody was observing him enter at this particular moment because of something he was going to do in there.'

Everybody, of course, was on the beach at this moment except those who had gone for expeditions. In about twenty minutes or so, Jackson himself would arrive on the beach in the course of his duties to aid Mr Rafiel to take his sea dip. If he wanted to do anything in the bungalow unobserved, now was a very good time. He had satisfied himself that Miss Marple was asleep on her bed, he had satisfied himself that there was nobody near at hand to observe his movements. Well, she must do her best to do exactly that.

Sitting down on her bed, Miss Marple removed her neat sandal shoes and replaced them with a pair of plimsolls. Then she shook her head, removed the plimsolls, burrowed in her suitcase and took out a pair of shoes the heel of one of which she had recently caught on a hook by the door. It was now in a slightly precarious state and Miss Marple adroitly rendered it even more precarious by attention with a nail file. Then she emerged with due precaution from her door walking in stockinged feet. With all the care of a Big Game Hunter approaching up-wind of a herd of antelope, Miss Marple gently circumnavigated Mr Rafiel's bungalow. Cautiously she manoeuvred her way around the corner of the house. She put on one of the shoes she was carrying, gave a final wrench to the heel of the other, sank gently to her knees and lay prone under the window. If Jackson heard anything, if he came to the window to look out, an old lady would have had a fall owing to the heel coming off her shoe. But evidently Jackson had heard nothing.

Very, very gently Miss Marple raised her head. The windows of the bungalow were low. Shielding herself slightly with a festoon of creeper she peered inside...

Jackson was on his knees before a suitcase. The lid of the suitcase was up and Miss Marple could see that it was a specially fitted affair containing compartments filled with various kinds of papers. Jackson was looking through the papers, occasionally drawing documents out of long envelopes. Miss Marple did not remain at her observation post for long. All she wanted was to know what Jackson was doing. She knew now. Jackson was snooping. Whether he was looking for something in particular, or whether he was just indulging his natural instincts, she had no means of judging. But it confirmed her in her belief that Arthur Jackson and Jonas Parry had strong affinities in other things than facial resemblance.

Her problem was now to withdraw. Very carefully she dropped down again and crept along the flower-bed until she was clear of the window. She returned to her bungalow and carefully put away the shoe and the heel that she had detached from it. She looked at them with affection. A good device which she could use on another day if necessary. She resumed her own sandal shoes, and went thoughtfully down to the beach again.

Choosing a moment when Esther Walters was in the water, Miss Marple moved into the chair Esther had vacated.

Greg and Lucky were laughing and talking with Señora de Caspearo and making a good deal of noise.

Miss Marple spoke very quietly, almost under her breath, without looking at Mr Rafiel.

'Do you know that Jackson snoops?'

'Doesn't surprise me,' said Mr Rafiel. 'Caught him at it, did you?'

'I managed to observe him through a window. He had one of your suitcases open and was looking through your papers.'

'Must have managed to get hold of a key to it. Resourceful fellow. He'll be disappointed though. Nothing he gets hold of in that way will do him a mite of good.'

'He's coming down now,' said Miss Marple, glancing up towards the hotel.

'Time for that idiotic sea dip of mine.'

He spoke again – very quietly.

'As for you – don't be too enterprising. We don't want to be attending *your* funeral next. Remember your age, and be careful. There's somebody about who isn't too scrupulous, remember.'

CHAPTER TWENTY

NIGHT ALARM

I

EVENING CAME – THE lights came up on the terrace – People dined and talked and laughed, albeit less loudly and merrily than they had a day or two ago – The steel band played.

But the dancing ended early. People yawned – went off to bed – The lights went out – There was darkness and stillness – The Golden Palm Tree slept…

'Evelyn. Evelyn!' The whisper came sharp and urgent.

Evelyn Hillingdon stirred and turned on her pillow.

'*Evelyn*. Please wake up.'

Evelyn Hillingdon sat up abruptly. Tim Kendal was standing in the doorway. She stared at him in surprise.

'Evelyn, *please*, could you come? It's – Molly. She's ill. I don't know what's the matter with her. I think she must have taken something.'

Evelyn was quick, decisive.

'All right, Tim. I'll come. You go back to her. I'll be with you in a moment.'

Tim Kendal disappeared. Evelyn slipped out of bed, threw on a dressing-gown and looked across at the other bed. Her husband, it seemed, had not been awakened. He lay there, his head turned away, breathing quietly. Evelyn hesitated for a moment, then decided not to disturb him. She went out of the door and walked rapidly to the main building and beyond it to the Kendals' bungalow. She caught up with Tim in the doorway.

Molly lay in bed. Her eyes were closed and her breathing was clearly not natural. Evelyn bent over her, rolled up an eyelid, felt her pulse and then looked at the bedside table. There was a glass there which had been used. Beside it was an empty phial of tablets. She picked it up.

'They were her sleeping pills,' said Tim, 'but that bottle was half full yesterday or the day before. I think she must have taken the lot.'

'Go and get Dr Graham,' said Evelyn, 'and on the way knock them up and tell them to make strong coffee. Strong as possible. Hurry.'

Tim dashed off. Just outside the doorway he collided with Edward Hillingdon.

'Oh, sorry, Edward.'

'What's happening here?' demanded Hillingdon. 'What's going on?'

'It's Molly. Evelyn's with her. I must get hold of the doctor. I suppose I ought to have gone to him first but I – I wasn't sure and I thought Evelyn would know. Molly would have hated it if I'd fetched a doctor when it wasn't necessary.'

He went off, running. Edward Hillingdon looked after him for a moment and then he walked into the bedroom.

'What's happening?' he said. 'Is it serious?'

'Oh, there you are, Edward. I wondered if you'd woken up. This silly child has been taking things.'

'Is it bad?'

'One can't tell without knowing how much she's taken. I shouldn't think it was too bad if we get going in time. I've sent for coffee. If we can get some of that down her –'

'But why should she do such a thing? You don't think –' He stopped.

'What don't I think?' said Evelyn.

'You don't think it's because of the inquiry – the police – all that?'

'It's possible, of course. That sort of thing could be very alarming to a nervous type.'

'Molly never used to seem a nervous type.'

'One can't really tell,' said Evelyn. 'It's the most unlikely people sometimes who lose their nerve.'

'Yes, I remember...' Again he stopped.

'The truth is,' said Evelyn, 'that one doesn't really know anything about anybody.' She added, 'Not even the people who are nearest to you...'

'Isn't that going a little too far, Evelyn – exaggerating too much?'

'I don't think it is. When you think of people, it is in the image you have made of them for yourself.'

'I know you,' said Edward Hillingdon quietly.

'You think you do.'

'No. I'm sure.' He added, 'And you're sure of me.'

Evelyn looked at him then turned back to the bed. She took Molly by the shoulders and shook her.

'We ought to be doing something, but I suppose it's better to wait until Dr Graham comes – Oh, I think I hear them.'

II

'She'll do now.' Dr Graham stepped back, wiped his forehead with a handkerchief and breathed a sigh of relief.

'You think she'll be all right, sir?' Tim demanded anxiously.

'Yes, yes. We got to her in good time. Anyway, she probably didn't take enough to kill her. A couple of days and she'll be as right as rain but she'll have a rather nasty day or two first.' He picked up the empty bottle. 'Who gave her these things anyway?'

'A doctor in New York. She wasn't sleeping well.'

'Well, well. I know all we medicos hand these things out freely nowadays. Nobody tells young women who can't sleep to count sheep, or get up and eat a biscuit, or write a couple of letters and then go back to bed. Instant remedies, that's what people demand nowadays. Sometimes I think it's a pity we give them to them. You've got to learn to put up with things in life. All very well to stuff a comforter into a baby's mouth to stop it crying. Can't go on doing that all a person's life.' He gave a small chuckle. 'I bet you, if you asked Miss Marple what she does if she can't sleep, she'd tell you she counted sheep going under a gate.' He turned back to the bed where Molly was stirring. Her eyes were open now. She looked at them without interest or recognition. Dr Graham took her hand.

'Well, well, my dear, and what have you been doing to yourself?'

She blinked but did not reply.

'Why did you do it, Molly, why? Tell me why?' Tim took her other hand.

Still her eyes did not move. If they rested on anyone it was on Evelyn Hillingdon. There might have been even a faint question in them but it was hard to tell. Evelyn spoke as though there had been the question.

'Tim came and fetched me,' she said.

Her eyes went to Tim, then shifted to Dr Graham.

'You're going to be all right now,' said Dr Graham, 'but don't do it again.'

'She didn't mean to do it,' said Tim quietly. 'I'm sure she didn't mean to do it. She just wanted a good night's rest. Perhaps the pills didn't work at first and so she took more of them. Is that it, Molly?'

Her head moved very faintly in a negative motion.

'You mean – you took them on purpose?' said Tim.

Molly spoke then. 'Yes,' she said.

'But why, Molly, why?'

The eyelids faltered. 'Afraid.' The word was just heard.

'Afraid? Of what?'

But her eyelids closed down.

'Better let her be,' said Dr Graham. Tim spoke impetuously.

'Afraid of what? The police? Because they've been hounding you, asking you questions? I don't wonder. Anyone might feel frightened. But it's just their way, that's all. Nobody thinks for one moment –' he broke off.

Dr Graham made him a decisive gesture.

'I want to go to sleep,' said Molly.

'The best thing for you,' said Dr Graham.

He moved to the door and the others followed him.

'She'll sleep all right,' said Graham.

'Is there anything I ought to do?' asked Tim. He had the usual, slightly apprehensive attitude of a man in illness.

'I'll stay if you like,' said Evelyn kindly.

'Oh no. No, that's quite all right,' said Tim.

Evelyn went back towards the bed. 'Shall I stay with you, Molly?'

Molly's eyes opened again. She said, 'No,' and then after a pause, 'just Tim.'

Tim came back and sat down by the bed.

'I'm here, Molly,' he said and took her hand. 'Just go to sleep. I won't leave you.'

She sighed faintly and her eyes closed.

The doctor paused outside the bungalow and the Hillingdons stood with him.

'You're sure there's nothing more I can do?' asked Evelyn.

'I don't think so, thank you, Mrs Hillingdon. She'll be better with her husband now. But possibly tomorrow – after all, he's got this hotel to run – I think someone should be with her.'

'D'you think she might – try again?' asked Hillingdon.

Graham rubbed his forehead irritably.

'One never knows in these cases. Actually, it's most unlikely. As you've seen for yourselves, the restorative treatment is extremely unpleasant. But of course one can never be absolutely certain. She may have more of this stuff hidden away somewhere.'

'I should never have thought of suicide in connection with a girl like Molly,' said Hillingdon.

Graham said dryly, 'It's not the people who are always talking of killing themselves, threatening to do so, who do it. They dramatise themselves that way and let off steam.'

'Molly always seemed such a happy girl. I think perhaps' –

Evelyn hesitated – 'I ought to tell you, Dr Graham.' She told him then about her interview with Molly on the beach the night that Victoria had been killed. Graham's face was very grave when she had finished.

'I'm glad you've told me, Mrs Hillingdon. There are very definite indications there of some kind of deep-rooted trouble. Yes. I'll have a word with her husband in the morning.'

III

'I want to talk to you seriously, Kendal, about your wife.'

They were sitting in Tim's office. Evelyn Hillingdon had taken his place by Molly's bedside and Lucky had promised to come and, as she expressed it, 'spell her' later. Miss Marple had also offered her services. Poor Tim was torn between his hotel commitments and his wife's condition.

'I can't understand it,' said Tim, 'I can't understand Molly any longer. She's changed. Changed out of all seeming.'

'I understand she's been having bad dreams?'

'Yes. Yes, she complained about them a good deal.'

'For how long?'

'Oh, I don't know. About – oh, I suppose a month – perhaps longer. She – we – thought they were just – well, nightmares, you know.'

'Yes, yes, I quite understand. But what's a much more serious sign is the fact that she seems to have felt afraid of someone. Did she complain about that to you?'

'Well, yes. She said once or twice that – oh, people were following her.'

'Ah! Spying on her?'

'Yes, she did use that term once. She said they were her enemies and they'd followed her here.'

'Did she have enemies, Mr Kendal? –'

'No. Of course she didn't.'

'No incident in England, anything you know about before you were married?'

'Oh no, nothing of that kind. She didn't get on with her family very well, that was all. Her mother was rather an eccentric woman, difficult to live with perhaps, but...'

'Any signs of mental instability in her family?'

Tim opened his mouth impulsively, then shut it again. He pushed a fountain pen about on the desk in front of him.

The doctor said:

'I must stress the fact that it would be better to tell me, Tim, if that is the case.'

'Well, yes, I believe so. Nothing serious, but I believe there was an aunt or something who was a bit batty. But that's nothing. I mean – well you get that in almost any family.'

'Oh yes, yes, that's quite true. I'm not trying to alarm you about that, but it just might show a tendency to – well, to break down or imagine things if any stress arose.'

'I don't really know very much,' said Tim. 'After all, people don't pour out all their family histories to you, do they?'

'No, no. Quite so. She had no former friend – she was not engaged to anyone, anyone who might have threatened her or made jealous threats? That sort of thing?'

'I don't know. I don't think so. Molly *was* engaged to some other man before I came along. Her parents were very against it, I understand, and I think she really stuck to the chap more out of opposition and defiance than anything else.' He gave a sudden half-grin. 'You know what it is when you're young. If people cut up a fuss it makes you much keener on whoever it is.'

Dr Graham smiled too. 'Ah yes, one often sees that. One should never take exception to one's children's objectionable friends. Usually they grow out of them naturally. This man, whoever he was, didn't make threats of any kind against Molly?'

'No, I'm sure he didn't. She would have told me. She said herself she just had a silly adolescent craze on him, mainly because he had such a bad reputation.'

'Yes, yes. Well, that doesn't sound serious. Now there's another thing. Apparently your wife has had what she describes as blackouts. Brief passages of time during which she can't account for her actions. Did you know about that, Tim?'

'No,' said Tim slowly. 'No. I didn't. She never told me. I did notice, you know, now you mention it, that she seemed rather vague sometimes and…' He paused, thinking. 'Yes, that explains it. I couldn't understand how she seemed to have forgotten the simplest things, or sometimes not to seem to know what time of day it was. I just thought she was absent-minded, I suppose.'

'What it amounts to, Tim, is just this. I advise you most strongly to take your wife to see a good specialist.'

Tim flushed angrily.

'You mean a mental specialist, I suppose?'

'Now, now, don't be upset by labels. A neurologist, a psychologist, someone who specialises in what the layman calls nervous breakdowns. There's a good man in Kingston. Or there's New York of course. There is something that is causing these nervous terrors of your wife's. Something perhaps for which she hardly knows the reason herself. Get advice about her, Tim. Get advice as soon as possible.'

He clapped his hand on the young man's shoulder and got up.

'There's no immediate worry. Your wife has good friends and we'll all be keeping an eye on her.'

'She won't – you don't think she'll try it again?'

'I think it most unlikely,' said Dr Graham.

'You can't be sure,' said Tim.

'One can never be sure,' said Dr Graham, 'that's one of the first things you learn in my profession.' Again he laid a hand on Tim's shoulder. 'Don't worry too much.'

'That's easy to say,' said Tim as the doctor went out of the door. 'Don't worry, indeed! What does he think I'm made of?'

Chapter Twenty-One

Jackson on Cosmetics

'YOU'RE SURE YOU don't mind, Miss Marple?' said Evelyn Hillingdon.

'No, indeed, my dear,' said Miss Marple. 'I'm only too delighted to be of use in any way. At my age, you know, one feels very useless in the world. Especially when I am in a place like this, just enjoying myself. No duties of any kind. No, I'll be delighted to sit with Molly. You go along on your expedition. Pelican Point, wasn't it?'

'Yes,' said Evelyn. 'Both Edward and I love it. I never get tired of seeing the birds diving down, catching up the fish. Tim's with Molly now. But he's got things to do and he doesn't seem to like her being left alone.'

'He's quite right,' said Miss Marple. 'I wouldn't in his place. One never knows, does one? When anyone has attempted anything of that kind – Well, go along, my dear.'

Evelyn went off to join a little group that was waiting for her. Her husband, the Dysons and three or four other people. Miss Marple checked her knitting requirements, saw that she had all she wanted with her, and walked over towards the Kendals' bungalow.

As she came up on to the loggia she heard Tim's voice through the half-open french window.

'If you'd only tell me *why* you did it, Molly. What made you? Was it anything I did? There must be some reason. If you'd only tell me.'

Miss Marple paused. There was a little pause inside before

Molly spoke. Her voice was flat and tired.

'I don't know, Tim, I really don't know. I suppose – something came over me.'

Miss Marple tapped on the window and walked in.

'Oh, there you are, Miss Marple. It is very good of you.'

'Not at all,' said Miss Marple. 'I'm delighted to be of any help. Shall I sit here in this chair? You're looking much better, Molly. I'm so glad.'

'I'm all right,' said Molly. 'Quite all right. Just – oh, just sleepy.'

'I shan't talk,' said Miss Marple. 'You just lie quiet and rest. I'll get on with my knitting.'

Tim Kendal threw her a grateful glance and went out. Miss Marple established herself in her chair.

Molly was lying on her left side. She had a half-stupefied, exhausted look. She said in a voice that was almost a whisper:

'It's very kind of you, Miss Marple. I – I think I'll go to sleep.'

She half turned away on her pillows and closed her eyes. Her breathing grew more regular though it was still far from normal. Long experience of nursing made Miss Marple almost automatically straighten the sheet and tuck it under the mattress on her side of the bed. As she did so her hand encountered something hard and rectangular under the mattress. Rather surprised she took hold of this and pulled it out. It was a book. Miss Marple threw a quick glance at the girl in the bed, but she lay there utterly quiescent. She was evidently asleep. Miss Marple opened the book. It was, she saw, a current work on nervous diseases. It came open naturally at a certain place which gave a description of the onset of persecution mania and various other manifestations of schizophrenia and allied complaints.

It was not a highly technical book, but one that could be easily understood by a layman. Miss Marple's face grew very grave as she read. After a minute or two she closed the book and stayed thinking. Then she bent forward and with care replaced the book where she had found it, under the mattress.

She shook her head in some perplexity. Noiselessly she rose

from her chair. She walked the few steps towards the window, then turned her head sharply over her shoulder. Molly's eyes were open but even as Miss Marple turned the eyes shut again. For a minute or two Miss Marple was not quite certain whether she might not have imagined that quick, sharp glance. Was Molly then only pretending to be asleep? That might be natural enough. She might feel that Miss Marple would start talking to her if she showed herself awake. Yes, that could be all it was.

Was she reading into that glance of Molly's a kind of slyness that was somehow innately disagreeable? One doesn't know, Miss Marple thought to herself, one really doesn't know.

She decided that she would try to manage a little talk with Dr Graham as soon as it could be managed. She came back to her chair by the bed. She decided after about five minutes or so that Molly was really asleep. No one could have lain so still, could have breathed so evenly. Miss Marple got up again. She was wearing her plimsolls today. Not perhaps very elegant, but admirably suited to this climate and comfortable and roomy for the feet.

She moved gently round the bedroom, pausing at both of the windows, which gave out in two different directions.

The hotel grounds seemed quiet and deserted. Miss Marple came back and was standing a little uncertainly before regaining her seat, when she thought she heard a faint sound outside. Like the scrape of a shoe on the loggia? She hesitated a moment then she went to the window, pushed it a little farther open, stepped out and turned her head back into the room as she spoke.

'I shall be gone only a very short time, dear,' she said, 'just back to my bungalow, to see where I could possibly have put that pattern. I was so sure I had brought it with me. You'll be quite all right till I come back, won't you?' Then turning her head back, she nodded to herself. 'Asleep, poor child. A good thing.'

She went quietly along the loggia, down the steps and turned sharp right to the path there. Passing along between the screen of some hibiscus bushes an observer might have been curious to see that Miss Marple veered sharply on to the flower-bed, passed round to the back of the bungalow and entered it again through the second door there. This led directly into a small room that Tim sometimes used as an unofficial office and from that into the sitting-room.

Here there were wide curtains semi-drawn to keep the room cool. Miss Marple slipped behind one of them. Then she waited. From the window here she had a good view of anyone who approached Molly's bedroom It was some few minutes, four or five, before she saw anything.

The neat figure of Jackson in his white uniform went up the steps of the loggia. He paused for a minute at the balcony there, and then appeared to be giving a tiny discreet tap on the door of the window that was ajar. There was no response that Miss Marple could hear. Jackson looked around him, a quick furtive glance, then he slipped inside the open doors. Miss Marple moved to the door which led into the adjoining bathroom. Miss Marple's eyebrows rose in slight surprise. She reflected a minute or two, then walked out into the passageway and into the bathroom by the other door.

Jackson spun round from examining the shelf over the wash-basin. He looked taken aback, which was not surprising.

'Oh,' he said, 'I – I didn't…'

'Mr Jackson,' said Miss Marple, in great surprise.

'I thought you'd be here somewhere,' said Jackson.

'Did you want anything?' inquired Miss Marple.

'Actually,' said Jackson, 'I was just looking at Mrs Kendal's brand of face cream.'

Miss Marple appreciated the fact that as Jackson was standing with a jar of face cream in his hand he had been adroit in mentioning the fact at once.

'Nice smell,' he said, wrinkling up his nose. 'Fairly good stuff, as these preparations go. The cheaper brands don't suit every skin. Bring it out in a rash as likely as not. The same thing with face powders sometimes.'

'You seem to be very knowledgeable on the subject,' said Miss Marple.

'Worked in the pharmaceutical line for a bit,' said Jackson. 'One learns to know a good deal about cosmetics there. Put stuff in a fancy jar, package it expensively, and it's astonishing what you could rook women for.'

'Is that what you –?' Miss Marple broke off deliberately.

'Well no, I didn't come in here to talk about cosmetics,' Jackson agreed.

'You've not had much time to think up a lie,' thought Miss Marple to herself. 'Let's see what you'll come out with.'

'Matter of fact,' said Jackson, 'Mrs Walters lent her lipstick to Mrs Kendal the other day. I came in to get it back for her. I tapped on the window and then I saw Mrs Kendal was fast asleep, so I thought it would be quite all right if I just walked across into the bathroom and looked for it.'

'I see,' said Miss Marple. 'And did you find it?'

Jackson shook his head. 'Probably in one of her handbags,' he said lightly. 'I won't bother. Mrs Walters didn't make a point of it. She only just mentioned it casually.' He went on, surveying the toilet preparations: 'Doesn't have very much, does she? Ah well, doesn't need it at her age. Good natural skin.'

'You must look at women with quite a different eye from ordinary men,' said Miss Marple, smiling pleasantly.

'Yes. I suppose various jobs do alter one's angle.'

'You know a good deal about drugs?'

'Oh yes. Good working acquaintance with them. If you ask me, there are too many of them about nowadays. Too many tranquillisers and pep pills and miracle drugs and all the rest of it. All right if they're given on prescription, but there are too many of them you can get without prescription. Some of them can be dangerous.'

'I suppose so,' said Miss Marple. 'Yes, I suppose so.'

'They have a great effect, you know, on behaviour. A lot of this teenage hysteria you get from time to time. It's not natural causes. The kids've been taking things. Oh, there's nothing new about it. It's been known for ages. Out in the East – not that I've ever been there – all sorts of funny things used to happen. You'd be surprised at some of the things women gave their husbands. In India, for example, in the bad old days, a young wife who married an old husband. Didn't want to get rid of him, I suppose, because she'd have been burnt on the funeral pyre, or if she wasn't burnt she'd have been treated as an outcast by the family. No catch to have been a widow in India in those days. But she could keep an elderly husband under drugs, make him semi-imbecile, give him hallucinations, drive him more or less off his head.' He shook his head. 'Yes, lot of dirty work.'

He went on: 'And witches, you know. There's a lot of interesting things known now about witches. Why did they always confess, why did they admit so readily that they *were* witches, that they had flown on broomsticks to the Witches' Sabbath?'

'Torture,' said Miss Marple.

'Not always,' said Jackson. 'Oh yes, torture accounted for a lot of it, but they came out with some of those confessions almost before torture was mentioned. They didn't so much confess as boast about it. Well, they rubbed themselves with ointment, you know. Anointing they used to call it. Some of the preparations, belladonna, atropine, all that sort of thing; if you rub them on the skin they give you hallucinations of levitation, of flying through the air. They thought it all was genuine, poor devils. And look at the Assassins – medieval people, out in Syria, the Lebanon, somewhere like that. They fed them Indian hemp, gave them hallucinations of Paradise and houris, and endless time. They were told that that was what would happen to them after death, but to attain it they had to go and do a ritual killing. Oh, I'm not putting it in fancy language, but that's what it came to.'

'What it came to,' said Miss Marple, 'is in essence the fact that people are highly credulous.'

'Well yes, I suppose you could put it like that.'

'They believe what they are told,' said Miss Marple. 'Yes indeed, we're all inclined to do that,' she added. Then she said sharply, 'Who told you these stories about India, about the doping of husbands with datura,' and she added sharply, before he could answer, 'Was it Major Palgrave?'

Jackson looked slightly surprised. 'Well – yes, as a matter of fact, it was. He told me a lot of stories like that. Of course most of it must have been before his time, but he seemed to know all about it.'

'Major Palgrave was under the impression that he knew a lot about everything,' said Miss Marple. 'He was often inaccurate in what he told people.' She shook her head thoughtfully. 'Major Palgrave,' she said, 'has a lot to answer for.'

There was a slight sound from the adjoining bedroom. Miss Marple turned her head sharply. She went quickly out of the bathroom into the bedroom. Lucky Dyson was standing just inside the window.

'I – oh! I didn't think you were here, Miss Marple.'

'I just stepped into the bathroom for a moment,' said Miss Marple, with dignity and a faint air of Victorian reserve.

In the bathroom, Jackson grinned broadly. Victorian modesty always amused him.

'I just wondered if you'd like me to sit with Molly for a bit,' said Lucky. She looked over towards the bed. 'She's asleep, isn't she?'

'I think so,' said Miss Marple. 'But it's really quite all right. You go and amuse yourself, my dear. I thought you'd gone on that expedition?'

'I was going,' said Lucky, 'but I had such a filthy headache that at the last moment I cried off. So I thought I might as well make myself useful.'

'That was very nice of you,' said Miss Marple. She reseated herself by the bed and resumed her knitting, 'but I'm *quite* happy here.'

Lucky hesitated for a moment or two and then turned away and went out. Miss Marple waited a moment then tiptoed back into the bathroom, but Jackson had departed, no doubt through the other door. Miss Marple picked up the jar of face cream he had been holding, and slipped it into her pocket.

Chapter Twenty-Two

A Man in her Life?

Getting a little chat in a natural manner with Dr Graham was not so easy as Miss Marple had hoped. She was particularly anxious not to approach him directly since she did not want to lend undue importance to the questions that she was going to ask him.

Tim was back, looking after Molly, and Miss Marple had arranged that she should relieve him there during the time that dinner was served and he was needed in the dining-room. He had assured her that Mrs Dyson was quite willing to take that on, or even Mrs Hillingdon, but Miss Marple said firmly that they were both young women who liked enjoying themselves and that she herself preferred a light meal early and so that would suit everybody. Tim once again thanked her warmly. Hovering rather uncertainly round the hotel and on the pathway which connected with various bungalows, among them Dr Graham's, Miss Marple tried to plan what she was going to do next.

She had a lot of confused and contradictory ideas in her head and if there was one thing that Miss Marple did not like, it was to have confused and contradictory ideas. This whole business had started out clearly enough. Major Palgrave with his regrettable capacity for telling stories, his indiscretion that had obviously been overheard and the corollary, his death within twenty-four hours. Nothing difficult about *that,* thought Miss Marple.

But afterwards, she was forced to admit, there was nothing *but* difficulty. Everything pointed in too many different directions at once. Once admit that you didn't believe a word that anybody had said to you, that nobody could be trusted, and that many of the persons with whom she had conversed here had regrettable resemblances to certain persons at St Mary Mead, and where did that lead you?

Her mind was increasingly focused on the victim. Someone was going to be killed and she had the increasing feeling that she ought to know quite well who that someone was. There had been *something*. Something she had heard? Noticed? Seen?

Something someone had told her that had a bearing on the case. Joan Prescott? Joan Prescott had said a lot of things about a lot of people. Scandal? Gossip? What exactly *had* Joan Prescott said?

Gregory Dyson, Lucky – Miss Marple's mind hovered over Lucky. Lucky, she was convinced with a certainty born of her natural suspicions, had been actively concerned in the death of Gregory Dyson's first wife. Everything pointed to it. Could it be that the predestined victim over whom she was worrying was Gregory Dyson? That Lucky intended to try her luck again with another husband, and for that reason wanted not only freedom but the handsome inheritance that she would get as Gregory Dyson's widow?

'But really,' said Miss Marple to herself, 'this is all pure conjecture. I'm being stupid. I know I'm being stupid. The truth must be quite plain, if one could just clear away the litter. Too much litter, that's what's the matter.'

'Talking to yourself?' said Mr Rafiel.

Miss Marple jumped. She had not noticed his approach. Esther Walters was supporting him and he was coming slowly down from his bungalow to the terrace.

'I really didn't notice you, Mr Rafiel.'

'Your lips were moving. What's become of all this urgency of yours?'

'It's still urgent,' said Miss Marple, 'only I can't just see what must be perfectly plain –'

'I'm glad it's as simple as that – Well, if you want any help, count on me.'

He turned his head as Jackson approached them along the path.

'So there you are, Jackson. Where the devil have you been? Never about when I want you.'

'Sorry, Mr Rafiel.'

Dexterously he slipped his shoulder under Mr Rafiel's. 'Down to the terrace, sir?'

'You can take me to the bar,' said Mr Rafiel. 'All right, Esther, you can go now and change into your evening togs. Meet me on the terrace in half an hour.'

He and Jackson went off together. Mrs Walters dropped into the chair by Miss Marple. She rubbed her arm gently.

'He *seems* a very light weight,' she observed, 'but at the moment my arm feels quite numb. I haven't seen you this afternoon at all, Miss Marple.'

'No, I've been sitting with Molly Kendal,' Miss Marple explained. 'She seems really very much better.'

'If you ask me there was never very much wrong with her,' said Esther Walters.

Miss Marple raised her eyebrows. Esther Walters's tone had been decidedly dry.

'You mean – you think her suicide attempt...'

'I don't think there *was* any suicide attempt,' said Esther Walters. 'I don't believe for a moment she took a real overdose and I think Dr Graham knows that perfectly well.'

'Now you interest me very much,' said Miss Marple. 'I wonder why you say that?'

'Because I'm almost certain that it's the case. Oh, it's a thing that happens very often. It's a way, I suppose, of calling attention to oneself,' went on Esther Walters.

'"You'll be sorry when I'm dead"?' quoted Miss Marple.

'That sort of thing,' agreed Esther Walters, 'though I don't think that was the motive in this particular instance. That's the sort of thing you feel like when your husband's playing you up and you're terribly fond of him.'

'You don't think Molly Kendal is fond of her husband?'

'Well,' said Esther Walters, 'do you?'

Miss Marple considered. 'I have,' she said, 'more or less assumed it.' She paused a moment before adding, 'Perhaps wrongly.'

Esther was smiling her rather wry smile.

'I've heard a little about her, you know. About the whole business.'

'From Miss Prescott?'

'Oh,' said Esther, 'from one or two people. There's a man in the case. Someone she was keen on. Her people were dead against him.'

'Yes,' said Miss Marple, 'I did hear that.'

'And then she married Tim. Perhaps she was fond of him in a way. But the other man didn't give up. I've wondered once or twice if he didn't actually follow her out here.'

'Indeed. But – who?'

'I've no idea who,' said Esther, 'and I should imagine that they've been very careful.'

'You think she cares for this other man?'

Esther shrugged her shoulders. 'I dare say he's a bad lot,' she said, 'but that's very often the kind who knows how to get under a woman's skin and stay there.'

'You never heard what kind of a man – what he did – anything like that?'

Esther shook her head. 'No. People hazard guesses, but you can't go by that type of thing. He may have been a married man. That may have been why her people disliked it, or he may have been a real bad lot. Perhaps he drank. Perhaps he tangled with the law – I don't know. But she cares for him still. That I know positively.'

'You've seen something, heard something?' Miss Marple hazarded.

'I know what I'm talking about,' said Esther. Her voice was harsh and unfriendly.

'These murders –' began Miss Marple.

'Can't you forget murders?' said Esther. 'You've got Mr Rafiel now all tangled up in them. Can't you just – let them be? You'll never find out any more, I'm sure of that.'

Miss Marple looked at her.

'You think you know, don't you?' she said.

'I think I do, yes. I'm fairly sure.'

'Then oughtn't you to tell what you know – do something about it?'

'Why should I? What good would it do? I couldn't prove anything. What would happen anyway? People get let off nowadays so easily. They call it diminished responsibility and things like that. A few years in prison and you're out again, as right as rain.'

'Supposing, because you don't tell what you know, somebody else gets killed – another victim?'

Esther shook her head with confidence. 'That won't happen,' she said.

'You can't be sure of it.'

'I am sure. And in any case I don't see who –' She frowned. 'Anyway,' she added, almost inconsequently, 'perhaps it *is* – diminished responsibility. Perhaps you can't help it – not if you are really mentally unbalanced. Oh, I don't know. By far the best thing would be if she went off with whoever it is, then we could all forget about things.'

She glanced at her watch, gave an exclamation of dismay and got up.

'I must go and change.'

Miss Marple sat looking after her. Pronouns, she thought, were always puzzling and women like Esther Walters were particularly prone to strew them about haphazardly. Was Esther Walters for some reason convinced that a *woman* had been responsible for the deaths of Major Palgrave and Victoria? It sounded like it. Miss Marple considered.

'Ah, Miss Marple, sitting here all alone – and not even knitting?'

It was Dr Graham for whom she had sought so long and so unsuccessfully. And here he was prepared of his own accord to sit down for a few minutes' chat. He wouldn't stay long, Miss

Marple thought, because he too was bent on changing for dinner, and he usually dined fairly early. She explained that she had been sitting by Molly Kendal's bedside that afternoon.

'One can hardly believe she has made such a good recovery so quickly,' she said.

'Oh well,' said Dr Graham, 'it's not very surprising. She didn't take a very heavy overdose, you know.'

'Oh, I understood she'd taken quite a half-bottle full of tablets.'

Dr Graham was smiling indulgently.

'No,' he said, 'I don't think she took that amount. I dare say she meant to take them, then probably at the last moment she threw half of them away. People, even when they think they want to commit suicide, often don't *really* want to do it. They manage not to take a full overdose. It's not always deliberate deceit, it's just the subconscious looking after itself.'

'Or, I suppose it might be deliberate. I mean, wanting it to appear that...' Miss Marple paused.

'It's possible,' said Dr Graham.

'If she and Tim had had a row, for instance?'

'They don't have rows, you know. They seem very fond of each other. Still, I suppose it can always happen once. No, I don't think there's very much wrong with her now. She could really get up and go about as usual. Still, it's safer to keep her where she is for a day or two –'

He got up, nodded cheerfully and went off towards the hotel. Miss Marple sat where she was a little while longer.

Various thoughts passed through her mind – The book under Molly's mattress – The way Molly had feigned sleep –

Things Joan Prescott and, later, Esther Walters, had said...

And then she went back to the beginning of it all – to Major Palgrave –

Something struggled in her mind. Something about Major Palgrave –

Something that if she could only remember –

CHAPTER TWENTY-THREE

THE LAST DAY

I

'AND THE EVENING *and the morning were the last day*,' said Miss Marple to herself.

Then, slightly confused, she sat upright again in her chair. She had dozed off, an incredible thing to do because the steel band was playing and anyone who could doze off during the steel band – Well, it showed, thought Miss Marple, that she was getting used to this place! What was it she had been saying? Some quotation that she'd got wrong. Last day? *First* day. That's what it ought to be. This wasn't the first day. Presumably it wasn't the last day either.

She sat upright again. The fact was that she was extremely tired. All this anxiety, this feeling of having been shamefully inadequate in some way... She remembered unpleasantly once more that queer sly look that Molly had given her from under her half-closed eyelids. What had been going on in that girl's head? How different, thought Miss Marple, everything had seemed at first. Tim Kendal and Molly, such a natural happy young couple. The Hillingdons so pleasant, so well-bred, such what is called 'nice' people. The gay hearty extrovert, Greg Dyson, and the gay strident Lucky, talking nineteen to the dozen, pleased with herself and the world... A quartet of people getting on so well together. Canon Prescott, that genial kindly man. Joan Prescott, an acid streak in her, but a very nice woman, and nice women had to have their gossipy distractions. They have to know what

is going on, to know when two and two make four, and when it
is possible to stretch them to five! There was no harm in such
women. Their tongues wagged but they were kind if you were
in misfortune. Mr Rafiel, a personality, a man of character, a man
that you would never by any chance forget. But Miss Marple
thought she knew something else about Mr Rafiel.

The doctors had often given him up, so he had said, but this
time, she thought, they had been more certain in their
pronouncements. Mr Rafiel knew that his days were numbered.

Knowing this with certainty, was there any action he might have
been likely to take?

Miss Marple considered the question.

It might, she thought, be important.

What was it exactly he had said, his voice a little too loud, a
little too sure? Miss Marple was very skilful in tones of voice.
She had done so much listening in her life.

Mr Rafiel had been telling her something that wasn't true.

Miss Marple looked round her. The night air, the soft
fragrance of flowers, the tables with their little lights, the women
with their pretty dresses, Evelyn in a dark indigo and white print,
Lucky in a white sheath, her golden hair shining. Everybody
seemed gay and full of life tonight. Even Tim Kendal was
smiling. He passed her table and said:

'Can't thank you enough for all you've done. Molly's
practically herself again. The doc says she can get up tomorrow.'

Miss Marple smiled at him and said that that was good hearing.
She found it, however, quite an effort to smile. Decidedly, she
was tired...

She got up and walked slowly back to her bungalow. She
would have liked to go on thinking, puzzling, trying to
remember, trying to assemble various facts and words and
glances. But she wasn't able to do it. The tired mind rebelled.
It said 'Sleep! You've got to go to sleep!'

Miss Marple undressed, got into bed, read a few verses of the
Thomas à Kempis which she kept by her bed, then she turned
out the light. In the darkness she sent up a prayer. One couldn't

do everything oneself. One had to have help. 'Nothing will happen tonight,' she murmured hopefully.

II

Miss Marple woke suddenly and sat up in bed. Her heart was beating. She switched on the light and looked at the little clock by her bedside. Two am. Two am and outside activity of some kind was going on. She got up, put on her dressing-gown and slippers, and a woollen scarf round her head. and went out to reconnoitre. There were people moving about with torches. Among them she saw Canon Prescott and went to him.

'What's happening?'

'Oh, Miss Marple? It's Mrs Kendal. Her husband woke up, found she'd slipped out of bed and gone out. We're looking for her.'

He hurried on. Miss Marple walked more slowly after him. Where had Molly gone? Why? Had she planned this deliberately, planned to slip away as soon as the guard on her was relaxed, and while her husband was deep in sleep? Miss Marple thought it was probable. But why? What was the reason? Was there, as Esther Walters had so strongly hinted, some other man? If so, who could that man be? Or was there some more sinister reason?

Miss Marple walked on, looking around her, peering under bushes. Then suddenly she heard a faint call:

'Here... This way...'

The cry had come from some little distance beyond the hotel grounds. It must be, thought Miss Marple, near the creek of water that ran down to the sea. She went in that direction as briskly as she could.

There were not really so many searchers as it had seemed to her at first. Most people must still be asleep in their bungalows. She saw a place on the creek bank where there were people standing. Someone pushed past her, almost knocking her down, running in that direction. It was Tim Kendal. A minute or two later she heard his voice cry out:

'Molly! My God, Molly!'

It was a minute or two before Miss Marple was able to join the little group. It consisted of one of the Cuban waiters, Evelyn Hillingdon, and two of the native girls. They had parted to let Tim through. Miss Marple arrived as he was bending over to look.

'Molly…' He slowly dropped on to his knees. Miss Marple saw the girl's body clearly, lying there in the creek, her face below the level of the water, her golden hair spread over the pale green embroidered shawl that covered her shoulders. With the leaves and rushes of the creek, it seemed almost like a scene from *Hamlet* with Molly as the dead Ophelia…

As Tim stretched out a hand to touch her, the quiet, common-sense Miss Marple took charge and spoke sharply and authoritatively.

'Don't move her, Mr Kendal,' she said. 'She mustn't be moved.'

Tim turned a dazed face up to her.

'But – I must – it's Molly. I must…'

Evelyn Hillingdon touched his shoulder.

'She's dead, Tim. I didn't move her, but I did feel her pulse.'

'Dead?' said Tim unbelievingly. 'Dead? You mean she's – *drowned* herself?'

'I'm afraid so. It looks like it.'

'But *why?*' A great cry burst from the young man. '*Why?* She was so happy this morning. Talking about what we'd do tomorrow. Why should this terrible death wish come over her again? Why should she steal away as she did – rush out into the night, come down here and drown herself? What despair did she have – what misery – why couldn't she *tell* me anything?'

'I don't know, my dear,' said Evelyn gently. 'I don't know.'

Miss Marple said:

'Somebody had better get Dr Graham. And someone will have to telephone the police.'

170

'The police?' Tim uttered a bitter laugh. 'What good will they be?'

'The police have to be notified in a case of suicide,' said Miss Marple.

Tim rose slowly to his feet.

'I'll get Graham,' he said heavily. 'Perhaps – even now – he could – do something.'

He stumbled away in the direction of the hotel.

Evelyn Hillingdon and Miss Marple stood side by side looking down at the dead girl.

Evelyn shook her head. 'It's too late. She's quite cold. She must have been dead at least an hour – perhaps more. What a tragedy it all is. Those two always seemed so happy. I suppose she was always unbalanced.'

'No,' said Miss Marple. 'I don't think she was unbalanced.'

Evelyn looked at her curiously. 'What do you mean?'

The moon had been behind a cloud, but now it came out into the open. It shone with a luminous silvery brightness on Molly's outspread hair...

Miss Marple gave a sudden ejaculation. She bent down, peering, then stretched out her hand and touched the golden head. She spoke to Evelyn Hillingdon, and her voice sounded quite different.

'I think,' she said, 'that we had better make sure.'

Evelyn Hillingdon stared at her in astonishment.

'But you yourself told Tim we mustn't touch anything?'

'I know. But the moon wasn't out. I hadn't seen –'

Her finger pointed. Then, very gently, she touched the blonde hair and parted it so that the roots were exposed...

Evelyn gave a sharp ejaculation.

'*Lucky!*'

And then after a moment she repeated:

'Not Molly... Lucky.'

Miss Marple nodded. 'Their hair was of much the same colour – but hers, of course, was dark at the roots because it was dyed.'

'But she's wearing Molly's shawl?'

'She admired it. I heard her say she was going to get one like it. Evidently she did.'

'So that's why we were – deceived…'

Evelyn broke off as she met Miss Marple's eyes watching her.

'Someone,' said Miss Marple, 'will have to tell her husband.'

There was a moment's pause, then Evelyn said:

'All right. I'll do it.'

She turned and walked away through the palm trees.

Miss Marple remained for a moment motionless, then she turned her head very slightly, and said:

'Yes, Colonel Hillingdon?'

Edward Hillingdon came from the trees behind her to stand by her side.

'You knew I was there?'

'You cast a shadow,' said Miss Marple.

They stood a moment in silence.

He said, more as though he were speaking to himself:

'So, in the end, she played her luck too far…'

'You are, I think, glad that she is dead?'

'And that shocks you? Well, I will not deny it. I am glad she is dead.'

'Death is often a solution to problems.'

Edward Hillingdon turned his head slowly. Miss Marple met his eyes calmly and steadfastly.

'If you think –' he took a sharp step towards her.

There was a sudden menace in his tone.

Miss Marple said quietly:

'Your wife will be back with Mr Dyson in a moment. Or Mr Kendal will be here with Dr Graham.'

Edward Hillingdon relaxed. He turned back to look down at the dead woman.

Miss Marple slipped away quietly. Presently her pace quickened.

Just before reaching her own bungalow, she paused. It was here that she had sat that day talking to Major Palgrave. It was here that he had fumbled in his wallet looking for the snapshot of a murderer...

She remembered how he had looked up, and how his face had gone purple and red... 'So ugly,' as Señora de Caspearo had said. 'He has the Evil Eye.'

The Evil Eye... Eye... *Eye...*

Chapter Twenty-Four

Nemesis

I

Whatever the alarms and excursions of the night, Mr Rafiel had not heard them.

He was fast asleep in bed, a faint thin snore coming from his nostrils, when he was taken by the shoulders and shaken violently.

'Eh – what – what the devil's this?'

'It's me,' said Miss Marple, for once ungrammatical, 'though I should put it a little more strongly than that. The Greeks, I believe, had a word for it. Nemesis, if I am not wrong.'

Mr Rafiel raised himself on his pillows as far as he could. He stared at her. Miss Marple, standing there in the moonlight, her head encased in a fluffy scarf of pale pink wool, looked as unlike a figure of Nemesis as it was possible to imagine.

'So you're Nemesis, are you?' said Mr Rafiel after a momentary pause.

'I hope to be – with your help.'

'Do you mind telling me quite plainly what you're talking about like this in the middle of the night.'

'I think we may have to act quickly. Very quickly. I have been foolish. Extremely foolish. I ought to have known from the very beginning what all this was about. It was so simple.'

'What was simple, and what are you talking about?'

'You slept through a good deal,' said Miss Marple. 'A body was found. We thought at first it was the body of Molly Kendal. It wasn't, it was Lucky Dyson. Drowned in the creek.'

'Lucky, eh?' said Mr Rafiel. 'And drowned? In the creek. Did she drown herself or did somebody drown her?'

'Somebody drowned her,' said Miss Marple.

'I see. At least I think I see. That's what you mean by saying it's so simple, is it? Greg Dyson was always the first possibility, and he's the right one. Is that it? Is that what you're thinking? And what you're afraid of is that he may get away with it.'

Miss Marple took a deep breath.

'Mr Rafiel, will you trust me? We have got to stop a murder being committed.'

'I thought you said it *had* been committed.'

'That murder was committed in error. Another murder may be committed any moment now. There's no time to lose. We must prevent it happening. We must go at once.'

'It's all very well to talk like that,' said Mr Rafiel. '*We*, you say? What do you think *I* can do about it? I can't even walk without help. How can you and I set about preventing a murder? You're about a hundred and I'm a broken-up old crock.'

'I was thinking of Jackson,' said Miss Marple. 'Jackson will do what you tell him, won't he?'

'He will indeed,' said Mr Rafiel, 'especially if I add that I'll make it worth his while. Is that what you want?'

'Yes. Tell him to come with me and tell him to obey any orders I give him.'

Mr Rafiel looked at her for about six seconds. Then he said:

'Done. I expect I'm taking the biggest risk of my life. Well, it won't be the first one.' He raised his voice. 'Jackson.' At the same time he picked up the electric bell that lay beside his hand and pressed the button.

Hardly thirty seconds passed before Jackson appeared through the connecting door to the adjoining room.

'You called and rang, sir? Anything wrong?' He broke off, staring at Miss Marple.

'Now, Jackson, do as I tell you. You will go with this lady, Miss Marple. You'll go where she takes you and you'll do exactly as she says. You'll obey every order she gives you. Is that understood?'

'I –'

'*Is that understood?*'

'Yes, sir.'

'And for doing that,' said Mr Rafiel, 'you won't be the loser. I'll make it worth your while.'

'Thank you, sir.'

'Come along, Mr Jackson,' said Miss Marple. She spoke over her shoulder to Mr Rafiel. 'We'll tell Mrs Walters to come to you on your way. Get her to get you out of bed and bring you along.'

'Bring me along where?'

'To the Kendals' bungalow,' said Miss Marple. 'I think Molly will be coming back there.'

II

Molly came up the path from the sea. Her eyes stared fixedly ahead of her. Occasionally, under her breath, she gave a little whimper...

She went up the steps of the loggia, paused a moment, then pushed open the window and walked into the bedroom. The lights were on, but the room itself was empty. Molly went across to the bed and sat down. She sat for some minutes, now and again passing her hand over her forehead and frowning.

Then, after a quick surreptitious glance round, she slipped her hand under the mattress and brought out the book that was hidden there. She bent over it, turning the pages to find what she wanted.

Then she raised her head as a sound of running footsteps came from outside. With a quick guilty movement she pushed the book behind her back.

Tim Kendal, panting and out of breath, came in, and uttered a great sigh of relief at the sight of her.

'Thank God. Where have you been, Molly? I've been searching everywhere for you.'

'I went to the creek.'

'You went –' he stopped.

'Yes. I went to the creek. But I couldn't wait there. I couldn't. There was someone in the water – and she was dead.'

'You mean – Do you know I thought it was *you*. I've only just found out it was Lucky.'

'I didn't kill her. Really, Tim, I didn't kill her. I'm sure I didn't. I mean – I'd remember if I did, wouldn't I?'

Tim sank slowly down on the end of the bed.

'You didn't – Are you sure that –? No. No, of course you didn't!' He fairly shouted the words. 'Don't start thinking like that, Molly. Lucky drowned herself. Of course she drowned herself. Hillingdon was through with her. She went and lay down with her face in the water –'

'Lucky wouldn't do that. She'd never do that. But *I* didn't kill her. I swear I didn't.'

'Darling, of course you didn't!' He put his arms round her but she pulled herself away.

'I hate this place. It ought to be all sunlight. It seemed to be all sunlight. But it isn't. Instead there's a shadow – a big black shadow… And I'm in it – and I can't get out –'

Her voice had risen to a shout.

'Hush, Molly. For God's sake, hush!' He went into the bathroom, came back with a glass.

'Look. Drink this. It'll steady you.'

'I – I can't drink anything. My teeth are chattering so.'

'Yes you can, darling. Sit down. Here, on the bed.' He put his arm round her. He approached the glass to her lips. 'There you are now. Drink it.'

A voice spoke from the window.

'Jackson,' said Miss Marple clearly. 'Go over. Take that glass from him and hold it tightly. Be careful. He's strong and he may be pretty desperate.'

There were certain points about Jackson. He was a man with

a great love for money, and money had been promised him by his employer, that employer being a man of stature and authority. He was also a man of extreme muscular development heightened by his training. His not to reason why, his but to do.

Swift as a flash he had crossed the room. His hand went over the glass that Tim was holding to Molly's lips, his other arm had fastened round Tim. A quick flick of the wrist and he had the glass. Tim turned on him wildly, but Jackson held him firmly.

'What the devil – let go of me. Let go of me. Have you gone mad? What are you doing?'

Tim struggled violently.

'Hold him, Jackson,' said Miss Marple.

'What's going on? What's the matter here?'

Supported by Esther Walters, Mr Rafiel came through the window.

'You ask what's the matter?' shouted Tim. 'Your man's gone mad, stark, staring mad, that's what's the matter. Tell him to let go of me.'

'No,' said Miss Marple.

Mr Rafiel turned to her.

'Speak up, Nemesis,' he said. 'We've got to have chapter and verse of some kind.'

'I've been stupid and a fool,' said Miss Marple, 'but I'm not being a fool now. When the contents of that glass that he was trying to make his wife drink have been analysed, I'll wager – yes, I'll wager my immortal soul that you'll find it's got a lethal dose of narcotic in it. It's the same pattern, you see, the same pattern as in Major Palgrave's story. A wife in a depressed state, and she tries to do away with herself, husband saves her in time. Then the second time she succeeds. Yes, it's the right pattern. Major Palgrave told me the story and he took out a snapshot and then he looked up and saw –'

'Over your right shoulder –' continued Mr Rafiel.

'No,' said Miss Marple, shaking her head. '*He didn't see anything over my right shoulder.*'

'What are you talking about? You told me...'

178

'I told you wrong. I was completely wrong. I was stupid beyond belief. Major Palgrave *appeared* to me to be looking over my right shoulder, glaring, in fact, at something – But he couldn't have *seen* anything, because he was looking through his left eye and his left eye was his glass eye.'

'I remember – he *had* a glass eye,' said Mr Rafiel. 'I'd forgotten – or I took it for granted. You mean he couldn't see anything?'

'Of course he could *see*,' said Miss Marple. 'He could *see* all right, but he could only see with one eye. The eye he *could* see with was his *right* eye. And so, you see, he must have been looking at something or someone not to the right of me but to the *left* of me.'

'Was there anyone on the left of you?'

'Yes,' said Miss Marple. 'Tim Kendal and his wife were sitting not far off. Sitting at a table just by a big hibiscus bush. They were doing accounts there. So you see the Major looked up. His glass left eye was glaring over my shoulder, but what he *saw* with his other eye was a man sitting by a hibiscus bush and the face was the same, only rather older, as the face in the snapshot. Also by a hibiscus bush. Tim Kendal had heard the story the Major had been telling and he saw that the Major had recognised him. So, of course, he had to kill him. Later, he had to kill the girl, Victoria, because she'd seen him putting a bottle of tablets in the Major's room. She didn't think anything of it at first because of course it was quite natural on various occasions for Tim Kendal to go into the guests' bungalows. He might have just been returning something to it that had been left on a restaurant table. But she thought about it and then she asked him questions and so he had to get rid of her. But this is the real murder, the murder he's been planning all along. He's a wife-killer, you see.'

'What damned nonsense, what –' Tim Kendal shouted.

There was a sudden cry, a wild angry cry. Esther Walters detached herself from Mr Rafiel, almost flinging him down, and rushed across the room. She pulled vainly at Jackson.

'Let go of him – let go of him. It's not true. Not a word of it's true. Tim – Tim darling, it's not true. You could never kill anyone, I know you couldn't. I know you wouldn't. It's that horrible girl you married. She's been telling lies about you. They're not true. None of them are true. I believe in you. I love you and trust in you. I'll never believe a word anyone says. I'll –'

Then Tim Kendal lost control of himself.

'For God's sake, you damned bitch,' he said, 'shut up, can't you? D'you want to get me hanged? Shut up, I tell you. Shut that big, ugly mouth of yours.'

'Poor silly creature,' said Mr Rafiel softly. 'So that's what's been going on, is it?'

Chapter Twenty-Five

Miss Marple uses her Imagination

'So that's what had been going on?' said Mr Rafiel.

He and Miss Marple were sitting together in a confidential manner.

'She'd been having an affair with Tim Kendal, had she?'

'Hardly an affair, I imagine,' said Miss Marple, primly. 'It was, I think, a romantic attachment with the prospect of marriage in the future.'

'What – after his wife was dead?'

'I don't think poor Esther Walters knew that Molly was going to die,' said Miss Marple. 'I just think she believed the story Tim Kendal told her about Molly having been in love with another man, and the man having followed her here, and I think she counted on Tim's getting a divorce. I think it was all quite proper and respectable. But she was very much in love with him.'

'Well, that's easily understood. He was an attractive chap. But what made *him* go for her – d'you know that too?'

'*You* know, don't you?' said Miss Marple.

'I dare say I've got a pretty fair idea, but I don't know how you should know about it. As far as that goes, I don't see how Tim Kendal could know about it.'

'Well, I really think I could explain all that with a little imagination, though it would be simpler if you told me.'

'I'm not going to tell you,' said Mr Rafiel. 'You tell me, since you're being so clever.'

'Well, it seems to me possible,' said Miss Marple, 'that as I have already hinted to you, your man Jackson was in the habit of taking a good snoop through your various papers from time to time.'

'Perfectly possible,' said Mr Rafiel, 'but I shouldn't have said there was anything there that could do him much good. I took care of that.'

'I imagine,' said Miss Marple, 'he read your will.'

'Oh I see. Yes, yes, I did have a copy of my will along.'

'You told me,' said Miss Marple, 'you told me – (as Humpty Dumpty said – very loud and clear) that you had *not* left anything to Esther Walters in your will. You had impressed that fact upon her, and also upon Jackson. It was true in Jackson's case, I should imagine. You have not left *him* anything, but you *had* left Esther Walters money, though you weren't going to let her have any inkling of the fact. Isn't that right?'

'Yes, it's quite right, but I don't know how *you* knew.'

'Well, it's the way you insisted on the point,' said Miss Marple. 'I have a certain experience of the way people tell lies.'

'I give in,' said Mr Rafiel. 'All right. I left Esther £50,000. It would come as a nice surprise to her when I died. I suppose that, knowing this, Tim Kendal decided to exterminate his present wife with a nice dose of something or other and marry £50,000 and Esther Walters. Possibly to dispose of her also in good time. But how did *he* know she was going to have £50,000?'

'Jackson told him, of course,' said Miss Marple. 'They were very friendly, those two. Tim Kendal was nice to Jackson and, quite, I should imagine, without ulterior motive. But amongst the bits of gossip that Jackson let slip I think Jackson told him that unbeknownst to herself, Esther Walters was going to inherit a fat lot of money, and he may have said that he himself hoped to induce Esther Walters to marry him though he hadn't had much success so far in taking her fancy. Yes, I think that's how it happened.'

'The things you imagine always seem perfectly plausible,' said Mr Rafiel.

'But I was stupid,' said Miss Marple, 'very stupid. Everything fitted in really, you see. Tim Kendal was a very clever man as well as being a very wicked one. He was particularly good at putting about rumours. Half the things I've been told here came from him originally, I imagine. There were stories going around about Molly wanting to marry an undesirable young man, but I rather fancy that the undesirable young man was actually Tim Kendal himself, though that wasn't the name he was using then. Her people had heard something, perhaps that his background was fishy. So he put on a high indignation act, refused to be taken by Molly to be "shown off" to her people and then he brewed up a little scheme with her which they both thought great fun. She pretended to sulk and pine for him. Then a Mr Tim Kendal turned up, primed with the names of various old friends of Molly's people, and they welcomed him with open arms as being the sort of young man who would put the former delinquent one out of Molly's head. I am afraid Molly and he must have laughed over it a good deal. Anyway, he married her, and with her money he bought out the people who ran this place and they came out here. I should imagine that he ran through her money at a pretty fair rate. Then he came across Esther Walters and he saw a nice prospect of more money.'

'Why didn't he bump me off?' said Mr Rafiel.

Miss Marple coughed.

'I expect he wanted to be fairly sure of Mrs Walters first. Besides – I mean…' She stopped, a little confused.

'Besides, he realised he wouldn't have to wait long,' said Mr Rafiel, 'and it would clearly be better for me to die a natural death. Being so rich. Deaths of millionaires are scrutinised rather carefully, aren't they, unlike mere wives?'

'Yes, you're quite right. Such a lot of lies as he told,' said Miss Marple. 'Look at the lies he got Molly herself to believe – putting that book on mental disorders in her way. Giving her drugs which would give her dreams and hallucinations. You know, your Jackson was rather clever over that. I think he recognised certain of Molly's symptoms as being the result of drugs. And he came into the bungalow that day to potter about a bit in the bathroom. That face cream he examined. He might have got some idea from the old tales of witches rubbing themselves with ointments that had belladonna in them. Belladonna in face cream could have produced just that result. Molly would have blackouts. Times she couldn't account for, dreams of flying through the air. No wonder she got frightened about herself. She had all the signs of mental illness, Jackson was on the right track. Maybe he got the idea from Major Palgrave's stories about the use of datura by Indian women on their husbands.'

'Major Palgrave!' said Mr Rafiel. 'Really, that man!'

'He brought about his own murder,' said Miss Marple, 'and that poor girl Victoria's murder, and he nearly brought about Molly's murder. But he recognised a murderer all right.'

'What made you suddenly remember about his glass eye?' asked Mr Rafiel curiously.

'Something that Señora de Caspearo said. She talked some nonsense about his being ugly, and having the Evil Eye; and I said it was only a glass eye, and he couldn't help that, poor man, and she said his eyes looked different ways, they were cross-eyes – which, of course, they were. And she said it brought bad luck. I knew – I *knew* that I had heard something that day that was important. Last night, just after Lucky's death, it came to me what it was! And then I realised there was no time to waste...'

'How did Tim Kendal come to kill the wrong woman?'

'Sheer chance. I think his plan was this: Having convinced everybody – and that included Molly herself – that she was mentally unbalanced, and after giving her a sizeable dose of the drug he was using, he told her that between them they were going to clear up all these murder puzzles. But she had got to help him. After everyone was asleep, they would go separately and meet at an agreed spot by the creek.

'He said he had a very good idea who the murderer was, and they would trap him. Molly went off obediently – but she was confused and stupefied with the drug she had been given, and it slowed her up. Tim arrived there first and saw what he thought was Molly. Golden hair and pale green shawl. He came up behind her, put his hand over her mouth, and forced her down into the water and held her there.'

'Nice fellow! But wouldn't it have been easier just to give her an overdose of narcotic?'

'Much easier, of course. But that *might* have given rise to suspicion. All narcotics and sedatives have been very carefully removed from Molly's reach, remember. And if she *had* got hold of a fresh supply, who more likely to have supplied it than her husband? But if, in a fit of despair, she went out and drowned herself whilst her innocent husband slept, the whole thing would be a romantic tragedy, and no one would be likely to suggest that she had been drowned deliberately. Besides,' added Miss Marple, 'murderers always find it difficult to keep things simple. They can't keep themselves from elaborating.'

'You seem convinced you know all there is to be known about murderers! So you believe Tim didn't know he had killed the wrong woman?'

Miss Marple shook her head.

'He didn't even look at her face, just hurried off as quickly as he could, let an hour elapse, then started to organise a search for her, playing the part of a distracted husband.'

'But what the devil was Lucky doing hanging about the creek in the middle of the night?'

Miss Marple gave an embarrassed little cough.

'It is possible, I think, that she was – er – waiting to meet someone.'

'Edward Hillingdon?'

'Oh *no*,' said Miss Marple. 'That's all over, I wondered whether – just possibly – she might have been waiting for Jackson.'

'Waiting for *Jackson?*'

'I've noticed her look at him once or twice,' murmured Miss Marple, averting her eyes.

Mr Rafiel whistled.

'My Tom Cat Jackson! I wouldn't put it past him! Tim must have had a shock later when he found he'd killed the wrong woman.'

'Yes, indeed. He must have felt quite desperate. Here was

Molly alive and wandering about. And the story he'd circulated
so carefully about her mental condition wouldn't stand up for a
moment once she got into the hands of competent mental
specialists. And once she told her damning story of his having
asked her to meet him at the creek, where would Tim Kendal
be? He'd only one hope – to finish off Molly as quickly as
possible. Then there was a very good chance that everyone would
believe that Molly, in a fit of mania, had drowned Lucky, and had
then, horrified by what she had done, taken her own life.'

'And it was then,' said Mr Rafiel, 'that you decided to play
Nemesis, eh?'

He leaned back suddenly and roared with laughter. 'It's a
damned good joke,' he said. 'If you knew what you looked like
that night with that fluffy pink wool all round your head, standing
there and saying you were Nemesis! I'll never forget it!'

Epilogue

THE TIME HAD come and Miss Marple was waiting at the airport for her plane. Quite a lot of people had come to see her off. The Hillingdons had left already. Gregory Dyson had flown to one of the other islands and the rumour had come that he was devoting himself to an Argentinian widow. Señora de Caspearo had returned to South America.

Molly had come to see Miss Marple off. She was pale and thin but she had weathered the shock of her discovery bravely and with the help of one of Mr Rafiel's nominees whom he had wired for to England, she was carrying on with the running of the hotel.

'Do you good to be busy,' Mr Rafiel observed. 'Keep you from thinking. Got a good thing here.'

'You don't think the murders –'

'People love murders when they're all cleared up,' Mr Rafiel had assured her. 'You carry on, girl, and keep your heart up. Don't distrust all men because you've met one bad lot.'

'You sound like Miss Marple,' Molly had said, 'she's always telling me Mr Right will come along one day.'

Mr Rafiel grinned at this sentiment. So Molly was there and the two Prescotts and Mr Rafiel, of course, and Esther – an Esther who looked older and sadder and to whom Mr Rafiel was quite often unexpectedly kind. Jackson also was very much to the fore, pretending to be looking after Miss Marple's baggage. He was all smiles these days and let it be known that he had come into money.

There was a hum in the sky. The plane was arriving. Things were somewhat informal here. There was no 'taking your place by Channel 8' or Channel 9. You just walked out from the little flower-covered pavilion on to the tarmac.

'Goodbye, darling Miss Marple.' Molly kissed her.

'Goodbye. Do try and come and visit us.' Miss Prescott shook her warmly by the hand.

'It has been a great pleasure to know you,' said the Canon. 'I second my sister's invitation most warmly.'

'All the best, Madam,' said Jackson, 'and remember any time you want any massage free, just you send me a line and we'll make an appointment.'

Only Esther Walters turned slightly away when the time came for goodbyes. Miss Marple did not force one upon her. Mr Rafiel came last. He took her hand.

'*Ave Caesar, nos morituri te salutamus,*' he said.

'I'm afraid,' said Miss Marple, 'I don't know very much Latin.'

'But you understand that?'

'Yes.' She said no more. She knew quite well what he was telling her.

'It has been a great pleasure to know you,' she said.

Then she walked across the tarmac and got into the plane.

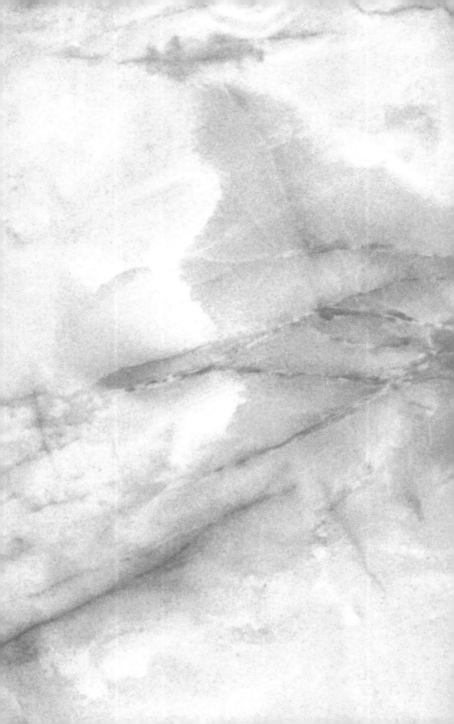